Modern Approaches to Targeted Drug Delivery

Modern Approaches to Targeted Drug Delivery

Editor: Laurence Denton

AMERICAN
MEDICAL PUBLISHERS
www.americanmedicalpublishers.com

AMERICAN
MEDICAL PUBLISHERS
www.americanmedicalpublishers.com

Cataloging-in-Publication Data

Modern approaches to targeted drug delivery / edited by Laurence Denton.
p. cm.
Includes bibliographical references and index.
ISBN 979-8-88740-273-4
1. Drug delivery systems. 2. Drug targeting. 3. Drug carriers (Pharmacy). 4. Drug delivery devices.
5. Pharmaceutical technology. I. Denton, Laurence.
RS199.5 .M63 2023
615.6--dc23

American Medical Publishers,
41 Flatbush Avenue,
1st Floor, New York,
NY 11217, USA

ISBN 979-8-88740-273-4 (Hardback)

Contents

Preface

This book has been an outcome of determined endeavour from a group of educationists in the field. The primary objective was to involve a broad spectrum of professionals from diverse cultural background involved in the field for developing new researches. The book not only targets students but also scholars pursuing higher research for further enhancement of the theoretical and practical applications of the subject.

Targeted drug delivery (TDD) is a process of delivering medication to a specific site like infected organ, tissue or cell. It comprises engineered technologies for the targeted delivery and controlled release of therapeutic agents. It is extensively used in the treatment of cancerous tumors. TDD is also beneficial in treating some other diseases, including cardiovascular diseases and diabetes. It aims to target, localize, prolong and have a protected drug interaction with the diseased tissue. There are various advantages of TDD, which include having a more uniform effect of the drug, reduction in the frequency of the dosages taken by the patient, reduced fluctuation in circulating drug levels, and reduction of drug side-effects. Different approaches, evaluations and advanced studies on targeted drug delivery have been included in this book. It aims to serve as a resource guide for students and researchers alike and contribute to the evolution of research on this area of study.

It was an honour to edit such a profound book and also a challenging task to compile and examine all the relevant data for accuracy and originality. I wish to acknowledge the efforts of the contributors for submitting such brilliant and diverse chapters in the field and for endlessly working for the completion of the book. Last, but not the least; I thank my family for being a constant source of support in all my research endeavours.

Editor

1

The Effect of Molecular Properties on Active Ingredient Release from Electrospun Eudragit Fibers

Kieran Burgess, Heyu Li, Yasmin Abo-zeid, Fatimah and Gareth R. Williams *

UCL School of Pharmacy, University College London, 29-39 Brunswick Square, London WC1N 1AX, UK; kieran.burgess.16@ucl.ac.uk (K.B.); heyu.li@ucl.ac.uk (H.L.); y.abozeid@ucl.ac.uk (Y.A.-z.); fatimah.14@ucl.ac.uk (F.)

* Correspondence: g.williams@ucl.ac.uk

Abstract: The formation of nanoscale fibers from pH-sensitive polymers is a route which has been widely explored for targeted drug delivery. In particular, the Eudragit L100 and S100 families of polymers have received significant attention for this purpose. However, while in some cases it is shown that making drug-loaded Eudragit polymers effectively prevents drug release in low-pH media where the polymer is insoluble, this is not always the case, and other studies have reported significant amounts of drug release at acidic pHs. In this study, we sought to gain insight into the factors influencing the release of active ingredients from Eudragit S100 (ES100) fibers. A family of materials was prepared loaded with the model active ingredients (AIs) benzoic acid, 1-naphthoic acid, 1-naphthylamine, and 9-anthracene carboxylic acid. Analogous systems were prepared with an AI-loaded core and an ES100 sheath. The resultant fibers were smooth and cylindrical in the majority of cases, and X-ray diffraction and differential scanning calorimetry showed them to comprise amorphous solid dispersions. When AI release from the monolithic fibers was probed, it was found that there was significant release at pH 1 in all cases except with 9-anthracene carboxylic acid. Analysis of the results indicated that both the molecular weight of the AI and its acidity/basicity are important in controlling release, with lower molecular weight AIs and basic species released more quickly. The same release trends are seen with the core/shell fibers, but AI release at pH 1 is attenuated. The most significant change between the monolithic and core/shell systems was observed in the case of 1-naphthylamine. Mathematical equations were devised to connect molecular properties and AI release under acidic conditions.

Keywords: electrospinning; Eudragit; nanofibers; drug release

---

1. Introduction

Electrospinning is a technique which has attracted great attention in the pharmaceutical technology field [1,2]. It most commonly involves the preparation of a polymer solution in a volatile solvent. This is loaded into a syringe and is slowly ejected through a narrow bore needle (the spinneret). A high voltage power supply is used to charge the needle, and the solution expelled towards a grounded collector plate. The application of the electrical energy causes drawing of the polymer solution into a fine jet, and ultimately results in the production of fibers with diameters typically on the nanoscale. The inclusion of a drug molecule in the solution generally yields drug-loaded fibers in the form of amorphous solid dispersions. In the simplest embodiment of the experiment, a single liquid is processed, but more advanced derivatives including coaxial electrospinning (which uses two needles nested concentrically one inside the other to process two liquids) and triaxial spinning (three needles, three solutions) have also been reported. The use of coaxial spinnerets results in core/shell structures, and triaxial spinnerets give three-compartment architectures.

Electrospun nanofibers have been explored for a wide range of drug delivery applications, including preparing fast-dissolving oral drug delivery systems designed for very rapid release in the mouth [3,4], extended release systems allowing the drug cargo to be freed over a number of hours or weeks [5–8], and systems able to respond to external stimuli such as temperature [9–12]. Given that the pH of the human gastrointestinal tract varies from 1–3 in the stomach, 6–8 in the small intestine, and 4–7 in the large intestine, materials able to respond to changes in pH are particularly useful for oral delivery systems. A range of polymers exist which are selectively soluble above or below a particular pH. One clinically used family of such polymers is the Eudragits, methacrylate-based polymers with tunable pH sensitivity. Eudragit L100-55 is soluble above pH 5.5, L100 above pH 6, and S100 above pH 7. This allows different sections of the intestinal tract to be targeted depending on the polymer chosen to fabricate a formulation. A number of authors have explored the electrospinning of Eudragits, as well as other pH-sensitive polymers such as shellac [13,14].

The studies in the literature exploring Eudragit have investigated both monolithic fibers from monoaxial electrospinning and core/shell materials. Shen et al. were the first to electrospin Eudragit, preparing L100-55 fibers loaded with diclofenac sodium [15]. They found that drug release at pH 1.0 was below 3%, confirming that pH-sensitive fibers can be produced. Other studies have built on this and reported similar conclusions, for instance with Eudragit fibers containing mebeverine HCl [16], ketoprofen [17], indomethacin [18] and helicid [19]. However, it is not always the case that simply making a drug-loaded Eudragit fiber formulation prevents drug release in the acidic pHs typical of the stomach. For instance, Karthikeyan et al. reported blend fibers of zein and Eudragit S100 (ES100) loaded with pantoprazole and aceclofenac gave 25% release of the latter after 2 h immersion in 0.1 M HCl [20]. The same has been shown to be true for spironolactone-loaded Eudragit FS fibers (up to 30% release at pH 1.2) [21], and 5-fluorouracil (5-FU)-loaded ES100 fibers, which showed some 80% release at pH 1 [22].

Analogous findings have been found when preparing core/shell systems. Whilst in some instances it is reported that drug release at pH 1–3 can be virtually completely obviated in fibers with a Eudragit shell and drug-loaded core (for instance containing a Gd-based contrast agent or indomethacin [23,24]), similar fibers containing 5-FU in the core release up to 70% of their drug loading under these conditions [22]. The reasons behind the different findings reported in the literature are not completely clear, but it seems that both the molecular weight and acidity or basicity of the drug incorporated are important. Most recently, Jia et al. prepared fibers with an ES100 shell and a poly(ethylene oxide) core containing either mebeverine HCl or indomethacin (model basic and acidic drugs with similar molecular weights (MWs)) [25]. It was observed that release of both the basic mebeverine and acidic indomethacin at pH 1.2 was restrained by the presence of the ES100 shell, but that there was a noticeably greater extent of release in the former case (up to 20%) than the latter (ca. 1%).

In this work, we sought to obtain a fundamental understanding of the factors underlying drug release from Eudragit fibers at acidic pHs. To do this, we assembled a training set of four model active ingredients (AIs; Figure 1). While none has any direct applications in drug delivery, the incremental variation in their structures is ideal for a fundamental study of this type. Benzoic acid (BA), 1-naphthoic acid (NA) and 9-anthracene carboxylic acid (ACA) all contain one carboxylic acid functional group and have similar pK_as (BA: 4.20; NA: 3.67; ACA: 3.68), but the number of aromatic rings in the series increases from one to three. 1-Naphthylamine (NAm) has an identical structure to NA except that the carboxylic acid is replaced by an amine group; the pK_a of NAm conjugate acid is very similar to that of NA at 3.92, and thus the influence of acidity/basicity can be elucidated through this molecule pair.

A series of ES100-based fibers was prepared containing the training set AIs, using both monoaxial electrospinning to generate monolithic composites and also coaxial spinning to produce core/shell systems with the AI confined to the core. The fibers were subject to a detailed examination of their physicochemical properties, and AI release explored at pH 1.0 and 6.8 following pharmacopoeia protocols. Correlations between molecular properties and the release profiles were sought.

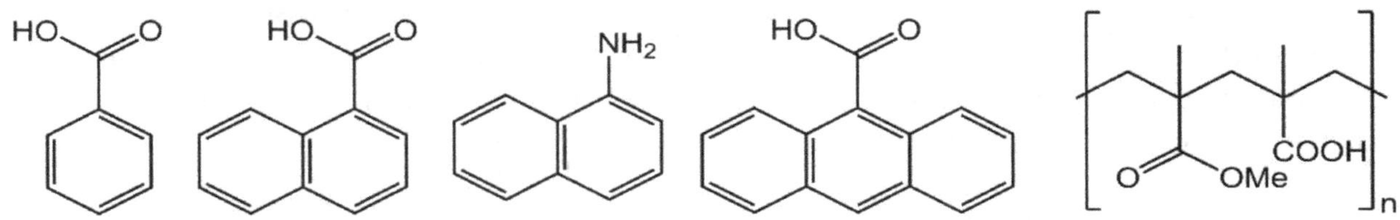

Benzoic acid (BA) 122 Da; 1-Naphthoic acid (NA) 172 Da; 1-Naphthylamine (NAm) 143 Da; 9-Anthracene carboxylic acid (ACA) 222 Da; ES100

Figure 1. The chemical structures of the active ingredients used in this work and their molecular weights, together with the structure of the polymer ES100. BA: Benzoic acid; NA: 1-naphthoic acid; NAm: 1-Naphthylamine; ACA: 9-anthracene carboxylic acid; ES100: Eudragit S100.

2. Materials and Methods

2.1. Materials

Benzoic acid (BA), 1-naphthoic acid (NA), 1-naphthylamine (NAm), 9-anthracene carboxylic acid (ACA), absolute ethanol and dimethylacetamide (DMAc) were purchased from Sigma-Aldrich (Gillingham, UK). Eudragit S100 (ES100) was a kind gift from Evonik GmbH (Darmstadt, Germany). Analytical grade hydrochloric acid and trisodium phosphate dodecahydrate were obtained from Fisher Scientific (Loughborough, UK). All water was deionised before use.

2.2. Methods

2.2.1. Monoaxial Electrospinning

Following a series of optimisation experiments, a solvent mixture of ethanol/water/DMAc (15/1/4 *v*/*v*/*v*) was selected as the most appropriate for electrospinning. A series of solutions was then prepared for monoaxial electrospinning (see Table 1). 1.2 g of ES100 and 0.1 g of the AI of interest were dissolved in 10 mL of the ethanol/water/DMAc solvent system. These were magnetically stirred for a minimum of 24 h to ensure a homogenous solution was formed.

Table 1. Details of the electrospun formulations prepared in this work.

ID	Active Ingredient (AI)	Theoretical Fiber AI Loading (% *w*/*w*) [a]	Observed Fiber AI Loading (% *w*/*w*) [b]	Entrapment Efficiency (%) [c]	Fiber Diameter (nm)
Monoaxial electrospinning					
S-BA	Benzoic acid	7.69	9.04 ± 0.13	118 ± 2	483 ± 145
S-NA	1-Naphthoic acid	7.69	7.05 ± 1.02	92 ± 13	129 ± 102
S-NAM	1-Naphthylamine	7.69	6.69 ± 0.27	91 ± 4	214 ± 105
S-ACA	9-Anthracene carboxylic acid	7.69	6.54 ± 0.38	85 ± 5	585 ± 158
Coaxial electrospinning					
C-BA	Benzoic acid	2.70	3.42 ± 0.27	127 ± 10	591 ± 189
C-NA	1-Naphthoic acid	2.70	2.38 ± 0.07	88 ± 2	664 ± 171
C-NAM	1-Naphthylamine	2.70	2.20 ± 0.37	81 ± 14	547 ± 124
C-ACA	9-Anthracene carboxylic acid	2.70	2.45 ± 0.16	91 ± 6	621 ± 140

[a] Calculated based on the relative masses of the polymer and drug in the system. [b] Determined experimentally through dissolution of the fibers (mean ± S.D.; $n = 3$). [c] Calculated as the percentage of the theoretical loading observed to be incorporated (mean ± S.D.; $n = 3$).

The solutions were loaded into a 5 mL Terumo syringe, with great care taken to avoid the formation of bubbles. The syringe was then fitted with a blunt-tipped metal needle (internal diameter 0.61 mm; Nordson EFD, Aylesbury, UK), and the positive electrode of a high-voltage power supply (HCP 35–35000, FuG Elektronik, Schechen, Germany) connected to the tip of the needle via a crocodile clip. The grounded collector comprised a flat piece of steel coated with aluminium foil. Liquid was dispensed using a syringe pump (KDS100, Cole Parmer, London, UK). Electrospinning was performed at ambient conditions (25 ± 3 °C; relative humidity 38 ± 6%), and processing parameters were as follows: voltage 16 kV; flow rate 0.5 mL h^{-1}; collection distance 18 cm. After fabrication, the fiber products were stored in a desiccator over silica beads.

2.2.2. Coaxial Electrospinning

A 12% *w*/*v* Eudragit S100 solution in ethanol/water/DMAc (15/1/4 *v*/*v*/*v*) was used as the shell liquid for coaxial electrospinning. The core solutions were the same as those used for monoaxial electrospinning (see Table 1). The applied voltage for coaxial spinning was 21 kV, the collection distance 18 cm, and experiments were performed under ambient conditions (25 ± 3 °C; relative humidity 38 ± 6%). The core and sheath solutions were independently dispensed through a coaxial spinneret (Linari Engineering, Pisa, Italy) using two separate KDS100 syringe pumps. The spinneret had internal/external diameters for the inner needle of 0.51/0.83 mm and for the outer needle at 1.37/1.83 mm. The core and shell flow rates were 0.4 and 0.8 mL/h respectively. After production, the fiber products were stored in a desiccator over silica beads.

2.3. *Characterisation*

2.3.1. Electron Microscopy

Small samples (ca. 0.5 × 0.5 cm) were cut from each fiber mat for scanning electron microscopy (SEM). These were sputter coated with gold and then imaged using a Quanta 200F instrument (FEI, Hillsboro, OR, USA). The fiber diameters were quantified at 100 points for each sample, using the ImageJ software (v1.48; National Institutes of Health, Bethesda, MD, USA). The coaxial materials were also studied with transmission electron microscopy (TEM) on a CM 120 Bio-Twin instrument (Philips, Amsterdam, The Netherlands). For this, fibers were directly spun onto carbon-coated TEM grids (TAAB, Aldermaston, UK).

2.3.2. Physical Form Characterisation

X-ray diffraction (XRD) patterns were collected on a MiniFlex 600 diffractometer (Rigaku, Tokyo, Japan) supplied with Cu Kα radiation. Data were collected over the 2θ range 3 to 35° at a rate of 5° min^{-1}. Differential scanning calorimetry (DSC) was performed on a Q2000 instrument (TA Instruments, New Castle, DE, USA). Samples weighing between 4–7 mg were placed into T-zero aluminium pans, sealed, and pinholed. Samples were equilibrated at 0 °C, heated to 100 °C at 10 °C min^{-1}, and then cooled to 0 °C again. A second heating run (to 200 °C in most cases) was finally performed at 10 °C min^{-1}. All DSC experiments were undertaken under a nitrogen purge of 50 mL min^{-1}. IR spectra were obtained with a Spectrum 100 spectrometer (Perkin Elmer, Waltham, MA, USA) over the wavenumber range 650–4000 cm^{-1} and with resolution of 1 cm^{-1}.

2.3.3. Active Ingredient Loading

After the fibers had been left to dry to remove any residual solvent, samples (ca. 10 mg) were cut from each sample and dissolved in a mixture of ethanol/water/DMAc (15/1/4 *v*/*v*/*v*). Calibration curves for each active ingredient (AI) were prepared using a 7315 spectrophotometer (Jenway, Stone, UK), and the AI loading determined (n = 3).

2.4. *Dissolution Studies*

Calibration curves were constructed for each AI at pH 1.0 (0.1 M HCl) and 6.8 (phosphate buffered saline; PBS) with the aid of a 7315 spectrophotometer (Jenway, Stone, UK). Dissolution studies were then undertaken following the USPII method on an automated instrument (Caleva, Dorchester, UK). The dissolution vessels were initially charged with 750 mL of 0.1 M HCl and equilibrated at 37 ± 0.5 °C under stirring at 50 rpm. Lids on each vessel prevented evaporation. Capsule sinkers were manually filled with ca. 60 mg of a fiber mat and placed into the vessel. Aliquots (5 mL) were periodically withdrawn from the vessels, and replaced with 5 mL of preheated 0.1 M HCl to maintain a constant volume. After 2 h of operation, 250 mL of preheated 0.2 M trisodium phosphate dodecahydrate was added to each vessel, yielding 1 L of a buffer at pH 6.8. Again, 5 mL aliquots were withdrawn at specific time points, and replenished with 5 mL of preheated PBS at pH 6.8. The AI concentrations in each aliquot were quantified with a 7315 spectrophotometer (Jenway, Stone, UK), and cumulative release percentages calculated from these.

3. Results

3.1. Monolithic Fibers

Scanning electron microscopy (SEM) images of the monolithic fibers are presented in Figure 2. In all cases, cylindrical fibers have clearly been formed. In the cases of S-BA and S-ACA, the fibers are homogenous and well formed, with diameters around 500–600 nm (see Table 1). In contrast, the S-NA and S-NAM materials clearly contain two populations of fibers, with a number of very small branched fibers visible, likely due to there being some jet instability during spinning. As a result, the average diameter is rather smaller for these fibers, at 129 ± 102 nm for S-NA and 214 ± 105 nm for S-NAM, and there is a proportionally greater deviation in the diameters.

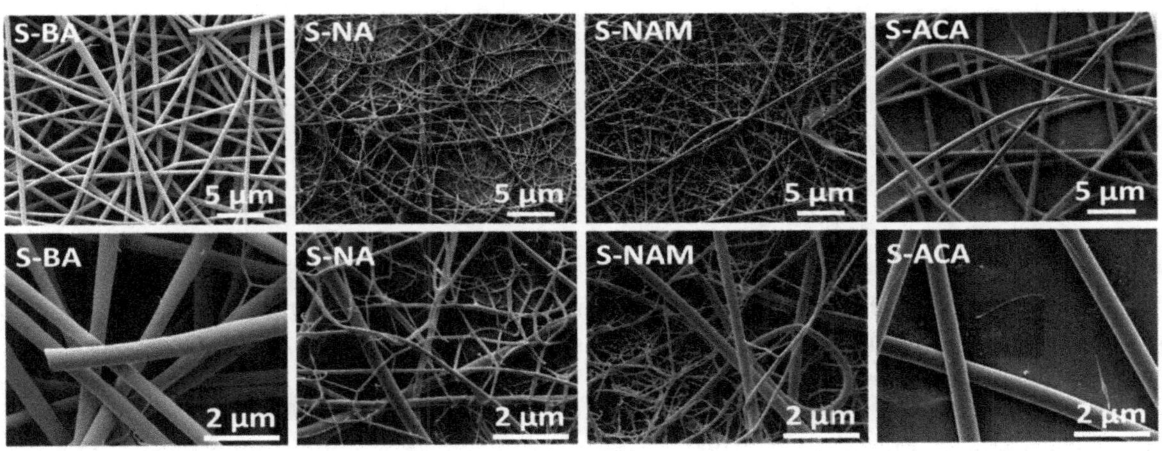

Figure 2. SEM images of the monolithic fibers (top: 10,000× magnification; bottom 40,000× magnification).

The physical form of the AI in the fibers was explored using XRD and DSC (Figure 3). The XRD data in Figure 3a demonstrate that the AIs are crystalline materials, with numerous Bragg reflections visible in their patterns. ES100 is amorphous, and only a broad halo is present in its pattern. No Bragg reflections can be observed for the fibers, showing them to be amorphous solid dispersions. The DSC data (Figure 3b,c) concur with these findings. While the AIs exhibit sharp melting endotherms in their thermograms, these are lacking for ES100 and all the fiber formulations. It should be noted that the DSC experiments were stopped at 200 °C with the fibers, since in preliminary experiments degradation was observed to start just above this temperature (data not shown). Thus, the melting of ACA would not be seen in the data even if crystalline material were present. However, T_g events are present between 100 and 125 °C for all the fibers, confirming their amorphous nature.

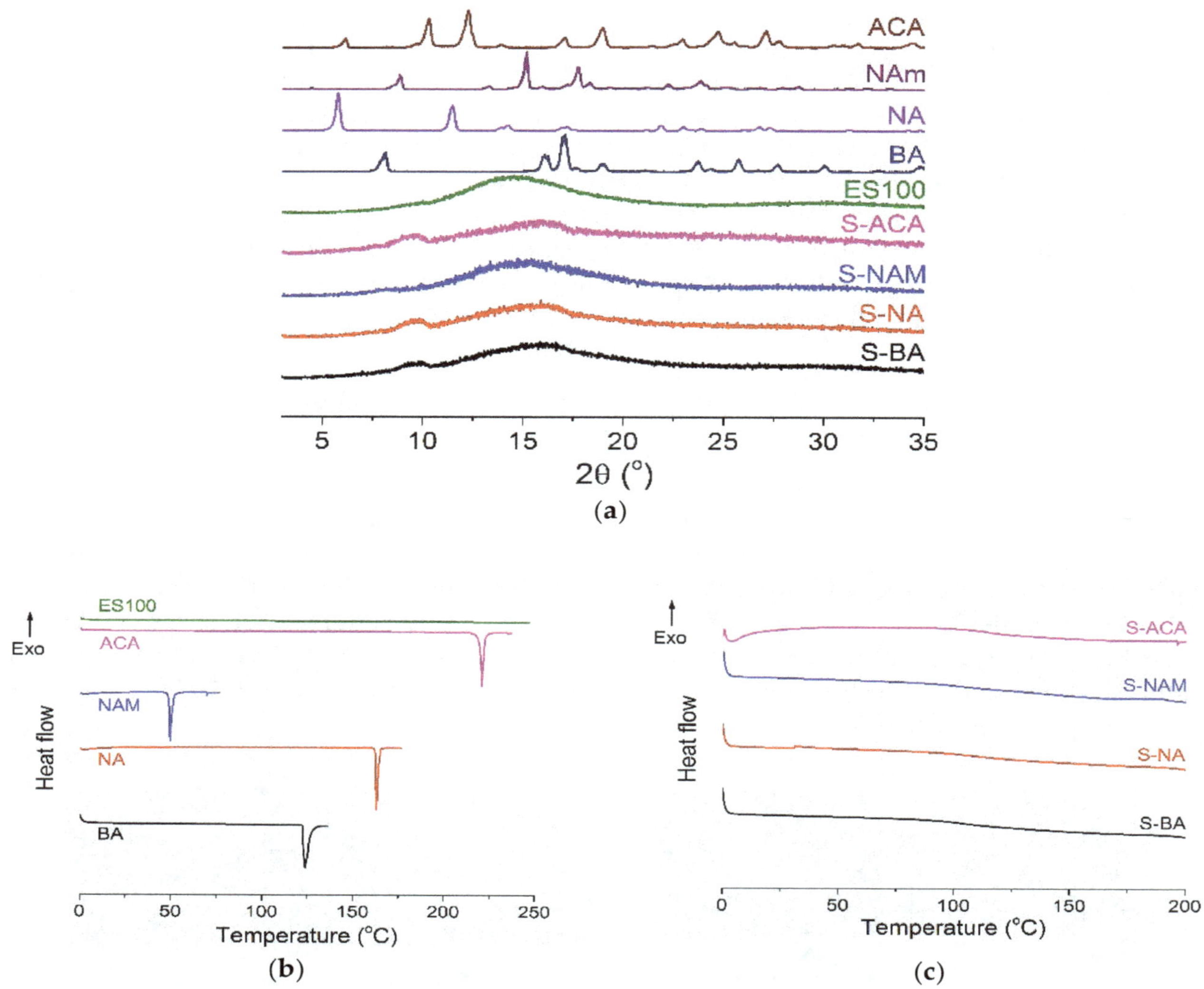

Figure 3. (**a**) XRD data and DSC data on (**b**) the raw materials and (**c**) formulations from monoaxial electrospinning. The data in (**a**) are normalized for ease of comparison.

IR spectra are given in Figure 4. ES100 has characteristic peaks at 2950–3000 cm^{-1} (CH_2 stretching), 1727 cm^{-1} (C=O stretching), and 1150–1275 cm^{-1} (C–O–C stretching). The spectra of the AI-loaded fibers are very similar to that of ES100, as expected given that the AI loading is relatively low (theoretical loading: 7.69%). However, some subtle changes can be observed. The C=O stretch of pure BA is found at 1678 cm^{-1}, and merges with the ES100 C=O stretch in the S-BA fibers to form a single peak at 1725 cm^{-1}. This shift might be attributed to the formation of intermolecular bonding interactions (e.g., H-bonding) between BA and ES100. Similarly, NA and ACA display a C=O stretch at 1667 and 1674 cm^{-1} while the S-NA and S-ACA fibers display single C=O bands at 1727 and 1726 cm^{-1} respectively. No shoulders are visible on these peaks, suggesting again that intermolecular interactions cause the bands to merge. In the case of S-NAM, the N–H stretching vibrations of NAm (at 3411 and 3341 cm^{-1}) are not visible in the fibers, which might be indicative of intermolecular bonding or simply the low AI loading in the formulations.

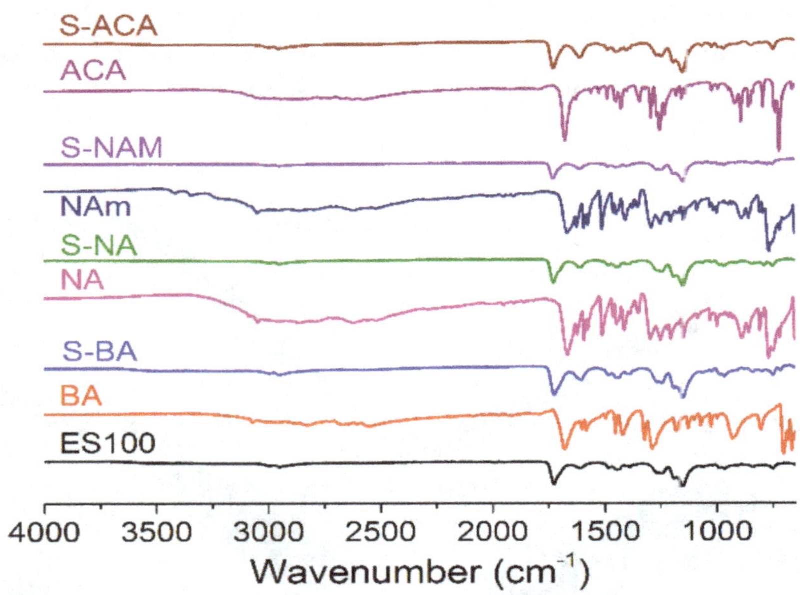

Figure 4. IR spectra of the monolithic fibers.

The AI loading (Table 1) is close to 100% of the theoretical content (>85% in all cases). The differences observed can be attributed to losses of AI during electrospinning (e.g., through small amounts of precipitation or adherence to the syringe walls), the presence of some residual solvent in the fibers, or small inaccuracies in the quantification method.

3.2. *Core/Shell Fibers*

Core/shell fibers were prepared with an ES100 shell and a core comprising ES100 and the AI. SEM images of these are given in Figure 5. The fibers are, in general, smooth and homogeneous, with average diameters of around 550–700 nm as detailed in Table 1. For C-BA and C-ACA there are a few very fine fibers present as well as the bulk at ca. 600 nm. For C-NA, what appear to be particles can be seen on the fiber surfaces, suggesting some phase separation may have occurred.

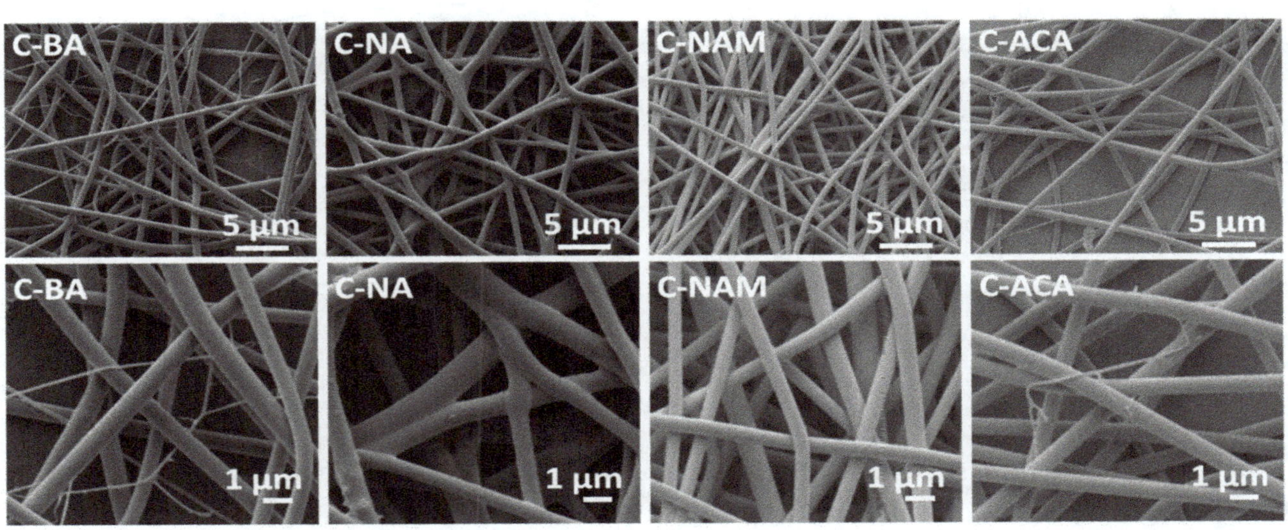

Figure 5. SEM images of the coaxial fibers.

TEM images of the fibers from coaxial electrospinning are depicted in Figure 6. The two solutions used for the core and shell are very similar in their composition, and hence the contrast between the core and shell is not particularly distinct. However, on close inspection it is clear that the fibers have separate core and shell compartments.

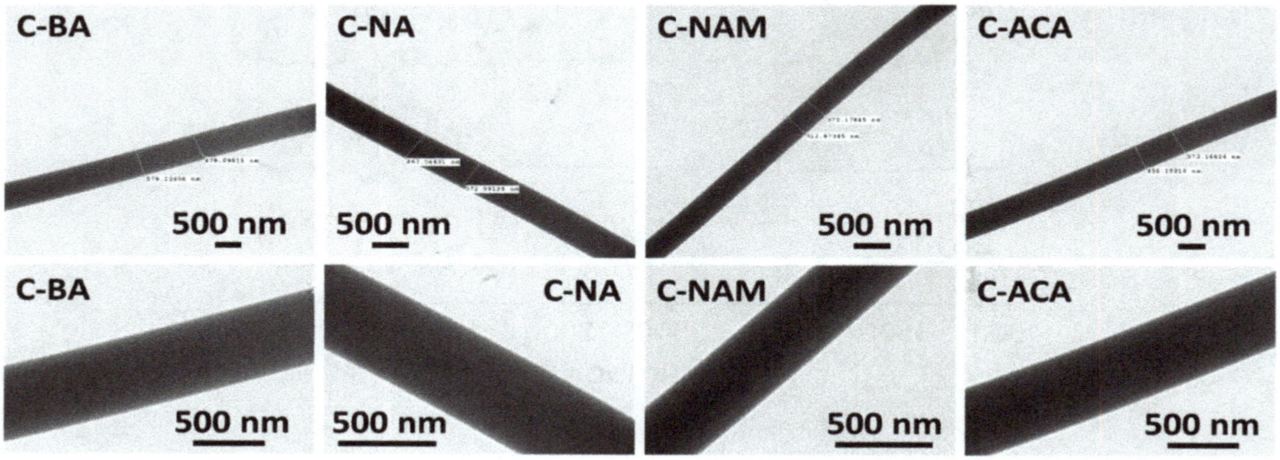

Figure 6. TEM images of the coaxial fibers.

The physical form of the AI in the fibers was probed using XRD and DSC (Figure 7). Similarly to the monolithic fibers, there is no evidence for any crystalline material being present in the products of coaxial electrospinning: the sharp Bragg reflections of the pure AIs are replaced by broad haloes in the XRD patterns of the fibers, consistent with amorphous AI-in-polymer dispersions. The DSC data are also typical of amorphous systems, with no melting endotherms visible but instead clear baseline changes corresponding to T_gs.

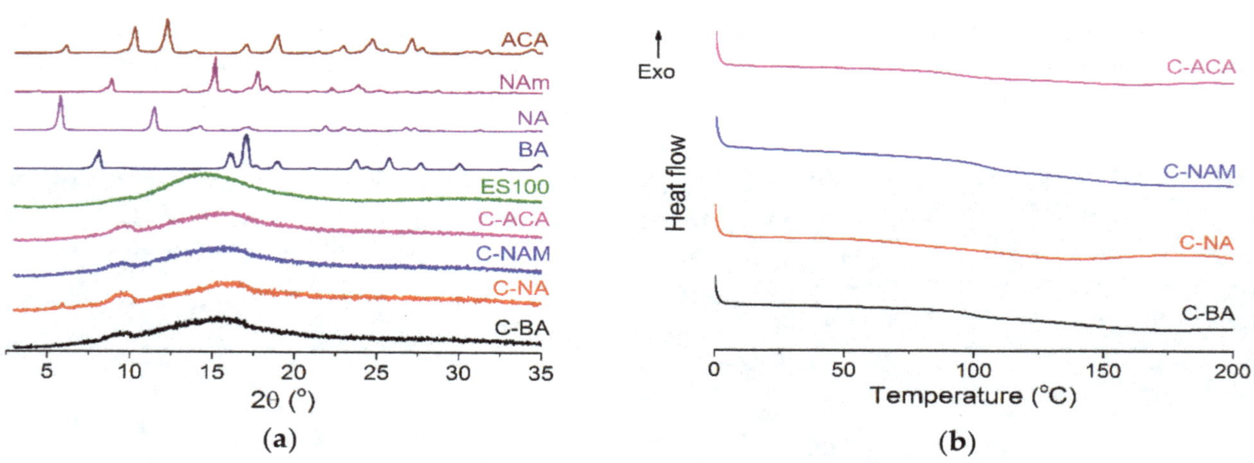

Figure 7. (**a**) XRD and (**b**) DSC data for the coaxial fibers. The data in (**a**) are normalized for ease of comparison.

IR spectra of the core/shell fibers (Figure 8) again are very similar to that of pure ES100, except with some small shifts in peak position (for instance, the C=O peak shifts from 1727 cm^{-1} in ES100 to 1725 cm^{-1} in C-BA and C-NA). Given the low AI loadings of these fibers (theoretical loading: 2.70%) it is not possible to draw any firm conclusions relating to physical form from the IR spectra alone, but it appears that intermolecular bonding may be operational here too.

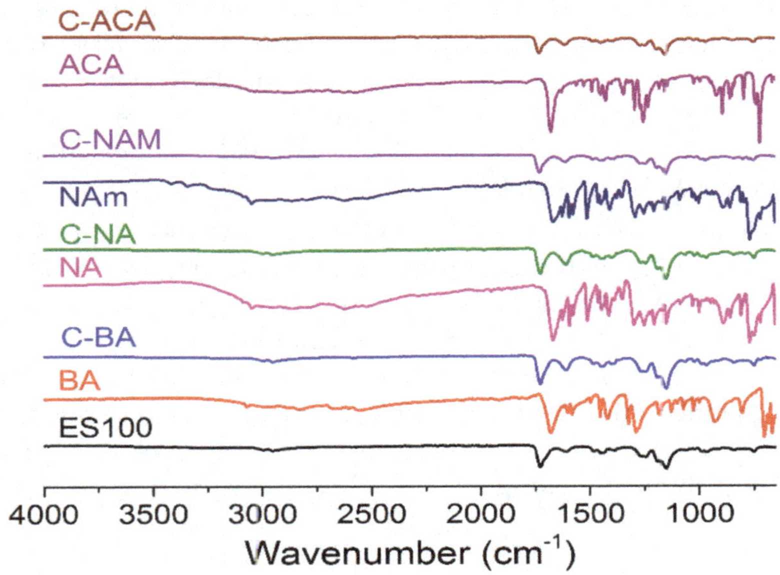

Figure 8. IR spectra of the coaxial fibers.

The AI loadings observed (see Table 1) are again close to 100% of the theoretical content (>80%), with the values close to those found in the monoaxial fibers.

3.3. AI Release

The AI release profiles for the monolithic fibers are shown in Figure 9a. It is clear that the simple fact of making fibers from ES100 does not prevent AI release at pH 1. This is because the AI is able to diffuse through the polymer matrix to reach solution. The extent to which this occurs depends on the nature of the molecule used as the AI: the amount of release in acidic pH decreases in the order S-BA (86.6 ± 1.9%) > S-NAM (59.4 ± 5.7%) > S-NA (25.5 ± 2.8%) > S-ACA (7.1 ± 4.5%). Both molecular weight (MW) and the acidity/basicity of the AIs are thus important: the lower MW BA (122 Da) releases more quickly and to a greater extent than the intermediate NAm (143 Da) and NA (172 Da) and higher MW ACA (222 Da). S-NAM releases markedly more than S-NA, presumably due to the basic nature of NAm favoring dissolution in the low pH environment in the former case.

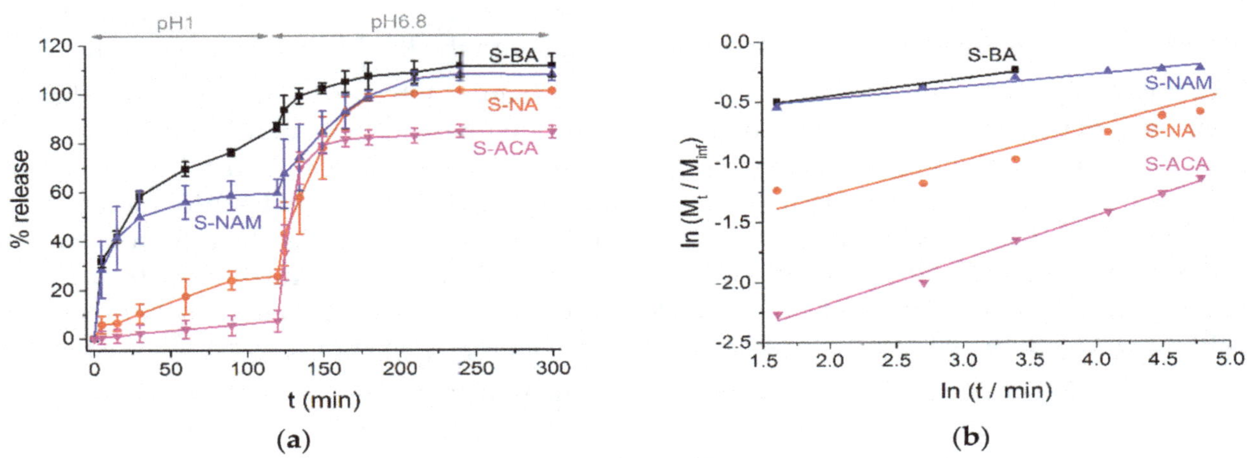

Figure 9. (**a**) AI release from the monolithic formulations, with data given as mean ± S.D. from three independent experiments; (**b**) fitting the Korsmeyer-Peppas model to the experimental data obtained at pH 1. Percentages are given relative to the theoretical AI loading in the fibers.

This hypothesis is supported by a Korsmeyer-Peppas analysis of the release data at pH 1 (Figure 9b and Table 2). This model takes the form $M_t/M_{inf} = kt^n$, where M_t is the amount of AI released at time t, M_{inf} is the theoretical AI loading of the fibers, k is a rate constant, and n is an exponent providing information on the reaction mechanism. For all the monolithic fibers, n is <0.45, indicating that Fickian diffusion is the predominant reaction mechanism. The calculated k values fall in the same order as the extent of release data, as would be expected.

Considering the release observed at pH 6.8, all the formulations rapidly release the majority of their remaining AI content after the pH is elevated, with maximum release attained after ca. 60 min immersion in PBS. S-BA, S-NA and S-NAM all reach approximately 100% release, while for S-ACA the plot levels off at around 84%. This can be attributed to the larger MW and lower solubility of ACA compared to the other AIs, as well as the reduced entrapment efficiency noted for S-ACA (calculated to be 85% of the theoretical loading). There are insufficient datapoints for a Peppas analysis of the release data at pH 6.8 but the slopes of plots of ln (M_t/M_{inf}) vs. ln t are much steeper than at acidic pH, indicating that polymer swelling and dissolution are the dominant release mechanisms in neutral conditions.

Table 2. Values extracted from Kormeyer-Peppas analysis of the AI release data at pH 1.

Formulation	n	k (min^{-1})
S-BA	0.14	0.48
S-NA	0.28	0.16
S-NAM	0.10	0.51
S-ACA	0.36	0.055
C-BA	0.11	0.47
C-NA	0.25	0.18
C-NAM	0.22	0.27
C-ACA	NC	NC

NC = not calculated. The release percentages obtained for C-ACA at pH 1 were all very close to zero, and hence mathematical analysis could not be undertaken.

AI release from the coaxial fibers shows similar trends to the monoaxial analogues (Figure 10a). The presence of a blank ES100 shell clearly reduces the amount of AI release seen at pH 1, with C-BA releasing only 57.4 ± 1.7% of its AI loading, cf. 86.6 ± 1.9% in the case of the monolithic systems. Similar results are seen for C-NAM vs. S-NAM (50.9 ± 2.8% and 59.4 ± 5.7% release, respectively) and the ACA-loaded formulations (C-ACA 1.5 ± 0.8%; S-ACA 7.1 ± 4.5%). C-NA and S-NA behave very similarly (C-NA 26.6 ± 1.5%; S-NA 25.5 ± 2.8%). It is evident in all cases bar ACA that a significant proportion of the AI is freed into acidic solution, even though the ES100 sheath is insoluble.

Korsmeyer-Peppas analysis of the pH 1 release data (Figure 10b and Table 2) indicates that, as for the monolithic materials, AI release is diffusion controlled, with $n < 0.45$. Looking at the rate constants (k), only for C-NAM is there any noticeable change from the monolithic fibers. This is potentially attributable to the basic nature of NAm: NAm has a pKa of 3.92, and so will be fully ionized at pH 1. This will cause it to be highly soluble, providing a thermodynamic driver for the molecules to diffuse out of the polymer matrix and into solution. The other three AIs are acidic, and will be 100% unionized at pH 1. It should be noted that the Korsmeyer-Peppas equation is really only suitable for release from monolithic systems however, and thus some caution must be exercised in considering the results.

When the pH is raised to 6.8, as for the monolithic materials the rate of AI release accelerates noticeably. Both C-NAM and C-NA release 100% of their AI cargo, while C-ACA releases around 81% of the theoretical loading (again consistent with the lower entrapment efficiency of this formulation (91%)). Interesting, C-BA behaves more similarly to the C-ACA material than the naphthalene analogues. It is not obvious why this should be, but it may be that BA forms strong H-bonds with the ES100 carrier as it dissolves, resulting in the formation of AI-polymer aggregates which are removed by filtration before the release percentage is quantified. The maximum extent of release in all cases is reached more slowly than for the monolithic systems, at around 2 h after the elevation of pH.

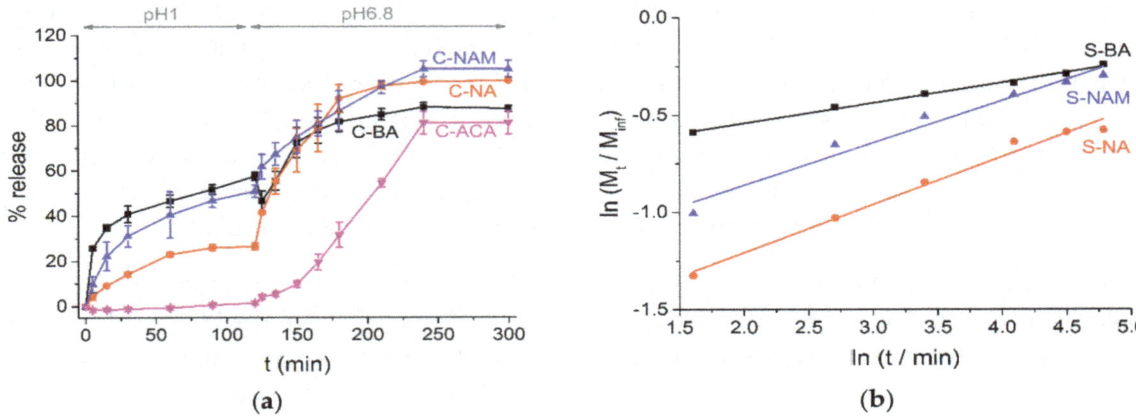

Figure 10. (**a**) AI release from the core/shell formulations, with data given as mean ± S.D. from three independent experiments; (**b**) fitting the Korsmeyer-Peppas model to the experimental data obtained at pH 1. Percentages are given relative to the theoretical AI loading in the fibers.

It proved possible to develop relationships between the molecular weight and the percentage release attained at pH 1 (Figure 11a). It should be noted that some caution is necessary in extracting these, since they are based on data from only a small number of formulations, but nevertheless some trends are clear. We attempted to fit both simple linear and exponential relationships to the percentage release data. For the monolithic fibers, the best fit to the data is obtained with an exponential relationship taking the form % release = $-6.07 + 92.7e^{-(MW-122)/51.3}$, whereas for the coaxial fibers a more simple linear equation gives the best fit: % release = 126 − 0.561MW. The influence of MW on the release percentage after 2 h at pH 1 is thus dulled by the addition of the blank polymer shell. Considering the Korsmeyer-Peppas rate constants (Figure 11b), an exponential equation of the form $k = 0.146 + 0.324e^{-(MW-122)/22.3}$ gives the best fit to the experimental data for the coaxial systems. In contrast, with the monolithic systems such a relationship can only be constructed for the three carboxylic acids, for which we find $k = 0.00372 + 0.476e^{-(MW-122)/44.9}$. The S-NAM datapoint clearly does not fit on this trendline, indicating that the basicity of the AI has a major influence on the rate constant in the case of the monolithic formulations.

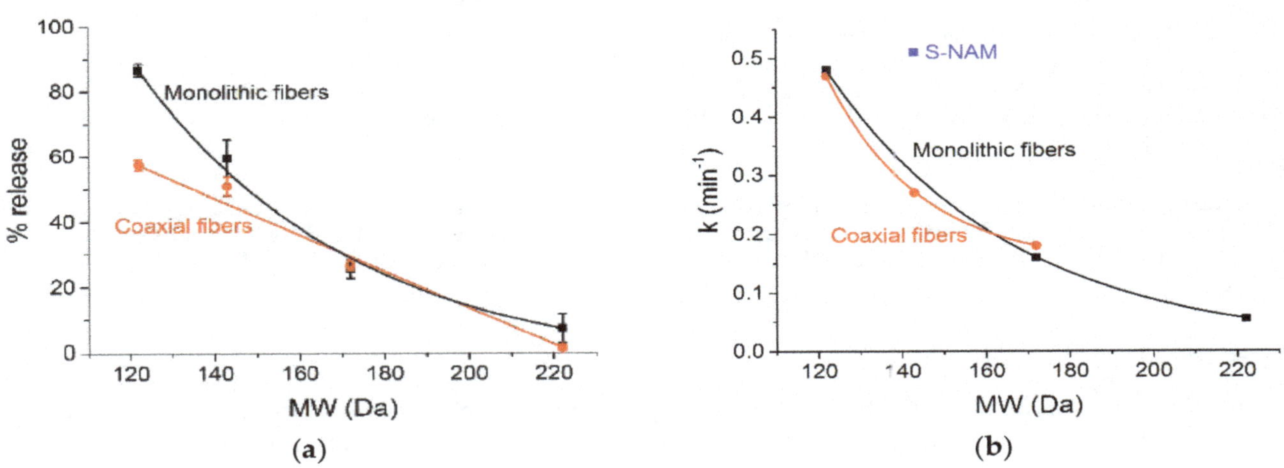

Figure 11. The relationships between AI MW and (**a**) percentage release after 2 h immersion in a pH 1 solution; and (**b**) the Korsmeyer-Peppas rate constant.

4. Discussion

We show in this work that both the molecular weight and the acidity/basicity of an AI are crucial in determining the extent to which release occurs from Eudragit S100 fibers in acidic media. The nanoscale nature of the fiber diameters means that they have very large surface area-to-volume ratios, and thus simply making a fiber from an insoluble polymer does not preclude AI release in conditions where the polymer is insoluble [22,26]. Rather, it is necessary to consider also the ability of the AI to diffuse through the matrix, and the thermodynamic solubility driver for this to happen. It has previously been speculated that lower molecular weight species and those which are more basic will release to a greater extent at acidic pHs [22,25], and in this work we confirm this to be the case.

For coaxial fibers with AI located in the core only, it is demonstrated that the molecular weight of the AI is a good predictor for the percentage and rate of release seen at pH 1, and mathematical relationships can be constructed linking these. For the monolithic fibers, the situation is more complex and although it is possible to elucidate a mathematical relationship between percentage release and AI MW, this does not hold true for the rate of release. For the latter, there is a clear linkage with the MW for the acidic carboxylate AIs considered, but this breaks down for the basic species included in the study. It thus appears that for the coaxial systems, the rate of diffusion through the polymer shell, which will be directly correlated with the MW of the AI, is the dominant factor governing release. For the monolithic analogues, while it is clear that diffusion through the polymer matrix is important, the solubility of the AI in the release milieu is also vital to consider.

5. Conclusions

We report new insights into the factors governing the release of active ingredients (AIs) from electrospun Eudragit S100 (ES100) fibers. Monolithic fibers loaded with benzoic acid, 1-naphthoic acid, 1-naphthylamine, and 9-anthracene carboxylic acid were generated, along with analogous systems with an AI-loaded core and an ES100 shell. The fibers were smooth and cylindrical in the main, and comprised amorphous solid dispersions. There was significant release at pH 1 with all of the monolithic fibers except for those containing 9-anthracene carboxylic acid. Both the molecular weight of the AI and its acidity/basicity are important in controlling release from such materials, with lower molecular weight AIs and basic species freed from the fibers more quickly. With the coaxial fibers, since the AI is present only in the core the acidity/basicity appears to be a less important factor, and the molecular weight, and thus the rate of diffusion through the polymer matrix, is found to be the rate limiting step in release. Mathematical equations could be constructed to predict the release obtained in acidic conditions with AIs of differing molecular properties.

Author Contributions: K.B., H.L, F. and G.R.W. conceived and designed the experiments; K.B. and Y.A.-z. performed the experiments; K.B., H.L., Y.A.-z., F. and G.R.W. analyzed the data; K.B. and G.R.W. wrote the manuscript.

Acknowledgments: We thank the China Scholarship Council for funding H.L.'s work in UCL, the British Council and Egyptian Sciences and Technology Development Fund for awarding a Newton-Mosharafa Researcher Links Travel Grant to Y.A.-z., and the Indonesia Endowment Fund for Education for the award of a PhD studentship to Fatimah.

References

1. Sebe, I.; Szabo, P.; Kallai-Szabo, B.; Zelko, R. Incorporating small molecules or biologics into nanofibers for optimized drug release: A review. *Int. J. Pharm.* **2015**, *494*, 516–530. [CrossRef] [PubMed]
2. Xie, J.; Jiang, J.; Davoodi, P.; Srinivasan, M.P.; Wang, C.H. Electrohydrodynamic atomization: A two-decade effort to produce and process micro-/nanoparticulate materials. *Chem. Eng. Sci.* **2015**, *125*, 32–57. [CrossRef] [PubMed]

3. Yu, D.G.; Shen, X.X.; Branford-White, C.; White, K.; Zhu, L.M.; Bligh, S.W. Oral fast-dissolving drug delivery membranes prepared from electrospun polyvinylpyrrolidone ultrafine fibers. *Nanotechnology* **2009**, *20*, 055104. [CrossRef] [PubMed]
4. Illangakoon, U.E.; Gill, H.; Shearman, G.C.; Parhizkar, M.; Mahalingam, S.; Chatterton, N.P.; Williams, G.R. Fast dissolving paracetamol/caffeine nanofibers prepared by electrospinning. *Int. J. Pharm.* **2014**, *477*, 369–379. [CrossRef] [PubMed]
5. Lu, H.; Wang, Q.; Li, G.; Qiu, Y.; Wei, Q. Electrospun water-stable zein/ethyl cellulose composite nanofiber and its drug release properties. *Mater. Sci. Eng. C* **2017**, *74*, 86–93. [CrossRef] [PubMed]
6. Meng, Z.X.; Zheng, W.; Li, L.; Zheng, Y.F. Fabrication, characterization and in vitro drug release behavior of electrospun PLGA/chitosan nanofibrous scaffold. *Mater. Chem. Phys.* **2011**, *125*, 606–611. [CrossRef]
7. Jia, X.; Zhao, C.; Li, P.; Zhang, H.; Huang, Y.; Li, H.; Fan, J.; Feng, W.; Yuan, X.; Fan, Y. Sustained release of VEGF by coaxial electrospun dextran/PLGA fibrous membranes in vascular tissue engineering. *J. Biomater. Sci. Polym. Ed.* **2011**, *22*, 1811–1827. [CrossRef] [PubMed]
8. Xie, J.; Wang, C.H. Electrospun micro- and nanofibers for sustained delivery of paclitaxel to treat C6 glioma in vitro. *Pharm. Res.* **2006**, *23*, 1817–1826. [CrossRef] [PubMed]
9. Li, H.; Williams, G.R.; Wu, J.; Lv, Y.; Sun, X.; Wu, H.; Zhu, L.M. Thermosensitive nanofibers loaded with ciprofloxacin as antibacterial wound dressing materials. *Int. J. Pharm.* **2017**, *517*, 135–147. [CrossRef] [PubMed]
10. Li, H.; Williams, G.R.; Wu, J.; Wang, H.; Sun, X.; Zhu, L.M. Poly(*N*-isopropylacrylamide)/poly(L-lactic acid-*co*-caprolactone) fibers loaded with ciprofloxacin as wound dressing materials. *Mater. Sci. Eng. C* **2017**, *79*, 245–254. [CrossRef] [PubMed]
11. Hu, J.; Li, H.-Y.; Williams, G.R.; Yang, H.-H.; Tao, L.; Zhu, L.-M. Electrospun poly(*N*-isopropylacrylamide)/ethyl cellulose nanofibers as thermoresponsive drug delivery systems. *J. Pharm. Sci.* **2016**, *105*. [CrossRef]
12. Lin, X.; Tang, D.; Cui, W.; Cheng, Y. Controllable drug release of electrospun thermoresponsive poly(*N*-isopropylacrylamide)/poly(2-acrylamido-2-methylpropanesulfonic acid) nanofibers. *J. Biomed. Mater. Res. A* **2012**, *100*, 1839–1845. [CrossRef] [PubMed]
13. Wang, X.; Yu, D.G.; Li, X.Y.; Bligh, S.W.; Williams, G.R. Electrospun medicated shellac nanofibers for colon-targeted drug delivery. *Int. J. Pharm.* **2015**, *490*, 384–390. [CrossRef] [PubMed]
14. Salehi, R.; Irani, M.; Eskandani, M.; Nowruzi, K.; Davaran, S.; Haririan, I. Interaction, controlled release, and antitumor activity of doxorubicin hydrochloride from pH-sensitive p(NIPAAm-MAA-VP) nanofibrous scaffolds prepared by green electrospinning. *Int. J. Polym. Mater.* **2014**, *63*, 609–619. [CrossRef]
15. Shen, X.; Yu, D.; Zhu, L.; Branford-White, C.; White, K.; Chatterton, N.P. Electrospun diclofenac sodium loaded Eudragit(R) L 100-55 nanofibers for colon-targeted drug delivery. *Int. J. Pharm.* **2011**, *408*, 200–207. [CrossRef] [PubMed]
16. Illangakoon, U.E.; Nazir, T.; Williams, G.R.; Chatterton, N.P. Mebeverine-loaded electrospun nanofibers: Physicochemical characterization and dissolution studies. *J. Pharm. Sci.* **2014**, *103*, 283–292. [CrossRef] [PubMed]
17. Yu, D.-G.; Williams, G.R.; Wang, X.; Liu, X.-K.; Li, H.-L.; Bligh, S.W.A. Dual drug release nanocomposites prepared using a combination of electrospraying and electrospinning. *RSC Adv.* **2013**, *3*, 4652. [CrossRef]
18. Akhgari, A.; Heshmati, Z.; Afrasiabi Garekani, H.; Sadeghi, F.; Sabbagh, A.; Sharif Makhmalzadeh, B.; Nokhodchi, A. Indomethacin electrospun nanofibers for colonic drug delivery: In vitro dissolution studies. *Colloids Surf. B* **2017**, *152*, 29–35. [CrossRef] [PubMed]
19. Yu, D.-G.; Liu, F.; Cui, L.; Liu, Z.-P.; Wang, X.; Bligh, S.W.A. Coaxial electrospinning using a concentric Teflon spinneret to prepare biphasic-release nanofibers of helicid. *RSC Adv.* **2013**, *3*, 17775–17783. [CrossRef]
20. Karthikeyan, K.; Guhathakarta, S.; Rajaram, R.; Korrapati, P.S. Electrospun zein/eudragit nanofibers based dual drug delivery system for the simultaneous delivery of aceclofenac and pantoprazole. *Int. J. Pharm.* **2012**, *438*, 117–122. [CrossRef] [PubMed]
21. Balogh, A.; Farkas, B.; Domokos, A.; Farkas, A.; Démuth, B.; Borbás, E.; Nagy, B.; Marosi, G.; Nagy, Z.K. Controlled-release solid dispersions of Eudragit®FS 100 and poorly soluble spironolactone prepared by electrospinning and melt extrusion. *Eur. Polym. J.* **2017**, *95*, 406–417. [CrossRef]
22. Illangakoon, U.E.; Yu, D.G.; Ahmad, B.S.; Chatterton, N.P.; Williams, G.R. 5-Fluorouracil loaded Eudragit fibers prepared by electrospinning. *Int. J. Pharm.* **2015**, *495*, 895–902. [CrossRef] [PubMed]

23. Jin, M.; Yu, D.G.; Wang, X.; Geraldes, C.F.; Williams, G.R.; Bligh, S.W. Electrospun contrast-agent-loaded fibers for colon-targeted MRI. *Adv. Healthcare Mater.* **2016**, *5*, 977–985. [CrossRef] [PubMed]
24. Jin, M.; Yu, D.G.; Geraldes, C.F.; Williams, G.R.; Bligh, S.W. Theranostic fibers for simultaneous imaging and drug delivery. *Mol. Pharm.* **2016**, *13*, 2457–2465. [CrossRef] [PubMed]
25. Jia, D.; Gao, Y.; Williams, G.R. Core/shell poly(ethylene oxide)/Eudragit fibers for site-specific release. *Int. J. Pharm.* **2017**, *523*, 376–385. [CrossRef] [PubMed]
26. Yu, D.G.; Li, X.Y.; Wang, X.; Yang, J.H.; Bligh, S.W.; Williams, G.R. Nanofibers fabricated using triaxial electrospinning as zero order drug delivery systems. *ACS Appl. Mater. Interfaces* **2015**, *7*, 18891–18897. [CrossRef] [PubMed]

2

Enhanced Delivery of Imatinib into Vaginal Mucosa via a New Positively Charged Nanocrystal-Loaded in Situ Hydrogel Formulation for Treatment of Cervical Cancer

Li-qian Ci [1,2,†], Zhi-gang Huang [1,†], Feng-mei Lv [2], Jun Wang [2], Ling-lin Feng [3], Feng Sun [4], Shui-juan Cao [5], Zhe-peng Liu [2], Yu Liu [1,*], Gang Wei [1] and Wei-yue Lu [1]

1. Department of Pharmaceutics, School of Pharmacy, Fudan University & Key Laboratory of Smart Drug Delivery (Fudan University), Ministry of Education, Shanghai 201203, China; ciliqian@foxmail.com (L.-q.C.); 16211030018@fudan.edu.cn (Z.-g.H.); weigang@shmu.edu.cn (G.W.); wylu@shmu.edu.cn (W.-y.L.)
2. School of Medical Instrument and Food Engineering, University of Shanghai for Science and Technology, Shanghai 200093, China; 15216806348@163.com (F.-m.L.); doudou19940424@163.com (J.W.); zhepengliu@126.com (Z.-p.L.)
3. NHC Key Laboratory of Reproduction Regulation (Shanghai Institute of Planned Parenthood Research), Fudan University, Room 904, No 1 Research Building, 2140 Xietu Road, Shanghai 200032, China; fenglinglinxin@163.com
4. Chinese Academy of Sciences Shanghai Institute of Materia Medica, Shanghai 201203, China; sunfengbbb@simm.ac.cn
5. Experimental Teaching Center, School of Pharmacy, Fudan University, Shanghai 201203, China; chaoshui2011@126.com

* Correspondence: liuyu@fudan.edu.cn
† Equally contributing authors.

Abstract: The present study was carried out to investigate the potential of cationic functionalization on imatinib nanocrystals to improve the mucoadhesiveness and, thus, delivery to the lesion of cervicovaginal tumors. Amino-group-functionalized imatinib nanocrystals (NC@PDA-NH_2) were prepared with near-spheroid shape, nanoscale size distribution, positive zeta potential, and relatively high drug content with the aid of the polydopamine-coating technique. Efficient interaction between NC@PDA-NH_2 and mucin was proven by mucin adsorption which was related to the positive zeta-potential value of NC@PDA-NH_2 and the change in the size distribution on mixing of NC@PDA-NH_2 and mucin. Cellular uptake, growth inhibition, and apoptosis induction in cervicovaginal cancer-related cells demonstrated the superiority of NC@PDA-NH_2 over unmodified nanocrystals. For practical intravaginal administration, NC@PDA-NH_2 was dispersed in Pluronic F127-based thermosensitive in situ hydrogel, which showed suitable gelation temperature and sustained-release profiles. In comparison with unmodified nanocrystals, NC@PDA-NH_2 exhibited extended residence on ex vivo murine vaginal mucosa, prolonged in vivo intravaginal residence, and enhanced inhibition on the growth of murine orthotopic cervicovaginal model tumors indicated by smaller tumor size, longer median survival time, and more intratumor apoptosis with negligible mucosal toxicity. In conclusion, cationic functionalization endowed NC@PDA-NH_2 significant mucoadhesiveness and, thus, good potential against cervicovaginal cancer via intravaginal administration.

Keywords: mucoadhesiveness; cervicovaginal tumors; cationic functionalization; imatinib; nanocrystals; in situ hydrogel

1. Introduction

Cervical cancer is the fourth most common cause of death from cancer in women [1]. With the development and popularization of regular Papanicolaou (Pap) tests, the majority of cervical cancer patients can be diagnosed in the early stages when the tumor is small in size and confined to the cervix. Nevertheless, the current treatment for early-stage cervical cancer usually involves significant adverse side effects. Surgery and radiation therapy are associated with increased risks of future negative gynecological and obstetric outcomes, including impaired sexual function, infertility, preterm delivery, and low birth weight. Systemic pharmacotherapy is generally the last option because only a negligible proportion of the drug reaches the vaginal mucosal epithelium. Now, clinicians are realizing that cervicovaginal tumors may represent the most important potential field needing good vaginal formulations [2]. Sustained and localized drug delivery in the female reproductive tract may avoid adverse effects associated with systemic administration, improve efficacy by assuring adequate local drug concentration, and allow convenient self-administration [3]. For example, the first tyrosine kinase inhibitor, imatinib, was reported to prevent the activation of platelet-derived growth factor receptor (PDGFR), which is often overexpressed in cervical cancer [4], thus inhibiting cervical cancer cell proliferation. In a study which screened carbo- and cisplatin, topotecan, paclitaxel, imatinib, gefitinib, cetuximab, and trastuzumab on freshly isolated tumor cells of 16 patients, 66% of tumor samples were sensitive to imatinib [5]. When administered orally, it worked effectively in the clinic, possibly due to its high plasma protein binding and insufficient drug delivery to the vaginal mucosal epithelium. It is reasonable to expect a positive outcome for imatinib if vaginal formulations with adequate vaginal mucosal delivery efficiency are available.

Recently, nanocrystals (NC) drew increasing interest in field of delivery of poorly soluble drugs [6–8] for their nanoscale and high drug content. These properties seem to be attractive for vaginal formulations. Only nanocrystals with suitable mucoadhesive modification can overcome the self-cleaning mechanism of the vagina, assure prolonged contact time with mucosa, and avoid multiple daily doses [9]. One of the most promising mucoadhesive strategies is cationic modification, which is based on the electrostatic interaction with negatively charged mucin in the mucus, as well as mucosal epithelial cells. The most exciting recent advance is positively charged 10-hydroxycamptothecin-loaded nanogels for intravesical instillation which successfully prolonged intravesical residence time, improved penetration into the vesical mucosa, and enhanced the anti-tumor efficacy in a murine orthotopic bladder cancer model [9]. Cationic functionalization was also applied in vaginal formulations. We previously synthesized a cationic derivative of Pluronic F127 to prepare a new type of thermosensitive/mucoadhesive in situ hydrogel, which significantly prolonged intravaginal drug residence and improved mucosal penetration [10]. Similar benefits were also reported for imiquimoid-loaded nanocapsules [11].

Being highly dispersed in nature, NCs are thermodynamically unstable, necessitating surface modification to prevent possible particle growth. In the meantime, surface modification can change the in vivo performance of nanocrystals. Polyethylene glycol (PEG)ylated paclitaxel nanocrystals showed good stability and in vivo tumor inhibition efficacy [12]. Albumin-stabilized paclitaxel nanocrystals showed enhanced uptake by SPARC$^+$ B16F10 melanoma cells and in vivo anti-tumor efficacy [13], and albumin-stabilized hydroxycamptothecin nanocrystals showed enhanced intratumor accumulation and prolonged survival time in MCF-7 model tumor-bearing mice [14]. Pluronic F68-stabilized paclitaxel nanocrystals exhibited elevated interaction with cancer cells and intratumor accumulation [15,16]. Pluronic F68 and soybean lecithin-stabilized 7-ethyl-10-hydroxycamptothecin nanocrystals inhibited the growth of MCF-7 model tumors more efficiently [17]. The abovementioned surface modification examples for nanocrystals are mainly based on either physical adsorption of stabilizers or chemical derivatization of the prototype drug.

Alternatively, polydopamine (PDA) coating may provide another choice. In a weak basic environment, dopamine can self-polymerize on the surface of solid materials to form a PDA layer which can subsequently react with thiol or amine groups at *o*-quinone moieties [18]. Since the pioneer work of Messersmith's group [19], this property of PDA attracted increasing interest for its good biocompatibility and capability of forming of nanostructures [20,21] or their surface functionalization [22,23]. Liang et al. recently reported the promising performance of tumor-targeting modified PDA-coated camptothecin nanocrystals [24].

Herein, positively charged polydopamine-coated imatinib nanocrystals (NC@PDA-NH_2) were prepared and characterized with respect to basic physicochemical properties, drug content and release, and in vitro interaction with mucin and cervical cancer-related cell lines. NC@PDA-NH_2 was further dispersed in a Pluronic F127-based in situ hydrogel vehicle to allow adequate interaction time between nanocrystals and mucosa. The NC@PDA-NH_2-loaded Pluronic F127-based in situ hydrogel (NC@PDA-NH_2/FG) was optimized based on rheological and release profiles and characterized with respect to ex vivo residence on mouse vaginal mucosa, in vivo intravaginal retention, and anti-tumor efficacy in a murine orthotopic cervicovaginal tumor model.

2. Methods

2.1. Materials and Animals

Imatinib (IMN), 1,1′-dioctadecyl-3,3,3′,3′-tetramethylindotricarbocyanine iodide (DiR), 2-(4-amidinophenyl)-6-indolecarbamindine dihydrochloride (DAPI), and 6-coumarin (C6) were purchased from Meilun Biotechnology Ltd. Co. (Dalian, Liaoning, China). Pluronic F127 (F127) was purchased from BASF Ltd. Co. (Ludwigshaften, Germany). Optical coherence tomography (OCT) was purchased from Sakura Finetek Inc. (Torrrance, CA, USA). Porcine gastric mucin (PGM) was purchased from Sigma-Aldrich Ltd. Co. (St Louis, MO, USA) and purified as described in previous literature [23]. All other chemicals were of analytical grade, purchased from Sinopharm Reagent Ltd. Co. (Shanghai, China) and used as received. Two cervical cancer-related cell lines, TC-1 and SiHa, were purchased from Fu-Heng Cell Center (Shanghai, China).

Female C57BL/6 mice were provided by Shanghai Laboratory Animal Center (Shanghai, China). All animals were allowed free access to standard food and tap water and acclimated for at least one week before use. All animal experiments were carried out in accordance with the guidelines evaluated and approved by the Ethics Committee of the School of Pharmacy, Fudan University (2015-O3-YJ-LY-0D approved on 4 March 2015).

2.2. Preparation of NC, NC@PDA, and NC@PDA-NH_2

NC@PDA-NH_2 was prepared by three steps. Firstly, a mixture of imatinib (3.5 mg) and stabilizers (3.8 mg TPGS and 7.5 mg citrate acid) was fully dissolved in 3 mL of ethanol in a round-bottom flask. Ethanol was evaporated with a rotary evaporator at 40 °C to form a thin film on the wall of the flask. Then, 5 mL of 35 mM $NaHCO_3$ aqueous solution was added to the film at room temperature. After hydration by gentle mixing, NCs were formed. Secondly, 5 mg of dopamine was added to 5 mL of the abovementioned NC suspension and incubated at room temperature for 10 min on a rotating rocker. Then, the suspension was centrifuged at 4448× g for 15 min at room temperature to remove unreacted dopamine and obtain NC@PDA. Thirdly, the pellet was re-suspended in 5 mL of pure water containing appropriate amounts of Boc-$NHCH_2CH_2$-NH_2 to react for at least 3 h. Then, the suspension was centrifuged at 4448× g for 15 min at room temperature to remove unreacted Boc-$NHCH_2CH_2$-NH_2 and was deprotected in 3 M HCl for 3 h to obtain NC@PDA-NH_2. DiR- or C6-labeled nanocrystals were similarly prepared except that DiR or C5 (5 μg/mL) was included in the initial mixture in the first step.

2.3. Characterization of NC, NC@PDA, and NC@PDA-NH_2

For determination of drug loading (DL) and encapsulation efficiency (EE), lyophilized nanocrystals with a premeasured mass were dissolved in acetonitrile (ACN), filtered with a 0.45-μm syringe filter, diluted if necessary, and submitted to HPLC analysis on an Agilent 1100 HPLC system (Palo Alto, CA, USA) equipped with an Xtimate ® C18 column (25 cm × 4.6 mm, particle size: 5 μm;

Welch Technology, Shanghai, China) with a mobile phase 45:55 (v/v) mixture of ACN/ammonium acetate buffer solution (10 mM, pH 10) at a flow rate 0.7 mL/min and a detection wavelength of 272 nm.

EE and DL were respectively calculated according to the following equations:

$$\mathrm{EE}(\%) = \frac{\text{Amount of drug in nanocrystals}}{\text{Total amount of feeding drug}} \times 100\%,$$

$$\mathrm{DL}(\%) = \frac{\text{Amount of drug in nanocrystals}}{\text{Total mass of nanocrystals}} \times 100\%.$$

In vitro release of imatinib from nanocrystals was investigated using the dialysis bag method with vaginal fluid simulant (VFS) as the release medium, prepared as reported previously [25] The morphology of various nanocrystals was observed using a transmission electron microscope (TEM, JEM-2100F, JEOL Co., Tokyo, Japan). The size distribution and zeta potential of nanocrystals were measured at 37 °C using dynamic light scattering (DLS) with a Zetasizer (ZS-10-82, Malvern Instruments Ltd. Co., Malvern, UK).

X-ray powder diffraction (XRPD) of nanocrystals was analyzed with a D2 Phaser diffractometer (BrukerCorp., Billerica, MA, USA) with a Cu-Kα radiation source and a LYNXEYE^{TM}-compound silicon strip detector. The powder patterns were obtained from 1 to 40° 2θ at a scan speed of 5°/min and a step size of 0.02°. The voltage and current used were 40 kV and 44 mA, respectively.

Differential scanning calorimetry (DSC) was carried out using a Perkin-Elmer Pyris 1 DSC instrument (Waltham, MA, USA) equipped with an intra-cooler 2P cooling accessory. Accurately weighed samples were separately sealed in standard aluminum pans and scanned from 20 to 300 °C at a heating rate of 10 °C/min with a nitrogen purge of 10 mL/min.

2.4. Interaction between Mucin and Nanocrystals

To investigate the change in the size distribution after mixing mucin and nanocrystals, purified PGM was mixed with NC@PDA-NH_2 or NC at the weight ratio of 2:1 in citrate buffer (0.1 M, pH 5, the physiological vaginal pH) for DLS measurements.

For determination of the adsorption amount (AA) of mucin by nanocrystals, purified PGM was mixed with NC@PDA-NH_2 with different positive surface charges (see Supplementary Materials) or NC at the weight ratio of 2:1 in citrate buffer (0.1 M, pH 5), incubated at 37 °C for 1 h and then centrifuged at 6672× g for 10 min (H1650-W centrifuge, Xiang-yi Instrument Inc., Changsha, China). The concentration of PGM in the supernatant was measured using Pierce® BCA Protein Assay Kits (Thermo Scientific, Rockford, IL, USA) to calculate AA according to the following equation:

$$\mathrm{AA} = \frac{\text{initial amount of PGM } - \text{ amount of PGM after adsorption}}{\text{Amount of nanocrystals}}.$$

2.5. Interaction of Nanocrystals with Cervicovaginal-Related Cell Lines

TC-1 and SiHa cells were grown in RPMI-1640 medium and DMEM medium, respectively, both containing 10% fetal bovine serum (FBS) and penicillin (100 IU/mL) and streptomycin (100 μg/mL).

For intracellular localization of nanocrystals, TC-1 cells were seeded in a 35-mm dish with a glass window (MatTek, Ashland, MA, USA) at a density of 4×10^4 cells per dish. After 24 h, the medium was replaced with fresh medium. Cells were incubated with LysoTracker Red DND-99 (25 nM) for 30 min and then incubated with C6-labeled NC@PDA-NH_2, NC, or free probe C6 for 2 h. Following washing with PBS, the cells were fixed with 4% paraformaldehyde in PBS for 20 min. After nucleus staining with DAPI, fluorescent images were taken with a Zeiss AXIO Observer Z1 confocal microscope (ZEISS LSM710, Zeiss, Athens, German). The fluorescence intensity of the cells was quantitatively analyzed using FCM analysis (BD FACSCalibur, Sparks, MD, USA) at the excitation wavelength (Ex) of 466 nm and emission wavelength (Em) of 504 nm using a Flow Cytometry System (BD FACSCalibur, Sparks, MD, USA).

For quantitative comparison of intracellular drug content, TC-1 cells were seeded in a 12-well plate at a density of 1.2×10^5 cells per well. After overnight incubation, the cell culture medium was replaced with fresh medium containing NC@PDA-NH_2, NC, or free imatinib (firstly dissolved in DMSO and then diluted in PBS) with the final concentration equivalent of imatinib at 120 μg/mL. After 4 h, cells were washed with PBS and collected for determination of the intracellular imatinib amount by HPLC as described in Section 2.3.

The cytotoxicity of NC@PDA-NH_2, NC, or free IMN on TC-1 or SiHa cells over a range of imatinib concentrations for 72 h was measured using the standard MTT method. Half maximal inhibitory concentration (IC_{50}) was calculated using GraphPad Prism 6 (La Jolla, CA, USA).

Apoptosis of TC-1 or SiHa cells induced by NC@PDA-NH_2, NC, or free IMN after incubation for 48 h was compared using flow cytometry after standard Annexin V-FITC/propidium iodide (PI) staining.

2.6. Preparation and Characterization of NC@PDA-NH_2/FG

NC@PDA-NH_2/FG was prepared by dissolving an appropriate amount of Pluronic F127 in the corresponding nanocrystal suspension at 4 °C. NC-loaded F127 in situ hydrogel (NC/FG) was prepared similarly. Free imatinib/FG was prepared using the thin film-cold method as described in previous literature [10].

The rheology of NC@PDA-NH_2/FG with three different F127 concentration was investigated using a rotatory rheometer (Bohlin Gemini Π, Malvern Instruments Ltd. Co., Malvern, UK) equipped with a parallel plate in the oscillation mode from 15–40 °C at a heating rate of 1 °C/min with a fixed frequency of 1 Hz and a fixed strain of 0.01. In vitro release of PC@PDA@NC/FG was evaluated using the membraneless method using vaginal fluid simulant (VFS) as the release medium. The concentration of imatinib in release samples was measured by HPLC as described in Section 2.3.

2.7. Ex Vivo and In Vivo Evaluation of the Mucoadhesiveness of NC@PDA-NH_2/FG

For suitable gelation temperature, a weight concentration of 17.5% of F127 was selected for further investigation. Ex vivo adhesion on murine vaginal mucosa, intramucosal penetration of fluorescent-labeled NC@PDA-NH_2/FG, NC/FG, and corresponding free probe/FG, and the intravaginal drug placement of NC@PDA-NH_2/FG, NC/FG, and free IMN/FG were compared with methods similar to our previous work [10] in healthy C57BL/6 female mice.

For ex vivo adhesion evaluation, C57BL/6 female mice were sacrificed with excess inhalation of ether to get the vagina mucosa. Onto the freshly prepared vagina mucosa which was smoothed out and fixed on a plastic card, 10 μL of corresponding tested formulation was dropped with a pipette. These tissues were kept at 37 °C under repeated flushing with 10 μL of VFS every 10 min with a pipette. Near-infrared fluorescent (NIR) images were obtained every hour for 8 h with a whole-mouse fluorescent imaging system (IVIS spectrum, PerkinElmer, Santa Clara, CA, USA) at Ex 748 nm and Em 780 nm.

For in vivo intramucosal penetration, 10 μL of tested formulation per mouse was intravaginally administered to female ICR mice by a microliter syringe with a blunt needle. Three mice were randomly selected from each group and sacrificed with excess inhalation of ether to get the vaginal tissue which was fixed in paraformaldehyde for 24 h, dehydrated in sucrose solution, embedded in OCT, sectioned on a freezing microtome, stained with DAPI, and observed under a fluorescence microscope (DMI 4000, Leica Camera Co., Wetzlar, Germany).

For quantitation of intravaginal drug placement, healthy mice (24 mice per group) were intravaginally administered with NC@PDA-NH2/FG, NC/FG, or free drug (suspended imatinib powder)/FG, as described in Section 2.5. At every pre-determined time point (immediately, 2 h, 4 h, 6 h, and 8 h after administration), six mice were randomly selected from each group to perform vaginal lavage in which the vagina was thoroughly lavaged by normal saline as previously reported. Imatinib concentration in the vaginal lavage and mucosa was determined as described in Section 2.3.

2.8. In Vivo Efficacy against the Orthotopic Cervicovaginal Tumor Model in Mice

An orthotopic cervicovaginal TC-1 tumor model was established in female C57BL/6 mice according to the method of Yang et al. [26]. Mice (6–8 weeks old) were subcutaneously treated with medroxyprogesterone acetate (2.5 mg per mouse per day) for a consecutive seven days prior to tumor inoculation. Then, mice were anesthetized to gently disrupt their cervicovaginal epithelia with a cytobrush. TC-1 cells were inoculated by vaginal instillation (1×10^5 cells per mouse) three days prior to day 0. Following day 0, intravaginal administration began. The formation and growth of tumor was preliminarily confirmed by palpation, as well as anatomical and histological examination, which found that TC-1 tumors grew along the length of the cervicovaginal tract and extended laterally toward surrounding tissues.

To compare the tumor growth inhibition effect of NC@PDA-NH_2/FG vs. NC/FG at three imatinib dosages (2, 4, and 8 mg/kg), 160 tumor-bearing mice were divided into eight groups (20 mice per group) including NC@PDA-NH_2/FG (8 mg/kg), NC@PDA-NH_2/FG (4 mg/kg), NC@PDA-NH_2/FG (2 mg/kg), NC/FG (8 mg/kg), NC/FG (4 mg/kg), NC/FG (2 mg/kg), free imatinib/FG (4 mg/kg), and normal saline intravaginally administered every other day. The animal number for each group was set at 20 to ensure that at least six animals survived by day 21 for all groups, especially for the normal saline control group. On day 21, mice were sacrificed for resection of uterus, cervix, and vagina to take photographs, weighing the tumors, and performing further microscopic examination for H&E staining or TUNEL assay (DeadEnd™ Fluorometric TUNEL system, Promega, Madison, WI, USA). The change in the body weight was also monitored.

2.9. Statistical Analysis

All statistical analysis was performed with GraphPad Prism 6. Data were analyzed with one-way ANOVA test to determine the difference of means among groups. The logrank (Mantel-Cox) test was used to compare survival curves. A value of $p < 0.05$ was considered statistically significant.

3. Results and Discussion

3.1. Preparation and Characterization of NC@PDA-NH_2

As depicted by Scheme 1, the core NCs were prepared by film hydration. Subsequently, dopamine was added to self-polymerize on the surface of NCs to obtain PDA-coated NCs (NC@PDA). The PDA coating provided the reacting platform for Boc-NH-CH_2CH_2-NH_2. Finally, the Boc groups were removed by acidic treatment to provide positive charges on the surface of NC@PDA-NH_2. NC@PDA-NH_2 could be prepared with a relative high drug content of 76.84 ± 1.78% (Table 1).

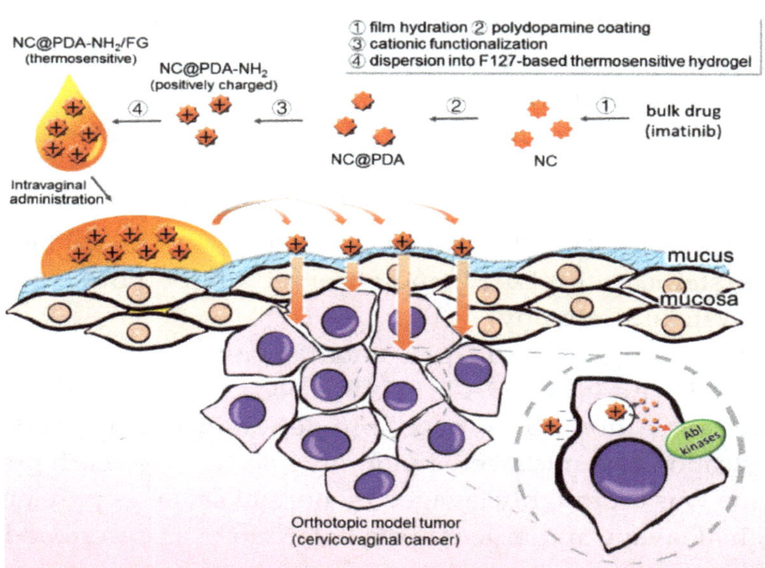

Scheme 1. Illustration of the preparation and in vivo fate of amino-group-functionalized polydopamine (PDA)-coated imatinib nanocrystals (NC) dispersed in F127 (FG) hydrogel (NC@PDA-NH_2/FG) in the orthotopic mouse cervicovaginal cancer model after intravaginal administration.

NC, NC@PDA, and NC@PDA-NH_2 all showed a near-spheroid shape (Figure 1A) with nanoscale size (Figure 1B). The zeta potentials of NC and NC@PDA were -14.9 ± 2.7 mV and -44.0 ± 3.4 mV, respectively, while that of NC@PDA-NH_2 was +27.2 $\pm$ 2.9 mV (Figure 1C), indicating the success of cationic modification. The size distribution of NC@PDA-NH_2 remained basically unchanged after one month, while the size of unmodified NC increased after only several days, which may be attributed to the electrostatic expulsion among positively charged NC@PDA-NH_2.

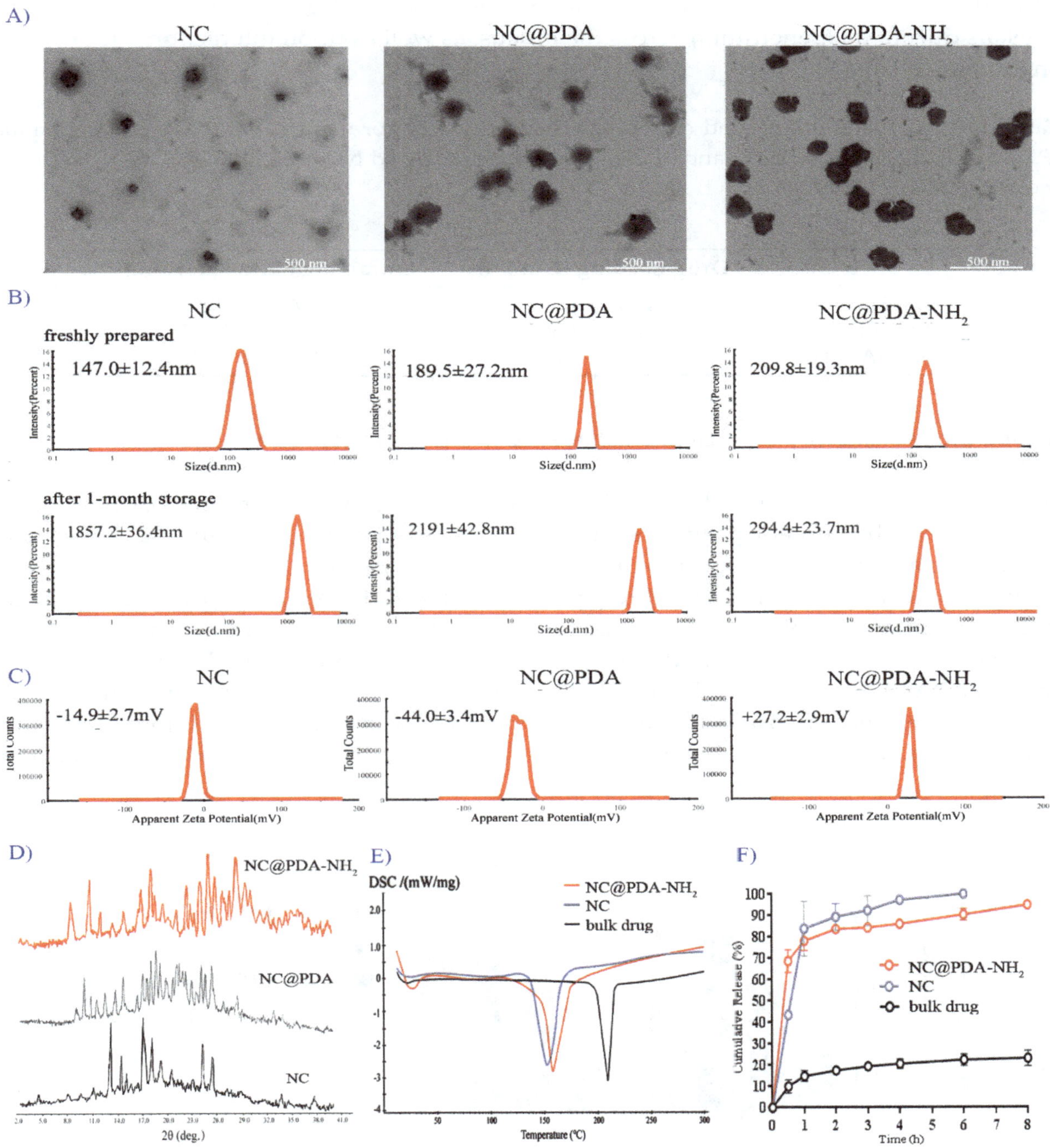

Figure 1. Characterization of NC, NC@PDA, and NC@PDA-NH_2. (**A**) TEM images. (**B**) size distribution measured by dynamic light scattering (DLS). Upper panels: freshly prepared; lower panels: after one month of storage. (**C**) Zeta-potential measured by DLS. (**D**) X-ray diffraction (XRD) patterns. (**E**) Differential scanning calorimetry (DSC) curves. (**F**) In vitro release profiles in vaginal fluid simulant (VFS) (n = 3, mean $\pm$ SD).

The XRPD patterns of bulk drug displayed peaks at 12.96°, 14.13°, 17.1°, 18.7°, 20.9°, 24.4°, and 25.2° (2θ), consistent with previous reports for I-type crystalline imatinib. By contrast, the patterns of NC and NC@PDA-NH_2 both showed distinct peaks at 15.0°, 17.2°, 18.1°, 18.7°, and 21.1°, characteristic of G-type crystalline [27] (Figure 1D). The DSC curves also indicated changes in the crystalline type from bulk drug to nanocrystals (Figure 1E).

In vitro release from NC and NC@PDA-NH_2 was much faster than that of bulk drug, perhaps related to their small size. This may be beneficial because most of the imatinib could remain in nanocrystals during the penetration across the mucus, as well as upon interaction with mucosa and entering tumor cells.

Table 1. Drug loading (DL) and entrapment efficiency (EE) for nanocrystal (NC), polydopamine (PDA)-coated NC (NC@PDA), and amino-group-functionalized NC@PDA (NC@PDA-NH_2) (n = 3, mean ± SD).

	Drug Loading (DL) (%)	Entrapment Efficiency (EE) (%)
NC	94.47 ± 2.85	94.45 ± 4.81
NC@PDA	82.72 ± 3.66	83.55 ± 12.01
NC@PDA-NH2	76.84 ± 1.78	87.11 ± 11.43

3.2. Cationic Functionalization Favored Interaction of Nanocrystals with Mucin

Adsorption of mucin is a widely used parameter in the evaluation of mucoadhesiveness [28]. NC@PDA-NH_2 with different positive surface charges was prepared (Figure S2, Supplementary Materials) and compared with respect to the capability of adsorbing mucin (Figure 2A). It is clear that the amount of mucin adsorption was directly correlated with the value of positive surface charge, indicating the important role of cationic functionalization in mucin adsorption by NC@PDA-NH_2. The interaction between NC@PDA-NH_2 and mucin was further proven by the increase in size after mixing NC@PDA-NH_2 and mucin (Figure 2B). A similar change in the particle size of mucin was also observed in the presence of positively charged polymers, including chitosan and amino-functionalized poloxamer 407, indicative of the interaction between positively charged polymers and mucin [29].

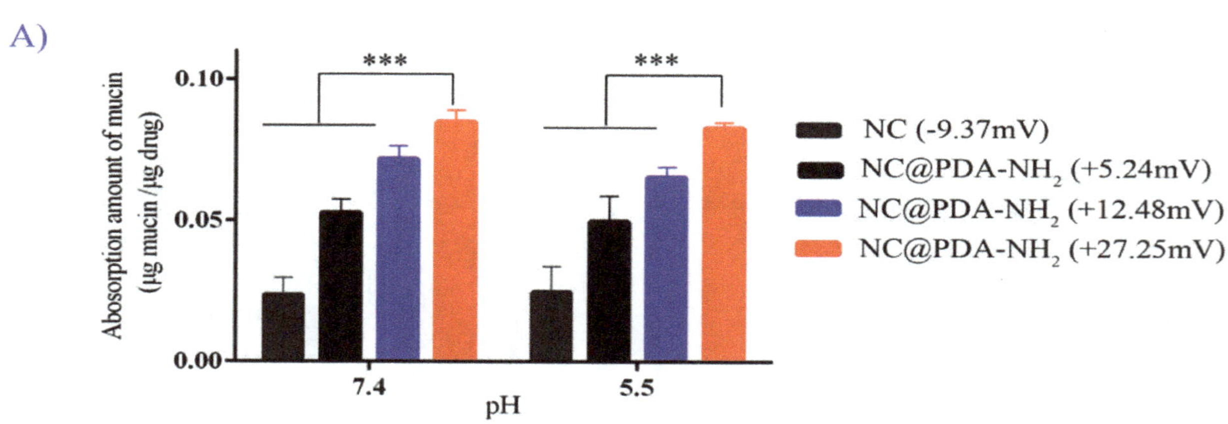

Figure 2. *Cont.*

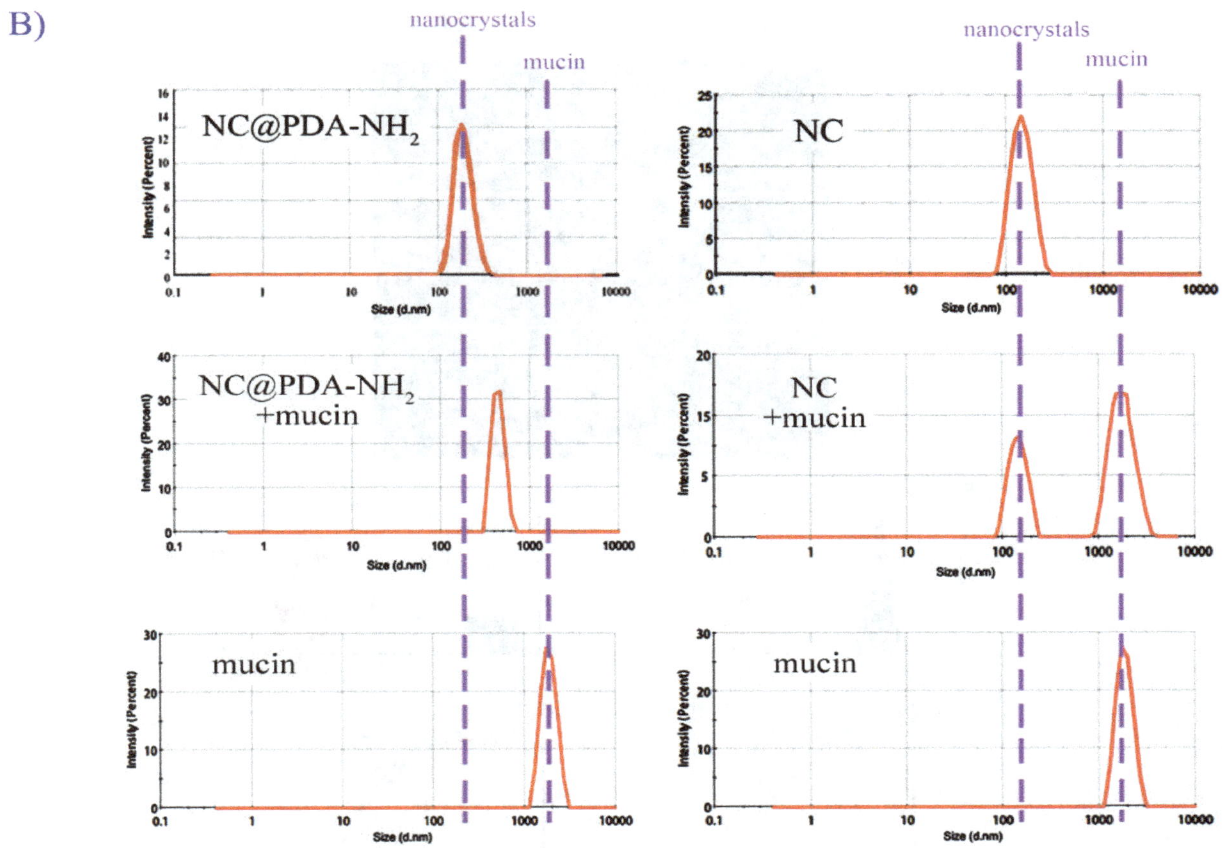

Figure 2. Interaction between NC@PDA-NH_2 and mucin. (**A**) Adsorption of mucin by NC@PDA-NH_2 with different surface charges or NC (n = 3, mean ± SD). (**B**) Change in size distribution of NC@PDA-NH_2 (or NC) after mixing with mucin. *** indicates $p < 0.001$.

3.3. Cationic Functionalization Favored Interaction of Nanocrystals with Cells

Investigation into the interaction between NC@PDA-NH_2 and cervical cancer-related cells was performed on TC-1 cells, which are immortalized murine epithelial cells transformed to express human papillomavirus (HPV)-16 E6/E7 and activated human c-Ha-ras oncogene, and exhibit similar genetic traits to human papillomavirus (HPV)-induced cervical tumors [26]. Both CLSM images (Figure 3A) and flow cytometry data (Figure 3B) demonstrated more cellular uptake of NC@PDA-NH_2 than NC, attributable to the electrostatic interaction between the positive charges on NC@PDA-NH_2 and the negative charges on the cell membrane. The intracellular fluorescent signal of NC@PDA-NH_2 overlapped with that of LysoTracker with a Pearson's correlation coefficient (R) of 0.80, suggesting possible involvement of the endocytosis pathway. Further investigation into the cellular uptake mechanism will be included in future work. Quantitative measurements of intracellular IMN concentration further confirmed that more imatinib entered cells after incubation with NC@PDA-NH_2 than NC or free imatinib (Figure 3C). The above enhanced cellular uptake was in accordance with the prolonged adhesion on the surface of cellular monolayers of positively charged liposomes than negatively charged or neutral liposomes [30].

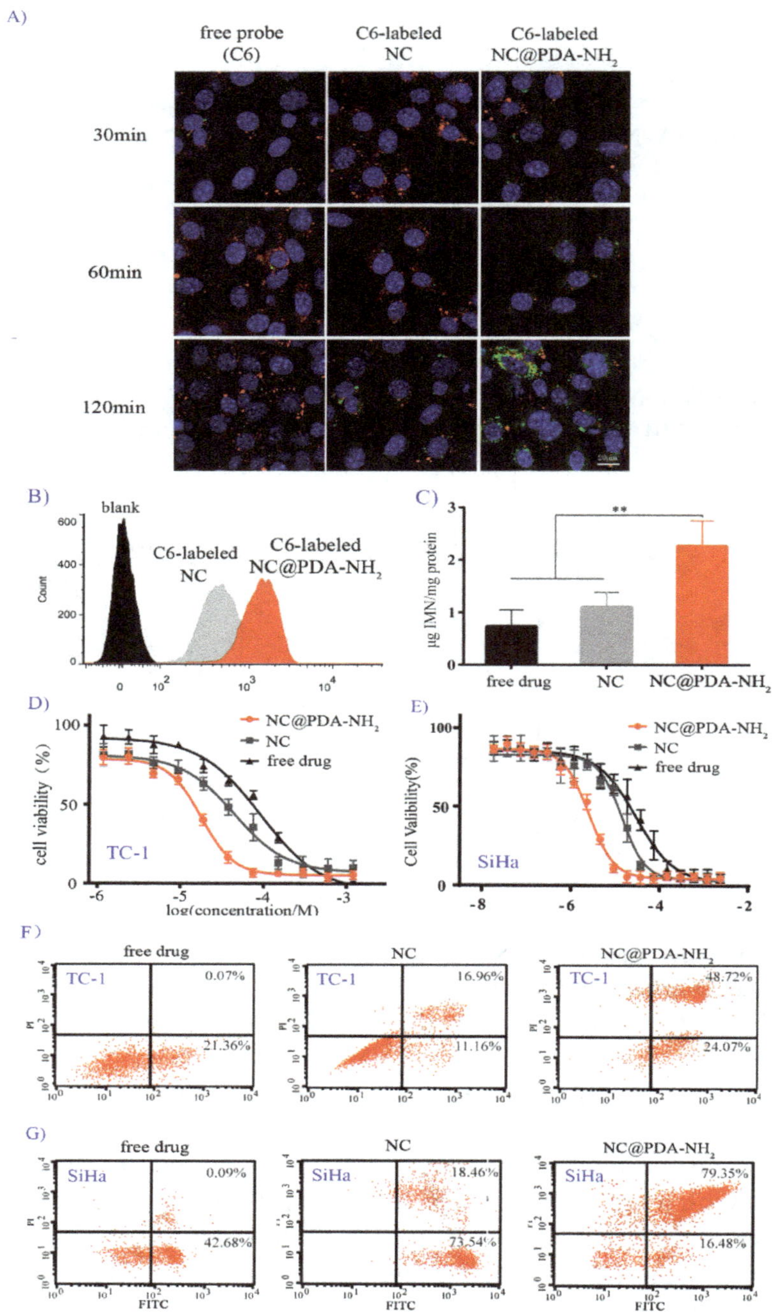

Figure 3. Cellular uptake and cytotoxicity in cervical cancer-related cell lines. (**A**) Representative CLSM images of TC-1 cells co-incubated with 6-coumarin (C6)-labeled NC@PDA-NH_2, NC, or free probe C6 (green signal). The nucleus was stained with 2-(4-amidinophenyl)-6-indolecarbamindine dihydrochloride (DAPI; blue) and the lysosomes were stained with LysoTracker Red. (**B**) Flow cytometry analysis on the fluorescent intensity of cells after co-incubation for 2 h with C6-labeled NC@PDA-NH_2, NC, or free probe in TC-1 cells. (**C**) Intracellular drug content after co-incubation for 72 h with NC@PDA-NH_2, NC, or free imatinib in TC-1 cells ($n = 5$, mean ± SD, ** represents $p < 0.01$). (**D,E**) In vitro cytotoxicity of NC@PDA-NH_2, NC, or free imatinib after 48 h of co-incubation in TC-1 cells (**D**) or SiHa cells (**E**). (**F,G**) Apoptotic cell populations determined by flow cytometry with Annexin V-FITC and propidium iodide (PI) staining after co-incubation with NC@PDA-NH_2, NC, or free imatinib in TC-1 cells (**E**) or SiHa cells (**G**). The lower-left (Q3), lower-right (Q4), upper-right (Q2), and upper-left (Q1) quadrants in each panel indicate the populations of normal, early, and late apoptotic, and apoptotic necrotic cells, respectively.

As shown by the MTT results (Figure 3D), enhanced cellular growth inhibition was observed with NC@PDA-NH_2. The IC_{50} values of NC@PDA-NH_2, NC, and free drug were 16.8 μM, 39.3 μM, and 84.9 μM, respectively. Such enhanced cellular growth inhibition of NC@PDA-NH2 compared to NC and free drug might be relevant with the different uptake and, thus, different intracellular drug accumulation.

More cellular apoptosis was also observed with NC@PDA-NH_2. NC@PDA-NH_2, NC, and free drug resulted in 24.07%, 11.16%, and 21.36% early apoptotic cells in the fourth quadrant (Q4) and 48.7%, 16.96%, and 0.07% late apoptotic cells in Q1, respectively. Similar trends were also observed in MTT and apoptosis results with another cervical cancer-related cell line (SiHa cells).

3.4. Cationic Functionalization Prolonged Intravaginal Retention and Enhanced Mucosal Penetration

Before ex vivo and in vivo application, NC@PDA-NH_2 was dispersed in Pluronic F127-based thermosensitive hydrogel (FG) to avoid leakage which might happen if administered as a simple aqueous dispersion, and enough time was allowed for nanocrystals to interact with the mucosa. Other vehicles for nanoparticles were also reported for vaginal use, such as hydroxypropyl methylcellulose/poly(vinyl alcohol) films [31] and poly(vinyl alcohol) nanofibers [32]. FG was also applied as a vaginal formulation vehicle with good safety for many therapeutic agents. Due to its lack of mucoadhesive properties, FG may serve as an ideal vehicle for the evaluation of NC@PDA-NH_2.

Consistent with previous reports on FG [33], the phase transition temperature and in vitro drug release rate of NC@PDA-NH_2-containing FG (NC@PDA-NH_2/FG) were both dependent on the concentration of Pluronic F127 (Figure 4). A concentration of 17.5% (*w*/*w*) was selected for Pluronic F127 to assure easy administration and moderate dispersion into vaginal fluid.

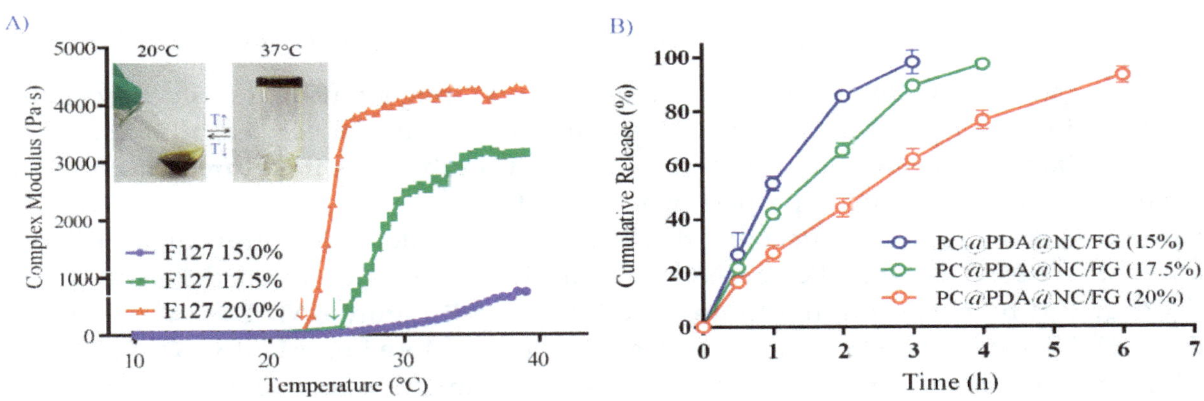

Figure 4. Rheological and in vitro release profiles of NC@PDA-NH_2/FG. (**A**) Temperature-dependent rheological profiles of NC@PDA-NH_2/FG with different F127 concentration (15.0%, 17.5%, and 20.0%, *w*/*w*). The red and green arrows denote the gelation temperature for 20.0% and 17.5%, respectively, while the thermal phase transition was not obvious for 15.0%. The insert is the typical photograph of NC@PDA-NH_2/FG (17.5%) at storage (20 °C) or body temperature (37 °C). (**B**) Release profiles from NC@PDA-NH_2/FG at different F127 concentration (15.0%, 17.5% and 20.0%, *w*/*w*) at 37 °C in VFS (n = 3, mean ± SD).

When dropped on ex vivo murine vagina mucosa and continuously flushed with VFS for 8 h, NC@PDA-NH_2/FG resulted in significantly longer residence of fluorescent signal than NC/FG or free probe/FG (Figure 5A,B). When observed microscopically, prolonged, more, and deeper fluorescence was found in the vaginal mucosa of mice administered with NC@PDA-NH_2/FG, suggesting improved accessibility and penetration into vaginal mucosa. Quantitative measurements of intravaginal imatinib amount further confirmed the superiority of NC@PDA-NH_2/FG with respect to intravaginal residence (Figure 5D).

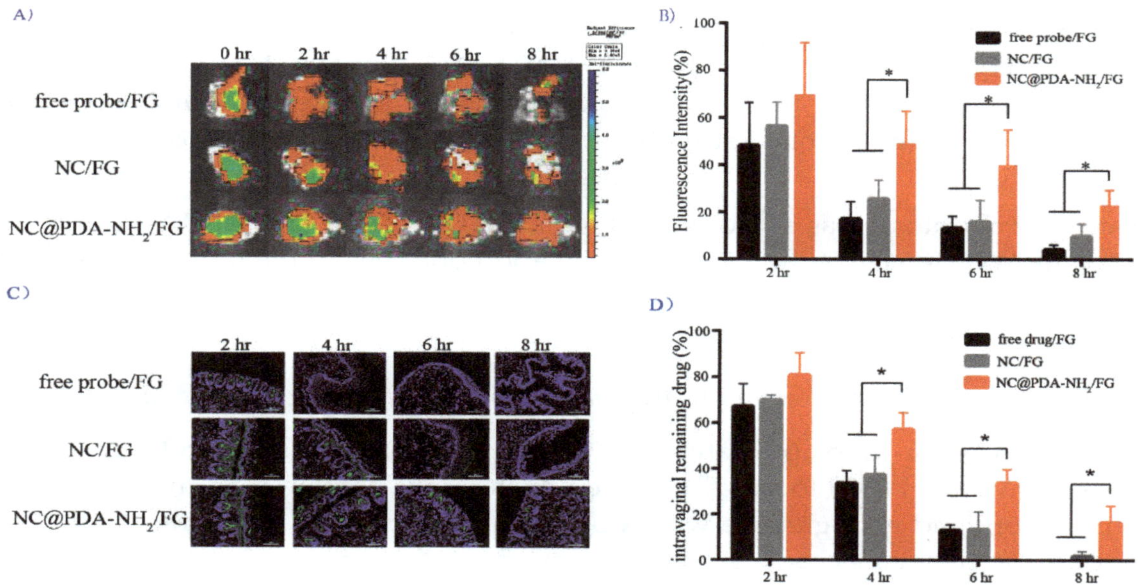

Figure 5. Ex vivo mucoadhesiveness and in vivo placement. (**A**) Typical fluorescent images, and (**B**) semi-quantitative fluorescent intensity (n = 6, mean ± SD) for the ex vivo residence of 1,1′-dioctadecyl-3,3,3′,3′-tetramethylindotricarbocyanine iodide (DiR)-labeled NC@PDA-NH_2/FG, NC/FG, or free probe DiR/FG on the surface of ex vivo vaginal mucosa of healthy mice during flushing by VFS at 37 °C. (**C**) Fluorescent microscopic images (green signal for C6, blue signal for DAPI; scale bar = 100 μm), and (**D**) intravaginal residence percentage of imatinib in healthy mice vaginally administered with NC@PDA-NH_2/FG, NC/FG, or free imatinib/FG (n = 6, mean ± SD); * indicates $p < 0.05$.

3.5. Cationic Functionalization Improved Tumor Inhibition in the Orthotopic TC-1 Cervical Cancer Model

The orthotopic TC-1 model was reported to represent a stringent model for cervicovaginal cancer within a short time frame and localized similarly to the anatomy of cervical tumors. In addition, this model is suitable for testing mucoadhesive formulations because it features the cervicovaginal mucus layer that acts as a barrier to particle penetration [26].

The tumor growth inhibition effect was firstly investigated after daily intravaginal administration treatment with NC@PDA-NH_2/FG or NC/FG for three weeks at three different doses (2, 4, and 8 mg/kg/2 d) by observing the tumor size by the end (Figure 6A). The inhibition effects of NC@PDA-NH_2/FG and NC/FG were both dose-dependent. More importantly, NC@PDA-NH_2/FG inhibited the growth of model tumors more effectively. This might be explained by more accessibility of NC@PDA-NH_2 to the vaginal mucosal as indicated by the semi-quantitative analysis of optical density of fluorescent microscopic images.

More and deeper fluorescence was found in the vaginal mucosa bearing model tumors for fluorescent-labeled NC@PDA-NH_2/FG (Figure 6B). Based on the Kaplan–Meier survival curves at the dosage of 4 mg/kg/2 d, NC@PDA-NH_2/FG prolonged the median survival time, 7.0-fold that of free drug/FG (35 d vs. 20 d) and 2.1-fold that of NC/FG group (35 d vs. 26 d). More apoptosis areas were also observed in the microscopic sections from the NC@PDA-NH_2/FG group than the NC/FG group (Figure 6E).

The safety of NC@PDA-NH_2/FG was evaluated by monitoring the change in the animal body weight during the abovementioned three-week treatment and histological examination of the vaginal mucosa by the end. As shown in Figure 6E, the body weight of mice in the NC@PDA-NH_2/FG group slowly increased, reflecting their relatively good health state. By contrast, the body weight continuously decreased in the free drug/FG or control groups (normal saline).

H&E staining sections (Figure 6F) also demonstrated the maximal anti-tumor efficiency and minimal mucosal toxicity for the NC@PDA-NH_2/FG group. The mucosal epithelium was destructed and compressed by the prosperous tumor tissues in the control group, while the mucosal epithelium partially recovered in the NC@PDA-NH_2/FG group.

As the TC-1 model tumor grew, elevated interstitial pressure within tumor tissue impaired intratumor penetration and made complete tumor eradication ultimately difficult for free drug [34]. It is encouraging that NC@PDA-NH_2/FG effectively suppressed the growth of TC-1 model tumors. Future studies using other murine cervical tumor models which are less aggressive and resemble the slow tumor progression in humans will further substantiate the effectiveness of NC@PDA-NH_2/FG.

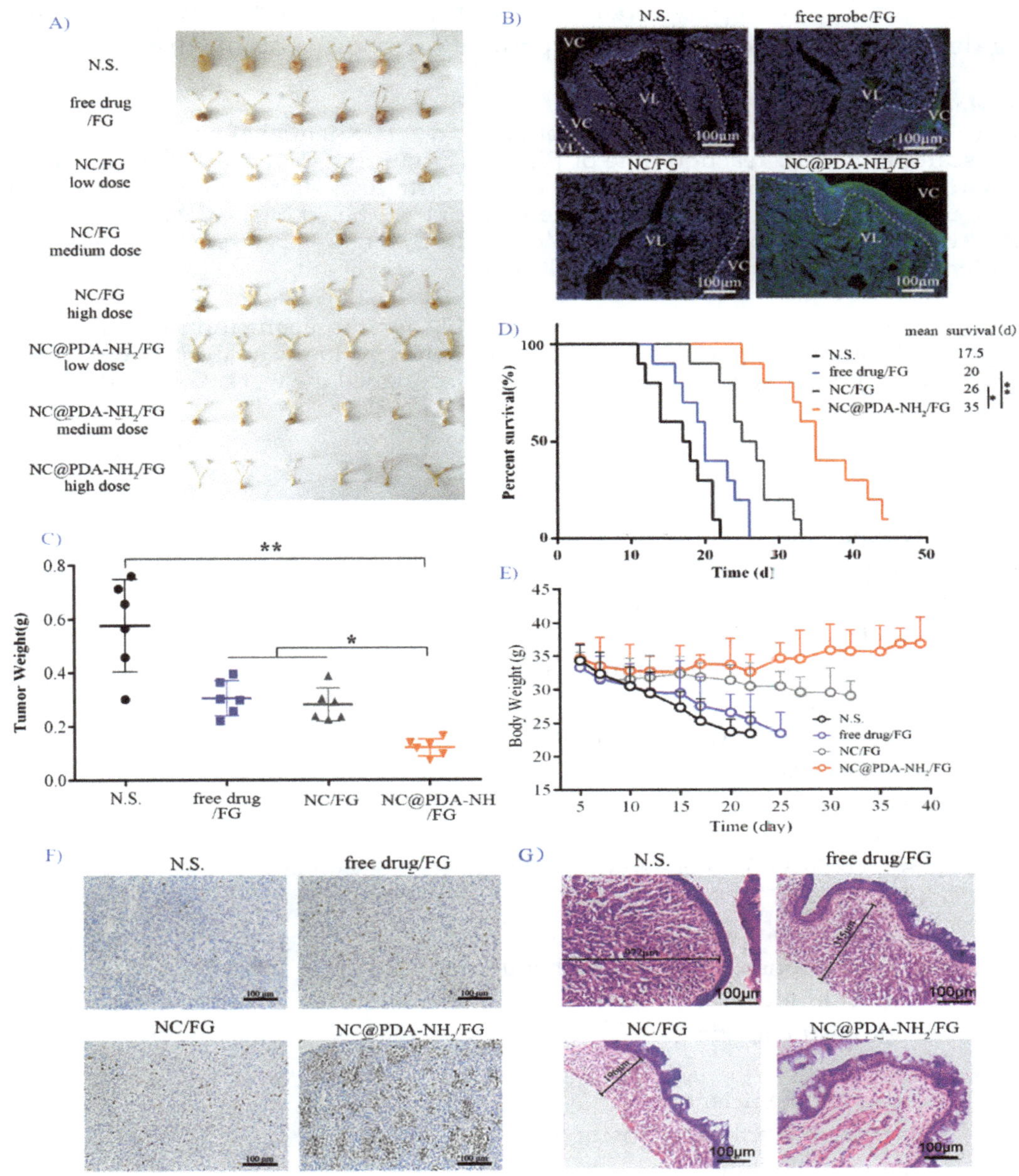

Figure 6. In vivo evaluation in orthotopic TC-1 cervicovaginal model tumor-bearing mice after intravaginal administration of different formulations every other day. (**A**) Dose-dependent inhibition on the tumor size after three-week treatment (dose: 2, 4, and 8 mg/kg/2 d). (**B**) Penetration of fluorescent signal into the vaginal mucosa (4 h after administration). (**C**) Tumor weights after treatment for three weeks (dose: 4 mg/kg/2 d; $n = 6$). (**D**) Survival time (dose: 4 mg/kg/2 d; $n = 10$). (**E**) Change in anima body weight (dose: 4 mg/kg/2 d; $n = 10$). (**F**) Representative immunohistochemical microphotographs of tumor sections stained for apoptosis after three-week treatment (dose: 4 mg/kg/2 d). (**G**) Representative H&E microphotographs of tumors and vagina after three-week treatment (dose: 4 mg/kg/2 d). * indicates $p < 0.05$, ** indicates $p < 0.01$.

4. Conclusions

In summary, positively charged NC@PDA-NH_2 significantly interacted with mucin in vitro and resulted in more cellular uptake, cellular growth inhibition efficacy, and induction of apoptosis. NC@PDA-NH_2/FG exhibited good ex vivo and in vivo mucoadhesiveness, as well as improved anti-tumor efficacy in the murine orthotopic cervicovaginal cancer tumor model. In conclusion, cationic functionalization endowed imatinib nanocrystals good potential as a novel mucoadhesive approach for intravaginal treatment of cervicovaginal cancer. Our work also reveals the good potential of surface functionalization based on polydopamine coating on nanocrystals, which appear to be a good nanoscale drug delivery system with high drug content for poorly soluble drugs.

Supplementary Materials:
Figure S1: Influence of reaction time on the size distribution and zeta potential of resulted nanocrystals measured by dynamic light scattering. Left: reaction time of PDA@NC with Boc-$NHCH_2CH_2NH_2$; right: deprotection time in acidic environment, Figure S2: NC@PDA-NH2 with different zeta potentials for comparison of mucin adsorption, Figure S3: Size distribution and zeta potentials of C6-labeled NC, NC@PDA, and NC@PDA-NH2, Figure S4: Typical chromatograph for imatinib (1 ug/mL, LLOQ), Figure S5: Typical chromatograph of vaginal lavage samples after intravaginal administration of NC@PDA-NH2/FG.

Author Contributions: L.-q.C. and Z.-g.H. were responsible for the acquisition of data. F.-m.L. and J.W. substantially helped in the animal experiments. L.-l.F. and F.S. helped in the analysis of data. S.-j.C. established the tumor-bearing animal model. Z.-p.L. drafted the work. Y.L. designed the work. G.W. and W.-y.L. substantively revised it.

Abbreviations

PDA	polydopamine
NC	nanocrystals
NC@PDA-NH2	cationic functionalized polydopamine-coated imatinib nanocrystals
NC@PDA	polydopamine-coated imatinib nanocrystals
F127	Pluronic F127
FG	Pluronic F127-based in situ hydrogel
TKI	tyrosine kinase inhibitors
IMN	imatinib
C6	6-coumarin
DiR	1,1′-dioctadecyl-3,3,3′,3′-tetramethylindotricarbocyanine iodide
OCT	optical coherence tomography
DAPI	2-(4-amidinophenyl)-6-indolecarbamindine dihydrochloride
PGM	porcine gastric mucin
DL	drug loading
EE	encapsulation efficiency
TEM	transmission electron microscope
DLS	dynamic light scattering
XRPD	X-ray powder diffraction
DSC	differential scanning calorimetry
VFS	vaginal fluid stimulant

References

1. Bernard, W.S.; Christopher, P.W. *World Cancer Report 2014*; World Health Organization: Switzerland, Geneva, 2014.
2. Major, I.; McConville, C. Vaginal drug delivery for the localised treatment of cervical cancer. *Drug Deliv. Transl. Res.* **2017**, *7*, 817–828. [CrossRef] [PubMed]

3. Cook, M.T.; Brown, M.B. Polymeric gels for intravaginal drug delivery. *J. Control. Release* **2018**, *270*, 145–157. [CrossRef] [PubMed]

4. Taja-Chayeb, L.; Chavez-Blanco, A.; Martínez-Tlahuel, J.; González-Fierro, A.; Candelaria, M.; Chanona-Vilchis, J.; Robles, E.; Dueñas-Gonzalez, A. Expression of platelet derived growth factor family members and the potential role of imatinib mesylate for cervical cancer. *Cancer Cell Int.* **2006**, *6*, 22. [CrossRef]

5. Kummel, S.; Heidecke, H.; Brock, B.; Denkert, C.; Hecktor, J.; Koninger, A.; Becker, I.; Sehouli, J.; Thomas, A.; Blohmer, J.U.; et al. Imatinib—A possible therapeutic option for cervical carcinoma: Results of a preclinical phase I study. *Gynakol. Geburtshilfliche Rundsch.* **2008**, *48*, 94–100.

6. Gao, L.; Liu, G.; Ma, J.; Wang, X.; Zhou, L.; Li, X. Drug nanocrystals: In vivo performances. *J. Control. Release* **2012**, *160*, 418–430. [CrossRef] [PubMed]

7. Müller, R.H.; Gohla, S.; Keck, C.M. State of the art of nanocrystals: Special features, production, nanotoxicology aspects and intracellular delivery. *Eur. J. Pharm. Biopharm.* **2011**, *78*, 1–9. [CrossRef] [PubMed]

8. Lu, Y.; Li, Y.; Wu, W. Injected nanocrystals for targeted drug delivery. *Acta Pharm. Sin. B* **2016**, *6*, 106–113. [CrossRef]

9. Guo, H.; Xu, W.; Chen, J.; Yan, L.; Ding, J.; Hou, Y.; Chen, X. Positively charged polypeptide nanogel enhances mucoadhesion and penetrability of 10-hydroxycamptothecin in orthotopic bladder carcinoma. *J. Control. Release* **2017**, *259*, 136–148. [CrossRef]

10. Ci, L.Q.; Huang, Z.G.; Liu, Y.; Liu, Z.P.; Wei, G.; Lu, W.Y. Amino-functionalized poloxamer 407 with both mucoadhesive and thermosensitive properties: Preparation, characterization and application in vaginal drug delivery system. *Acta Pharm. Sin. B* **2017**, *7*, 593–602. [CrossRef]

11. Frank, L.A.; Chaves, P.S.; D'Amore, C.M.; Contri, R.V.; Frank, A.G.; Beck, R.C.; Pohlmann, A.R.; Buffon, A.; Guterres, S.S. The use of chitosan as cationic coating or gel vehicle for polymeric nanocapsules: Increasing penetration and adhesion of imiquimod in vaginal tissue. *Eur. J. Pharm. Biopharm.* **2017**, *114*, 202–212. [CrossRef]

12. Zhang, H.; Hu, H.; Zhang, H.; Dai, W.; Wang, X.; Wang, X.; Zhang, Q. Effects of PEGylated paclitaxel nanocrystals on breast cancer and its lung metastasis. *Nanoscale* **2015**, *7*, 10790–10800. [CrossRef] [PubMed]

13. Park, J.; Sun, B.; Yeo, Y. Albumin-coated nanocrystals for carrier-free delivery of paclitaxel. *J. Control. Release* **2017**, *263*, 90–101. [CrossRef] [PubMed]

14. Zhang, L.; Wei, W.; Ma, G. HSA induced HCPT nanocrystal for high-performance antitumor therapy. *J. Control. Release* **2017**, *259*, e82. [CrossRef]

15. Gao, W.; Chen, Y.; Thompson, D.H.; Park, K.; Li, T. Impact of surfactant treatment of paclitaxel nanocrystals on biodistribution and tumor accumulation in tumor-bearing mice. *J. Control. Release* **2016**, *237*, 168–176. [CrossRef] [PubMed]

16. Gao, W.; Lee, D.; Meng, Z.; Li, T. Exploring intracellular fate of drug nanocrystals with crystal-integrated and environment-sensitive fluorophores. *J. Control. Release* **2017**, *267*, 214–222. [CrossRef] [PubMed]

17. Chen, M.; Li, W.; Zhang, X.; Dong, Y.; Hua, Y.; Zhang, H.; Gao, J.; Zhao, L.; Li, Y.; Zheng, A. In vitro and in vivo evaluation of SN-38 nanocrystals with different particle sizes. *Int. J. Nanomed.* **2017**, *12*, 5487–5500. [CrossRef]

18. Zhang, C.; Gong, L.; Xiang, L.; Du, Y.; Hu, W.; Zeng, H.; Xu, Z. Deposition and Adhesion of Polydopamine on the Surfaces of Varying Wettability. *ACS Appl. Mater. Interfaces* **2017**, *9*, 30943–30950. [CrossRef]

19. Lee, H.; Dellatore, S.M.; Miller, W.M.; Messersmith, P.B. Mussel-Inspired Surface Chemistry for Multifunctional Coatings. *Science* **2007**, *318*, 426–430. [CrossRef]

20. Liu, Y.; Ai, K.; Liu, J.; Deng, M.; He, Y.; Lu, L. Dopamine-melanin colloidal nanospheres: An efficient near-infrared photothermal therapeutic agent for in vivo cancer therapy. *Adv. Mater.* **2013**, *5*, 1353–1359. [CrossRef]

21. Li, Y.; Jiang, C.; Zhang, D.; Wang, Y.; Ren, X.; Ai, K.; Chen, X.; Lu, L. Targeted polydopamine nanoparticles enable photoacoustic imaging guided chemo-photothermal synergistic therapy of tumor. *Acta Biomater.* **2017**, *47*, 124–134. [CrossRef]

22. Zeng, X.; Tao, W.; Liu, G.; Mei, L. Polydopamine-based surface modification of copolymeric nanoparticles as a targeted drug delivery system for cancer therapy. *J. Control. Release* **2017**, *259*, e150–e151. [CrossRef]

23. Xue, P.; Sun, L.; Li, Q.; Zhang, L.; Guo, J.; Xu, Z.; Kan, Y. PEGylated polydopamine-coated magnetic nanoparticles for combined targeted chemotherapy and photothermal ablation of tumour cells. *Colloids Surf. B Biointerfaces* **2017**, *160*, 11–21. [CrossRef] [PubMed]
24. Zhan, H.; Jagtiani, T.; Liang, J.F. A new targeted delivery approach by functionalizing drug nanocrystals through polydopamine coating. *Eur. J. Pharm. Biopharm.* **2017**, *114*, 221–229. [CrossRef] [PubMed]
25. Owen, D.H.; Katz, D.F. A vaginal fluid simulant. *Contraception* **1999**, *59*, 91–95. [CrossRef]
26. Yang, M.; Yu, T.; Wang, Y.Y.; Lai, S.K.; Zeng, Q.; Miao, B.; Tang, B.C.; Simons, B.W.; Ensign, L.M.; Liu, G.; et al. Vaginal delivery of paclitaxel via nanoparticles with nonmucoadhesive surfaces suppresses cervical tumor growth. *Adv. Healthc. Mater.* **2014**, *3*, 1044–1052. [CrossRef] [PubMed]
27. Novartis, A.G. Crystalline F, G, H, I and K type of Imatinib Mesylate. CN Patent 2006800440007.7, 26 November 2008.
28. Prosperi-Porta, G.; Kedzior, S.; Muirhead, B.; Sheardown, H. Phenylboronic-acid-based polymeric micelles for mucoadhesive anterior segment ocular drug delivery. *Biomacromolecules* **2016**, *17*, 1449–1457. [CrossRef]
29. Nikogeorgos, N.; Efler, P.; Kayitmazer, A.B.; Lee, S. "Bio-glues" to enhance slipperiness of mucins: Improved lubricity and wear resistance of porcine gastric mucin (PGM) layers assisted by mucoadhesion with chitosan. *Soft Matter* **2015**, *11*, 489–498. [CrossRef]
30. Adamczak, M.I.; Hagesaether, E.; Smistad, G.; Hiorth, M. An in vitro study of mucoadhesion and biocompatibility of polymer coated liposomes on HT29-MTX mucus-producing cells. *Int. J. Pharm.* **2016**, *498*, 225–233. [CrossRef]
31. Büyükköroğlu, G.; Şenel, B.; Başaran, E.; Yenilmez, E.; Yazan, Y. Preparation and in vitro evaluation of vaginal formulations including siRNA and paclitaxel-loaded SLNs for cervical cancer. *Eur. J. Pharm. Biopharm.* **2016**, *109*, 174–183. [CrossRef]
32. Ci, T.; Yuan, L.; Bao, X.; Hou, Y.; Wu, H.; Sun, H.; Cao, D.; Ke, X. Development and anti-*Candida* evaluation of the vaginal delivery system of amphotericin B nanosuspension-loaded thermogel. *J. Drug Target.* **2018**, *26*, 829–839. [CrossRef] [PubMed]
33. Liu, Y.; Yang, F.J.; Feng, L.L.; Yang, L.; Chen, L.Y.; Wei, G.; Lu, W.Y. In vivo retention of poloxamer-based in situ hydrogels for vaginal application in mouse and rat models. *Acta Pharm. Sin. B* **2017**, *7*, 502–509. [CrossRef] [PubMed]
34. Lin, K.Y.; Guarnieri, F.G.; Staveley-O'Carroll, K.F.; Levitsky, H.I.; August, J.T.; Pardoll, D.M.; Wu, T.C. Treatment of Established Tumors with a Novel Vaccine That Enhances Major Histocompatibility Class II Presentation of Tumor Antigen. *Cancer Res.* **1996**, *56*, 21–26. [PubMed]

3

Carbamazepine Gel Formulation as a Sustained Release Epilepsy Medication for Pediatric Use

Saeid Mezail Mawazi [1,2], Sinan Mohammed Abdullah Al-Mahmood [3], Bappaditya Chatterjee [1,4], Hazrina AB. Hadi [1] and Abd Almonem Doolaanea [1,5,*]

1 Department of Pharmaceutical Technology, Kulliyyah of Pharmacy, International Islamic University Malaysia, Kuantan 25200, Malaysia; saeidmezail@yahoo.com (S.M.M.); bdpharmaju@gmail.com (B.C.); hazrina.hadi@gmail.com (H.A.H.)
2 School of Pharmacy, PICOMS International University College, Batu Muda, Batu caves, Kuala Lumpur 68100, Malaysia
3 Pharmacy College, Al-Kitab University, Kirkuk 36010, Iraq; sinan.almawla@gmail.com
4 Department of Pharmaceutics, SPPSPTM, SVKM's NMIMS (Deemed to be University), Mumbai 400056, India
5 IKOP Sdn Bhd, Kulliyyah of Pharmacy, International Islamic University Malaysia, Kuantan 25200, Malaysia
* Correspondence: abdalmonemdoolaanea@yahoo.com;

Abstract: This study aimed to develop a carbamazepine (CBZ) sustained release formulation suitable for pediatric use with a lower risk of precipitation. The CBZ was first prepared as sustained release microparticles, and then the microparticles were embedded in alginate beads, and finally, the beads were suspended in a gel vehicle. The microparticles were prepared by a solvent evaporation method utilizing ethyl cellulose as a sustained release polymer and were evaluated for particle size, encapsulation efficiency, and release profile. The beads were fabricated by the dropwise addition of sodium alginate in calcium chloride solution and characterized for size, shape, and release properties. The gel was prepared using iota carrageenan as the gelling agent and evaluated for appearance, syneresis, drug content uniformity, rheology, release profile, and stability. The microparticles exhibited a particle size of 135.01 ± 0.61 μm with a monodisperse distribution and an encapsulation efficiency of 83.89 ± 3.98%. The beads were monodispersed with an average size of 1.4 ± 0.05 mm and a sphericity factor of less than 0.05. The gel was prepared using a 1:1 ratio (gel vehicle to beads) and exhibited no syneresis, good homogeneity, and good shear-thinning properties. The release profile from the beads and from the gel was not significantly affected, maintaining similarity to the tablet form. The gel properties were maintained for one month real time stability, but the accelerated stability showed reduced viscosity and pH with time. In conclusion, CBZ in a gel sustained release dosage form combines the advantages of the suspension form in terms of dosing flexibility, and the advantages of the tablet form in regards to the sustained release profile. This dosage form should be further investigated in vivo in animal models before being considered in clinical trials.

Keywords: gel; sustained release; carbamazepine; epilepsy; pediatric

1. Introduction

Carbamazepine (CBZ) is an epilepsy treatment used by patients of different age groups, including pediatrics and especially children below six years old. However, the sustained release dosage is only available as a solid oral dosage form (tablet or capsule). Children below six years old usually have difficulty swallowing solid oral dosage forms [1–3]. The United States Food and Drug Administration (FDA) and European Medical Agency (EMA) have encouraged developers to make sustained release formulations for pediatric use [4–6]. CBZ can be given as a suspension for children in 2–4 doses per day, but several side effects have been reported due to precipitation of the suspension [7–9]. This highlights the need for a new formulation that can provide a sustained release and avoid precipitation of CBZ. This study aimed to achieve these goals. Making a sustained release formulation suitable for children with swallowing difficulties (below six years old) is challenging. Based on EMA guidelines, currently only solution and suspension formulations are suitable for this age group [4–6]. While a sustained release form is difficult to develop, the suspension dosage form was considered.

Carbamazepine (CBZ) is an anticonvulsant drug used for the treatment of neuralgia, trigeminal, epilepsy, and bipolar disorder. CBZ is a white-yellowish, bitter tasting powder that is insoluble in water [10,11]. The FDA approved carbamazepine formulations include chewable tablets (Tegretol®), a suspension (Tegretol®), sustained release capsules (Carbatrol®), and sustained release tablets (Tegretol®-XR) [7]. Following a twice a day dosage regimen, the suspension provides higher peak levels and lower trough levels than those obtained from conventional tablets for the same dosage regimen. On the other hand, following a thrice daily dosage regimen, the CBZ suspension affords steady-state plasma levels comparable to CBZ tablets given twice a day when administered at the same total mg daily dose [7]. Following a twice daily dosage regimen, CBZ extended-release tablets afford steady-state plasma levels comparable to conventional CBZ tablets given four times a day, when administered at the same total mg daily dose [7]. CBZ is prescribed for children under 6 years of age at a dose of 10 to 20 mg/kg/day twice a day or three times a day. The dose is increased weekly to achieve an optimal clinical response, and administration may be increased to three times a day or four times a day. As such, the suspension dosage form allows dosing flexibility. However, it lacks the property of sustained release. This is available only in the solid oral dosage forms, like tablets and capsules. There is still a need for a sustained release CBZ formulation to be developed that provides both the required release profile and dosing flexibility.

The International Conference on Harmonisation of Technical Requirements for Registration of Pharmaceuticals for Human Use (ICH) has classified five different age groups: preterm new-borns infants, new-born infants (0–27 days), infants and toddlers (28 days–23 months), children (2–11 years), and adolescents (12 to 16–18 years, depending on the region) [12,13]. Due to the anatomy of their buccal cavity development, this young population is usually unable to swallow capsules or tablets. However, children may be able to swallow small tablets but not larger tablets. According to the Guideline on Development of Medicines for Paediatric Use, the acceptability of the tablets depends on their age and the size of the tablets [5,6]. For children from 2 to 5 years old (pre-school), the preferred dosage forms are solutions and suspensions, with the ability to swallow tablets smaller than 5 mm [5]. However, overdose caused by suspension sedimentation is one of the common reported issues with CBZ suspensions.

Most of the CBZ sustained release formulations have been developed as tablets. Only a few formulations have been attempted for paediatric use. Among them, nanoparticles and microparticles are the most reported, despite the authors not claiming their suitability for the paediatric population [14–20]. However, as multiparticulate systems with a size that can be swallowed by children younger than six years old, those dosage forms might be useful [21].

There are several types of polymers or coating materials, such as celluloses (like ethyl cellulose, methyl cellulose, carboxymethyl cellulose), gums (like gum Arabic), carrageenans (kappa carrageenan, iota carrageenan, and lambda carrageenan), and alginates (sodium alginate). Ethyl cellulose (EC) is the most stable polymer among the cellulose derivatives. It can resist alkalis in both concentrated and diluted solutions. It only adsorbs a very small amount of water from the moist air or from aqueous solutions during immersion [22]. There are three types of carrageenan—kappa carrageenan, iota carrageenan, and lambda carrageenan. Iota carrageenan is the only type that shows no syneresis [23]. Sodium alginate is a natural polysaccharide polymer that is soluble in cold and hot water. It is biocompatible, non-toxic, and widely used in pharmaceutical beads, microparticles, nano-particles, and sustained release preparations [24]. Beads of alginate are easily prepared by crosslinking with divalent cations, such as calcium.

Oral gel is a fundamental solution for dysphagic patients and is frequently prescribed for geriatrics [25,26]. The gel has the advantage of preventing precipitation due high viscosity. In addition, when the gel is shear-thinned, it allows flexible dosing because it flows easily upon application of suitable stress, like withdrawal by syringe. Gel formulations have been developed for some drugs already, such as paracetamol [27]. Gel formulations can be designed for immediate release or sustained release [28]. One study described a CBZ oral gel and performed a comparison study between different gelling agents and a stability study for those gelling agents, but the release was almost completed in 1 h (immediate release dosage form) [25,26]. There is no existing report on a sustained release gel formulation for CBZ.

In this study, a CBZ sustained release formulation suitable for pediatric use, especially for children below six years old, was developed based on multiparticulate systems (microparticles and beads). These particles were embedded in a gel as the final dosage form. The in vitro release properties were compared with those of commercial CBZ sustained release tablets.

2. Materials and Methods

2.1. Materials

Carbamazepine (CBZ) was purchased from Anuja Healthcare Limited (Punjab, India). Ethyl cellulose (EC) was bought from DOW chemicals (Louisiana, Greensburg, PA, USA). Polyvinyl alcohol (PVA), dichloromethane, and other chemicals were procured from Merck (Hohenbrunn, Germany). Sodium alginate was purchased from FMC (Philadelphia, PA, USA). Calcium chloride was obtained from Merck (Darmstadt, Germany). Iota carrageenan and honey powder were sourced from the Modernist Pantry (Portsmouth, NH, US). Propyl paraben was bought from Parchem (New Rochelle, NY, USA).

2.2. Preparation and Characterization of CBZ-Loaded Microparticles

CBZ was encapsulated in ethyl cellulose microspheres using the solvent evaporation technique. Briefly, 200 mg of CBZ and 200 mg of EC were dissolved in 10 mL dichloromethane to create the oil phase. The aqueous phase was prepared by dissolving PVA in water at 1% *w/v* concentration. Ten mL of the oil phase was added to 30 mL of the aqueous phase (ratio of 1:3) and mixed at 6000 rpm using a homogenizer for 180 s. The mixture was added to 120 mL of the dispersion medium of distilled water (ratio 1:3 emulsion to dispersion medium) and stirred for 3 h at room temperature to evaporate the organic solvent. Microparticles were collected by filtration then washed three times with distilled water [29,30].

The particle size of the CBZ-loaded microparticles was evaluated by suspending the microparticles in distilled water, followed by the measurement using a laser diffraction particle sizer (BT-9300H, Liaoning, China). Polydispersity of the microparticles was evaluated by calculating the span value (Equation (1)).

$$\text{Span value} = (D90 - D10)/D50, \tag{1}$$

where D10: 10% of the particles are smaller than this diameter; D50: 50% of the particles are smaller than this diameter; D90: 90% of the particles are smaller than this diameter [31].

The particle morphology was observed under a light stereomicroscope (Nikon SMZ745, Tokyo, Japan) attached to a Nikon special lens (Nikon DS-Fi2, Tokyo, Japan).

The presence of CBZ in the microparticles was confirmed by attenuated total reflectance Fourier transform infrared (ATR-FTIR) spectroscopy. Ethyl cellulose, CBZ, and CBZ microparticles were scanned in the range 4000–400 cm^{-1} using a Perkin-Elmer FTIR spectrometer (Perkin Elmer Corp., Norwalk, CT, USA).

The amount of CBZ encapsulated in the microparticles was determined by adding 10 mg of microparticles into 100 mL phosphate buffer at pH 6.8 and stirring at 200 rpm using an incubator shaker (INNOVA 4000, GMI, Ramsey, MN, USA) at 37 ± 0.05 °C for 4 h. Then, the sample was filtered (Whatman filter paper grade 1) and analyzed ($n = 3$) at 286 nm using a UV-spectrophotometer (SHIMADZU UV-1800, Kyoto, Japan). Encapsulation efficiency was calculated by dividing the actual amount of CBZ in the microparticles by the theoretical amount.

2.3. Encapsulation of CBZ-Loaded Microparticles in Alginate Beads

A quantity of the microparticles equivalent to 200 mg of CBZ was suspended in 5 mL of 2% *w/v* sodium alginate solution using a magnetic stirrer. The electrospray apparatus was assembled using a high voltage power supply from Genvolt (Shropshire, UK) and a syringe pump from Shenchen Pump (Baoding, China), and a stainless-steel needle. The microparticle-in-alginate suspension was extruded into 1% *w/v* calcium chloride solution using the electrospray at a 1 mL/min flow rate, with a 10 cm distance between the needle head and calcium chloride solution, and 4000 kV. Alginate beads were formed instantly by means of crosslinking between the alginate and calcium ions. The beads were collected using a metal mesh and washed using distilled water.

The particle size of 10 beads was determined using a digital microscope, U500 Shenzhen (Guangdong, China). The sphericity factor (SF) was used as an indication of the shape of the beads and calculated using Equation (2).

$$\text{Sphericity factor (SF)} = (D_{max} - D_{min})/(D_{max} + D_{min}), \quad (2)$$

where D_{max} is the longest diameter and D_{min} is the shortest diameter of the same bead.

The EE of the CBZ in the alginate beads was measured to ensure the loading of CBZ-loaded microparticles inside the beads. An indirect method was utilized by measuring the un-encapsulated amount of CBZ. Un-encapsulated CBZ leaks into calcium chloride solution either as soluble CBZ or as microparticles. Soluble CBZ was quantified using a spectrophotometer at a 286 nm wavelength. Meanwhile, measurement at 600 nm was also conducted and used to measure the turbidity in the calcium chloride solution resulting from the presence of microparticles that have not been embedded in the beads.

2.4. Loading of CBZ Alginate Beads in a Gel Vehicle

The gel vehicle was prepared by heating 40 mL of distilled water up to 90 °C, followed by addition of the gelling agent under continuous stirring. After complete dissolving and cooling, propyl paraben sodium was added as preservative then the solution was made up to 50 mL with distilled water. Two types of carrageenan (iota or kappa) at two concentrations (1 and 2.5% *w/v*) were used as gelling agents. CBZ alginate beads containing 2000 mg CBZ (about 50 mL as volume) were added into the gel vehicle at 40 °C, then left to cool down at room temperature to produce the gel formulation. The final gel formulation was prepared in two ratios—1 to 1 and 1 to 2 volume ratios of beads to iota carrageenan jelly. Therefore, the volume fraction of the alginate beads in the final gel was 1/2 (for the 1 to 1 ratio) and 1/3 (for the 1 to 2 ratio).

2.5. Characterization of CBZ Oral Gel

2.5.1. Physical Appearance and Syneresis

Visual observation of the fabricated CBZ-oral gels was undertaken to assess their clarity, smell, texture, and the presence of any foreign particles. The texture of the prepared gels was tested by rubbing them between two fingers to check their grittiness and stickiness.

Water separation from the gel is known as syneresis, which is a common problem associated with jellies during their storage [32–34] (Brinker and Scherer, 2013). Iota and kappa carrageenan gels at two different concentrations (1% and 2.5% *w/v*) were stored at room temperature (25 ± 2 °C) and in the refrigerator (8 ± 3 °C) for 24 h to observe syneresis, if any [25].

2.5.2. Homogeneity

A homogeneity test was carried out to ensure the distribution uniformity of CBZ beads in the gel. Beads prepared from 5 mL alginate suspension were added into 5 mL or 10 mL 2.5% *w/v* iota carrageenan gel to yield a ratio of 1:1 or 1:2. Three 1 mL aliquots from the gel (upper, middle and lower regions) were individually dissolved in 100 mL of phosphate buffer (pH 6.8) under continuous shaking at 200 rpm using an incubator shaker (Innova 4000, GMI, Ramsey, MN, USA) at 37 for 4 h. The samples were filtered and analyzed at 286 nm using a spectrophotometer (Shimadzu UV-1800, Kyoto, Japan) [35].

2.5.3. Rheology

Iota carrageenan gelling agent was first tested for rheology using a HAAKE Mars rheometer (Thermo-Scientific, Waltham, MA, USA). The data were then digitally analyzed by Haake Rheo-Win 3.61.0000 software (Thermo-Scientific, Waltham, MA, USA). The test was conducted at 25 °C ± 0.05 °C using a PP35 Ti spindle of 35 mm diameter and 1 mm gap. The test was conducted at an increasing shear rate (γ) from 0.01 to 100 s^{-1} at 1 Hz frequency, then a constant shear rate of 100 s^{-1} for 30 s, then a decreasing shear rate from 100 to 0.015 in 120 s [36]. The results were represented graphically as apparent viscosity (η), and shear stress (τ) vs. shear rate (γ). The same test was repeated after loading the CBZ alginate beads in the gel vehicle. Rheological modelling for each of the gels was fitted to either the Herschel Bulkley or Ostwald De Waele model.

2.6. *In Vitro Drug Release*

The sustained release properties of the CBZ gel formulation were evaluated and compared with the commercially available 200 mg Tegretol®-XR sustained release tablet (Novartis), by calculating the similarity factor (F2) using Equation (3). In addition, the release profiles of CBZ powder, CBZ microparticles, and CBZ-alginate beads were also compared in order to observe the effect of each preparation step on the release properties.

$$f_2 = 50log\left\{\left[1 + \frac{1}{\rho}\sum_{j=1}^{\rho}\left(u_{Tj} - u_{Rj}\right)^2\right]^{-\frac{1}{2}} \times 100\right\}, \quad (3)$$

where F2 is the similarity factor, R_t and T_t are the dissolved cumulative percentage of test and reference samples at selected (t) time points respectively, and n is the number of time points [37–39].

The release profile tests were conducted with a USP-II dissolution apparatus using a 900 mL volume of dissolution medium at 37 ± 0.5 °C and a rotating speed of 100 rpm. At a predetermined time, point (1, 3, 6, 12, and 24 h), 5 mL of dissolution medium was taken ($n = 3$) and replaced with an equal volume of fresh medium. The samples were filtered and analyzed spectrophotometrically at the wavelength of 286 nm.

For CBZ powder, CBZ microparticles and CBZ-alginate beads, the dissolution test was adopted from United States Pharmacopeia (USP), since these formulations can be considered solid dosage forms [40]. However, CBZ gel is a new dosage form not described in USP. Therefore, to compare it with commercial formulations, the dissolution was conducted using the two stage general dissolution method (HCl and phosphate buffer stages).

The Tegretol®-XR sustained release tablets containing 200 mg CBZ were immersed in HCl for the first 2 h, then the disintegrated tablet was filtered using Whatman filter paper no. 1. The tablet particles were collected easily, then transferred directly into phosphate buffer (pH 6.8) to continue the dissolution test for up to 24 h. For the CBZ gel, an amount containing 200 mg CBZ was immersed in HCl for 2 h. In another dissolution vessel, a similar quantity was added into the phosphate buffer pH 6.8 and the test was run for 24 h. The readings from 2 h were deducted from all subsequent readings.

2.7. Stability Study

The CBZ gel formulation, packed in glass containers, was evaluated for physical stability at 30 ± 2 °C with 70 ± 5% RH (real time stability conditions) and 40 ± 2 °C with 70 ± 5% RH (accelerated stability conditions) for 30 days (Countries, 2005). At different time points (0, 7, 15, and 30 days), various quality attributes were evaluated, including pH, physical appearance, syneresis, viscosity, and assay. The viscosity was evaluated using a Brookfield® viscometer (DVII+, Massachusetts, USA) with a spindle number (CPE51) at room temperature (25 °C ± 5 °C) and a rotating speed of 50 rpm [32].

2.8. Statistical Analysis

Statistical analysis was completed using a fractional factorial design for the preparation of all formulations, and a t-test for the stability study of the gel utilizing Minitab software (version 17.1.0; Minitab Inc., State College, PA, USA). When the *p*-value is less than 0.05 the null hypothesis will be rejected, and it will be considered as significant. When *p*-value is more than 0.05, the results will be considered as not significant and the null hypothesis will be accepted.

3. Results

3.1. CBZ-Loaded Microparticles

CBZ was successfully encapsulated in ethyl cellulose microparticles using the solvent evaporation method. The microparticles exhibited a particle size of 135.01 ± 0.61 μm with a monodisperse distribution (Figure 1), a span value of 1.28, and an encapsulation efficiency (EE) of 83.89 ± 3.98%. ATR-FTIR spectra confirmed the presence of CBZ in the microparticles, where CBZ peaks were clearly seen in the microparticle spectrum as presented in Figure 1c.

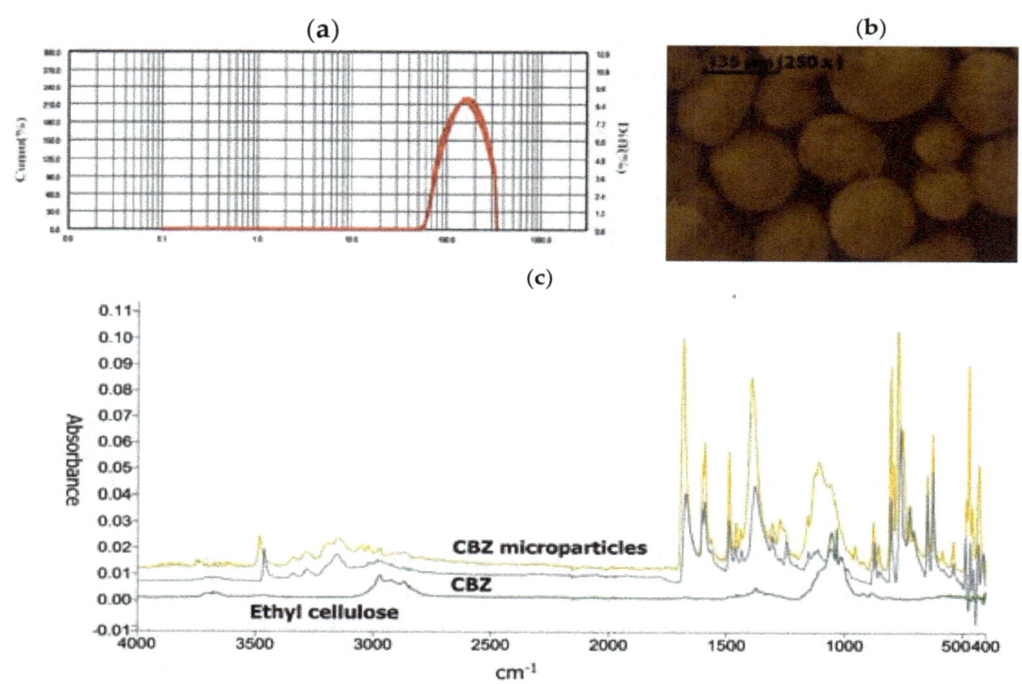

Figure 1. CBZ-loaded microparticle characterization. (**a**) Particle size distribution measured by laser diffraction, (**b**) morphology of the particles under a light microscope, (**c**) ATR-FTIR spectra of ethyl cellulose, CBZ and CBZ-loaded microparticles.

3.2. CBZ-Loaded Microparticles in Alginate Beads

Alginate beads were formed instantly upon contact of alginate solution containing CBZ-loaded microparticles with calcium chloride solution. The beads were spherical (Figure 2) with a size of 1.4 ± 0.05 mm and a sphericity factor of less than 0.05, which is considered spherical [41]. Spectrophotometric measurements revealed that only 0.38 ± 0.01% of the CBZ was un-encapsulated and dissolved in the calcium chloride solution. No CBZ-loaded microparticles were detected in the calcium chloride solution, whereby the turbidity of the solution did not change. This reveals that the encapsulation efficiency of CBZ in the beads was 99.62 ± 0.01%.

(a) (b)

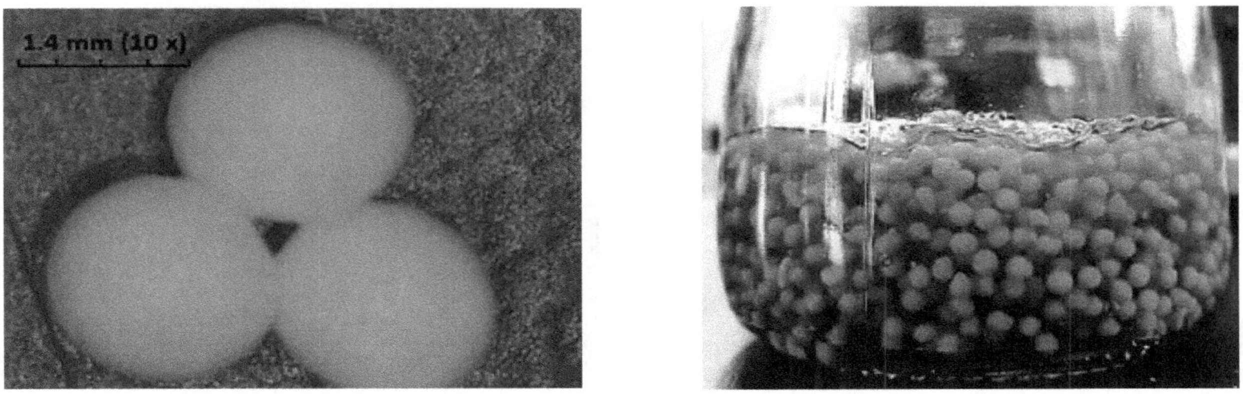

Figure 2. (**a**) CBZ-alginate beads, (**b**) CBZ-gel prepared at a 1:1 ratio of beads to iota carrageenan gel.

3.3. CBZ Oral Gel

3.3.1. Physical Appearance and Syneresis

CBZ gel prepared from iota carrageenan were transparent, non-sticky, of acceptable consistency, and without any feeling of grittiness. No syneresis was seen with any of the iota carrageenan gels, while all the kappa carrageenan gels exhibited syneresis except for the 2.5% gel stored in the refrigerator.

3.3.2. Homogeneity

Table 1 shows the assay results of CBZ from samples taken from different locations of the gel. The average value of the three locations was 100%. The ratio of 1:1 shows very close agreement between the three locations, while in the 1:2 ratio the CBZ was not homogenously distributed. The lower layer had a high concentration of CBZ compared to the upper layer due to precipitation of the CBZ-alginate beads in the bottom of the gel container.

Table 1. Homogeneity of CBZ gel.

Sample Location	Beads to Gel Ratio	CBZ Assay (%)
Up	(1:1)	100.9 ± 1.3
Middle	(1:1)	99.9 ± 1.1
Bottom	(1:1)	99.2 ± 1.9
Up	(1:2)	65.4 ± 2.4
Middle	(1:2)	96.5 ± 3.3
Bottom	(1:2)	138.0 ± 4.5

3.3.3. Rheology

The rheology profile for 2.5% *w*/*v* iota carrageenan gel exhibited a non-Newtonian profile, where the shear stress increased non-linearly with the shear rate. The gel fits the Herschel Bulkley model (R = 0.9981) with clear yield shear stress (Figure 3). However, after incorporating CBZ-alginate beads at a 1:1 loading ratio, the gel did not fit any model and exhibited a degree of thixotropy. The rheology profile of the gel containing the beads was disrupted with spikes. This was because the bead size was more than 1 mm and the gap between the upper and lower spindles was 1 mm. When the spindle rotated, it smashed and compressed the beads. Therefore, the measurement of gel rheology was interrupted with the presence of beads in the gel. The overall trend represents the gel where it appeared to have a shear thinning property with a degree of thixotropy, but the spikes in the graph came from the beads.

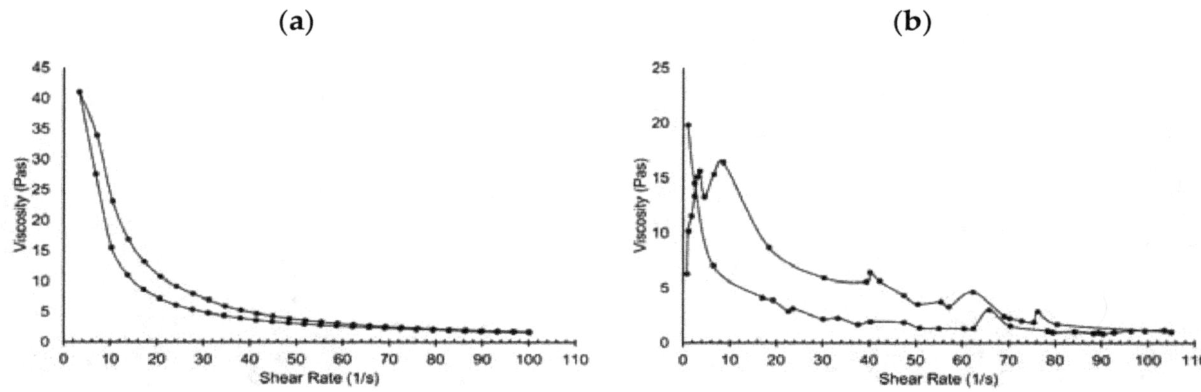

Figure 3. Rheology profile of 2.5% *w/v* iota-carrageenan gel, (**a**) without CBZ-alginate beads, (**b**) with CBZ-alginate beads.

3.4. In vitro Drug Release

CBZ oral gel exhibited a sustained release profile for 24 h (Figure 4). The release was comparable to the release from commercial Tegretol®-XR tablets, with a similarity factor of $f_2 = 74$. At t50 % the percentage of CBZ release from the microparticles was 71.05%, was 74.12% from the beads, was 68.94% from the gel, and was 68.25% from the commercial Tegretol®-XR tablets. These results revealed that the prepared CBZ gel was comparable to the commercial tablet.

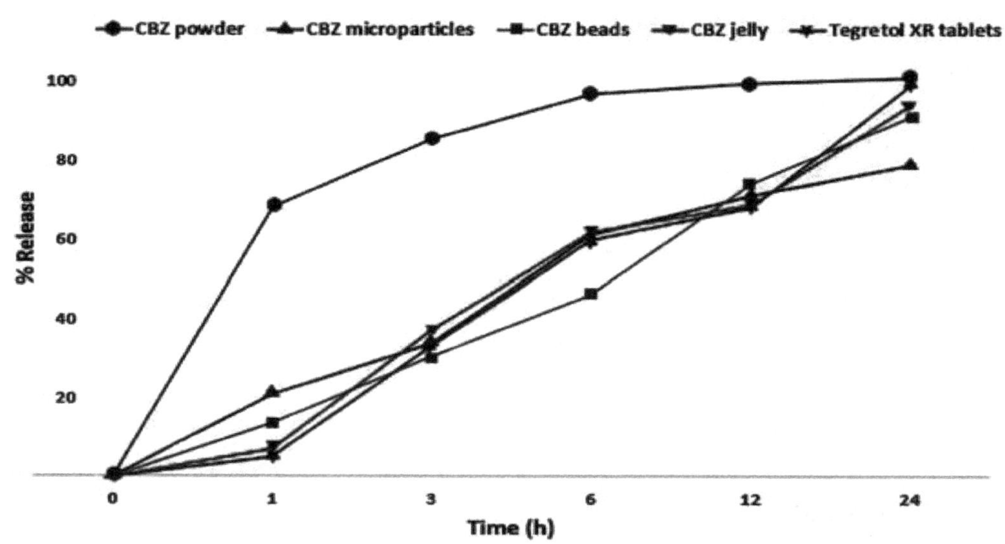

Figure 4. In vitro CBZ release (mean ± 1.86, $n = 3$) from CBZ gel in comparison with Tegretol®-XR tablets, CBZ powder, CBZ microparticles, and CBZ beads.

Release kinetic fitting is shown in Table 2. CBZ microparticles fitted best into the Higuchi model, suggesting a diffusion controlled mechanism. This was expected as the polymer used in the microparticle preparation was ethyl cellulose, which is not a fast degrading polymer. Therefore, the CBZ will release by diffusing through the microparticle matrix. On the other hand, CBZ beads and CBZ gel fitted best into first order kinetics. The presence of an alginate matrix around the microparticles, then the gel around the beads, slowed down the release.

Table 2. Fitting of the release profiles into different kinetic models.

Model	R2			
	CBZ Microparticles	CBZ Beads	CBZ Gel	CBZ Tablets (Tegretol®-XR)
Zero Order	0.7190	0.8828	0.8143	0.8601
First Order	0.8555	0.9968	0.9759	0.9301
Higuchi	0.9222	0.9842	0.9482	0.9591
Korsmeyer Peppas	0.6973	0.7677	0.8121	0.8457
Hixson Crowell	0.8116	0.9760	0.9527	0.9748

3.5. Stability Study

The appearance and texture of the gel in terms of stickiness did not change during the stability study (Table 3). No syneresis was observed within the stability period. The pH slightly dropped with time in both real time and accelerated conditions, but the change was not significantly different, with a p-value of 0.25. Viscosity of the gel stored at 40 °C decreased significantly, while no significant change was observed for the sample stored at 30 °C.

Table 3. Stability study of CBZ gel.

Test	Initial (0) Days	7 Days	15 Days	30 Days
	Real Time Conditions (30 ± 2 °C/70 ± 5% RH)			
Appearance	Transparent with embedded white beads	No change	No change	No change
Syneresis	No	No	No	No
pH	5.7 ± 0.0	5.4 ± 0.1	5.1 ± 0.0	4.5 ± 0.5
Viscosity (mPa.s)	644 ± 271	552 ± 239	676 ± 173	899 ± 208
	Accelerated Conditions (40 ± 2 °C/70 ± 5% RH)			
Appearance	Transparent with embedded white beads	No change	No change	No change
Syneresis	No	No	No	No
pH	5.8 ± 0.1	5.4 ± 0.0	4.6 ± 0.1	5.0 ± 1.8
Viscosity (mPa.s)	357 ± 37	325 ± 5	253 ± 92	180 ± 22

4. Discussion

CBZ was first encapsulated in microparticles using an ethyl cellulose polymer, a well-known polymer for sustained release formulations [42–46]. The microparticles exhibited good sustained release properties, comparable to those of commercial tablets that are given twice daily. However, CBZ-loaded microparticles precipitate when suspended in a liquid vehicle. In addition, microparticles, as relatively large particles, give an unpleasant gritty feeling.

To overcome the precipitation issue of the microparticles, gel was proposed as a vehicle for the microparticles. Gels have high viscosity and do not flow in the normal conditions of temperature and stress, so precipitation is avoided. However, the grittiness of the microparticles may not be overcome. In addition, CBZ may slowly leak out from the microparticles into the gel during long-term storage, resulting in loss of the sustained release properties. To solve this issue, another layer of coating was considered, using alginate beads. Upon crosslinking of alginate with calcium ions, rubbery gel beads are formed with no gritty texture. Alginate beads were prepared to encapsulate the CBZ-loaded microparticles. The beads were spherical in shape, within the recommended size for pediatric use (1–6 years old), and effectively entrapped the microparticles inside them. Since the targeted sustained release profile was obtained from the microparticles, the beads should have little effect on the release profile. The required or the target release profile was found to be similar to the release profile of commercial sustained release tablets, as stated in the United States Pharmacopeia (USP39)—10–35% in 3 h, 35–65% in 6 h, 65–90% in 12 h, and not less than (NLT) 75% in 24 h [47]. A kinetic release study showed that the all prepared formulations followed first order release mechanisms, as the coefficient correlation (R^2) was equal to 0.989 for the CBZ microparticles, 0.976 for the CBZ beads, 0.948 for the CBZ gel, and 0.948 for the Tegretol®-XR tablets. The first order model explained that the release of CBZ based on its dosage form was CBZ-concentration dependent. This means that the release of the drug can be increased when the concentration of that drug is increased in the dosage form over time [48–50]. The release study confirmed that the release of CBZ from the beads was comparable to that of the microparticles and was still similar to that of the commercial tablet.

The last step was to suspend the beads in the gel vehicle. This was performed at a temperature slightly higher than the solidifying temperature of the gelling agent. In comparing kappa and iota carrageenan at two concentrations, iota carrageenan gave the needed properties: no syneresis, homogenous, and with shear-thinning properties. During gel preparation the beads tended to precipitate due to the low viscosity of the hot gel. This is why homogeneity was better at a higher concentration of the beads, where the gel amount was just enough to suspend the beads. The shear-thinning property is needed for this medicated gel in order to allow easy dispensing. Iota carrageenan gel fits the Herschel-Bulkley model, which means it has yield stress—the state of the gel does not change until a specific stress is applied. The gel has high viscosity during storage to prevent bead precipitation, but the viscosity decreases upon applying stress like syringe withdrawal. This allows flexible dosing based on body weight, like a normal CBZ suspension. Similar to the beads, the iota carrageenan gel vehicle was found to have no significant effect on the release properties of CBZ-loaded microparticles. Consequently, the sustained release profile from the final formulation (CBZ-loaded microparticles-in-beads-in-gel) was similar to that of the FDA-approved Tegretol®-XR tablet.

The physical stability study showed that the gel formulation maintained its properties for 30 days when stored at 30 °C. However, the gel viscosity decreased when it was stored at 40 °C. This highlights the importance of storage conditions for this formulation. The pH of the gel was slightly acidic after preparation and showed a decreasing trend during the stability period. Using an ANOVA as the statistical analysis, the change in pH value was found to be not significant, possibly due to the large standard deviation of some points. The change in pH might be attributed to the fact that carrageenans are susceptible to acid-catalyzed hydrolysis [51]. Since the gel was slightly acidic after preparation, the hydrolysis of iota carrageenan might occur and accelerate at a higher temperature, leading to a further drop in pH. This explains the faster drop in pH under the accelerated stability condition (40 °C) compared to the real-time condition (30 °C). Such a change in pH is important to avoid. Iota carrageenan undergoes rapid and extensive loss of viscosity and gelation potential when solutions below pH 5 are heated. The loss of viscosity and gelation potential is primarily due to cleavage of the (1→3) glycosidic linkages [51]. For the gel dosage form, viscosity is critical and should be maintained. The pH of the formulation can be controlled by adding suitable buffering systems.

Based on these preliminary results of the stability study, the gel might need to be stored in the fridge (5 ± 3 °C). A scale up study is recommended to ensure suitability of the preparation method for large scale production. Further investigations are needed, but they are recommended to be done for a larger scale preparation.

5. Conclusions

A carbamazepine sustained release new dosage form designed for pediatric use was prepared and analyzed in this study. This dosage form was based on encapsulation of carbamazepine in microparticles to obtain the required sustained release profile. The microparticles were then embedded in alginate beads, which, in turn, were suspended in iota carrageenan gel. The developed formulation has the advantages of a suspension formulation, that is, flexible dosing and being easy to swallow. It also overcomes the issue of carbamazepine precipitation that is seen in the suspension formulation, which leads to overdose. Carbamazepine sustained release gel has the potential to make the advantages of a sustained release dosage form to pediatric patients accessible, especially children below six years old who have no current option for such a formulation.

6. Patents

The gel as dosage form was patented under the file number (PI 2017704458/Malaysia), under the patent name "A sustained-release drug composition".

Author Contributions: Conceptualization, A.A.D. and S.M.A.A.-M.; Methodology, S.M.M.; Formal Analysis, A.A.D. and S.M.M.; Investigation, S.M.M.; Data Curation, S.M.M. and B.C.; Writing—Original Draft Preparation, S.M.M.; Writing—Review & Editing, S.M.M., S.M.A.A.-M., B.C., H.A.H., and A.A.D.

Acknowledgments: The authors would like to thank Muhammad Taher and the department of pharmaceutical technology at IIUM for technical and facilitation support.

References

1. Zajicek, A.; Fossler, M.J.; Barrett, J.S.; Worthington, J.H.; Ternik, R.; Charkoftaki, G.; Lum, S.; Breitkreutz, J.; Baltezor, M.; Macheras, P. A report from the pediatric formulations task force: Perspectives on the state of child-friendly oral dosage forms. *AAPS J.* **2013**, *15*, 1072–1081. [CrossRef]
2. Standing, J.F.; Tuleu, C. Paediatric formulations—Getting to the heart of the problem. *Int. J. Pharm.* **2005**, *300*, 56–66. [CrossRef]
3. Schiele, J.T.; Quinzler, R.; Klimm, H.-D.; Pruszydlo, M.G.; Haefeli, W.E. Difficulties swallowing solid oral dosage forms in a general practice population: Prevalence, causes, and relationship to dosage forms. *Eur. J. Clin. Pharmacol.* **2013**, *69*, 937–948. [CrossRef] [PubMed]
4. European Medicines Agency. *ICH E11 (R1) Guideline on Clinical Investigation of Medicinal Products in the Pediatric Population*; European Medicines Agency: Amsterdam, The Netherlands, 2017.
5. Nunn, T. *Age Appropriate Formulations—Paediatric Needs*; National Institute for Health Research: Southampton, UK, 2011.
6. Nunn, T.; Williams, J. Formulation of medicines for children. *Br. J. Clin. Pharmacol.* **2005**, *59*, 674–676. [CrossRef] [PubMed]
7. Wolters Kluwer Health, A.S.O. H.-S.P. Cerner Multum and Micromedex from Truven Health Carbamazepine. Available online: https://www.drugs.com/cdi/carbamazepine.html (accessed on 8 September 2018).
8. Yuan, H.G.; Kalfas, G.; Ray, W.H. Suspension polymerization. *J. Macromol. Sci. Part C Polym. Rev.* **1991**, *31*, 215–299. [CrossRef]
9. Costenbader, V.; Markson, S. School suspension: A study with secondary school students. *J. Sch. Psychol.* **1998**, *36*, 59–82. [CrossRef]
10. Bloomer, D.; Dupuis, L.; MacGregor, D.; Soldin, S. Palatability and relative bioavailability of an extemporaneous carbamazepine oral suspension. *Clin. Pharm.* **1987**, *6*, 646–649.
11. Richard, D.; Mycek, J.; Harvey, R.; Champe, P. Lippincott's illustrated reviews: Pharmacology. *Philadelphia* **2006**, *3*, 413–415.
12. Magalhães, J.; Rodrigues, A.T.; Roque, F.; Figueiras, A.; Falcão, A.; Herdeiro, M.T. Use of off-label and unlicenced drugs in hospitalised paediatric patients: A systematic review. *Eur. J. Clin. Pharmacol.* **2015**, *71*, 1–13. [CrossRef]
13. Ernest, T.B.; Elder, D.P.; Martini, L.G.; Roberts, M.; Ford, J.L. Developing paediatric medicines: Identifying the needs and recognizing the challenges. *J. Pharm. Pharmacol.* **2007**, *59*, 1043–1055. [CrossRef]
14. Krishnan, V.; Xu, X.; Barwe, S.P.; Yang, X.; Czymmek, K.; Waldman, S.A.; Mason, R.W.; Jia, X.; Rajasekaran, A.K. Dexamethasone-loaded block copolymer nanoparticles induce leukemia cell death and enhance therapeutic efficacy: A novel application in pediatric nanomedicine. *Mol. Pharm.* **2012**, *10*, 2199–2210. [CrossRef] [PubMed]

15. Dumont, M.F.; Yadavilli, S.; Sze, R.W.; Nazarian, J.; Fernandes, R. Manganese-containing Prussian blue nanoparticles for imaging of pediatric brain tumors. *Int. J. Nanomed.* **2014**, *9*, 2581.
16. Basha, R.; Sabnis, N.; Heym, K.; Bowman, W.P.; Lacko, A.G. Targeted nanoparticles for pediatric leukemia therapy. *Front. Oncol.* **2014**, *4*, 101. [CrossRef] [PubMed]
17. Machado, M.C.; Cheng, D.; Tarquinio, K.M.; Webster, T.J. Nanotechnology: Pediatric applications. *Pediatr. Res.* **2010**, *67*, 500. [CrossRef] [PubMed]
18. Deutschmann, A.; Schlagenhauf, A.; Leschnik, B.; Hoffmann, K.M.; Hauer, A.; Muntean, W. Increased procoagulant function of microparticles in pediatric inflammatory bowel disease: Role in increased thrombin generation. *J. Pediatr. Gastroenterol. Nutr.* **2013**, *56*, 401–407. [CrossRef] [PubMed]
19. Chicella, M.; Branim, B.; Lee, K.R.; Phelps, S.J. Comparison of microparticle enzyme and fluorescence polarization immunoassays in pediatric patients not receiving digoxin. *Ther. Drug Monit.* **1998**, *20*, 347–351. [CrossRef] [PubMed]
20. Elsayh, K.I.; Zahran, A.M.; El-Abaseri, T.B.; Mohamed, A.O.; El-Metwally, T.H. Hypoxia biomarkers, oxidative stress, and circulating microparticles in pediatric patients with thalassemia in Upper Egypt. *Clin. Appl. Thromb. Hemost.* **2014**, *20*, 536–545. [CrossRef] [PubMed]
21. Albertini, B.; Di Sabatino, M.; Melegari, C.; Passerini, N. Formulating SLMs as oral pulsatile system for potential delivery of melatonin to pediatric population. *Int. J. Pharm.* **2014**, *469*, 67–79. [CrossRef] [PubMed]
22. Roy, D.; Semsarilar, M.; Guthrie, J.T.; Perrier, S. Cellulose modification by polymer grafting: A review. *Chem. Soc. Rev.* **2009**, *38*, 2046–2064. [CrossRef] [PubMed]
23. Blakemore, W.R.; Harpell, A.R. Carrageenan. In *Food Stabilisers, Thickeners and Gelling Agents*; Blackwell Publishing: Hoboken, NJ, USA, 2009; pp. 73–94.
24. Sosnik, A. Alginate Particles as Platform for Drug Delivery by the Oral Route: State-of-the-Art. *ISRN Pharm.* **2014**, *2014*, 926157. [CrossRef] [PubMed]
25. Prakash, K.; Satyanarayana, V.; Nagiat, H.; Fathi, A.; Shanta, A.; Prameela, A. Formulation development and evaluation of novel oral jellies of carbamazepine using pectin, guar gum, and gellan gum. *Asian J. Pharm.* **2014**, *8*, 241. [CrossRef]
26. Imai, K. Alendronate sodium hydrate (oral jelly) for the treatment of osteoporosis: Review of a novel, easy to swallow formulation. *Clin. Interv. Aging* **2013**, *8*, 681. [CrossRef] [PubMed]
27. Miyazaki, S.; Takahashi, A.; Itoh, K.; Ishitani, M.; Dairaku, M.; Togashi, M.; Mikami, R.; Attwood, D. Preparation and evaluation of gel formulations for oral sustained delivery to dysphagic patients. *Drug Dev. Ind. Pharm.* **2009**, *35*, 780–787. [CrossRef] [PubMed]
28. Satyanarayana, A.D.; Kulkarni, K.P.; Shivakumar, G.H. Gels and jellies as a dosage form for dysphagia patients: A review. *Curr. Drug Ther.* **2011**, *6*, 79–86. [CrossRef]
29. Rosca, I.D.; Watari, F.; Uo, M. Microparticle formation and its mechanism in single and double emulsion solvent evaporation. *J. Control. Release* **2004**, *99*, 271–280. [CrossRef] [PubMed]
30. Chen, X.; Young, T.J.; Sarkari, M.; Williams, R.O., III; Johnston, K.P. Preparation of cyclosporine A nanoparticles by evaporative precipitation into aqueous solution. *Int. J. Pharm.* **2002**, *242*, 3–14. [CrossRef]
31. Craig, D.; Barker, S.; Banning, D.; Booth, S. An investigation into the mechanisms of self-emulsification using particle size analysis and low frequency dielectric spectroscopy. *Int. J. Pharm.* **1995**, *114*, 103–110. [CrossRef]
32. Suda, N.; Shinzato, R.; Kiyokawa, M.; Kaneuchi, M.; Sugawara, M.; Kohri, N. Development of acetylcysteine jelly for the prevention of radiocontrast-induced reductions in renal function and its evaluation. *Jpn. J. Pharm. Health Care Sci.* **2005**, *31*, 355–359. [CrossRef]
33. Christensen, B.E. Alginates as biomaterials in tissue engineering. In *Carbohydrate Chemistry: Chemical and Biological Approaches*; Royal Society of Chemistry: London, UK, 2011; Volume 37, pp. 227–258.
34. Brinker, C.J.; Scherer, G.W. *Sol-Gel Science: The Physics and Chemistry of Sol-Gel Processing*; Academic Press: Cambridge, MA, USA, 2013.
35. Garud, N.; Garud, A. Preparation and in-vitro evaluation of metformin microspheres using non-aqueous solvent evaporation technique. *Trop. J. Pharm. Res.* **2012**, *11*, 577–583. [CrossRef]
36. Watanabe, A.; Hanawa, T.; Sugihara, M. Application of glycerogelatin as oral dosage form for the elderly. *J. Pharm. Sci. Technol. Jpn.* **1994**, *54*, 77.
37. Shah, V.P.; Tsong, Y.; Sathe, P.; Liu, J.-P. In vitro dissolution profile comparison—Statistics and analysis of the similarity factor, f2. *Pharm. Res.* **1998**, *15*, 889–896. [CrossRef] [PubMed]

38. Liu, J.-P.; Ma, M.-C.; Chow, S.-C. Statistical evaluation of similarity factor f2 as a criterion for assessment of similarity between dissolution profiles. *Drug Inf. J.* **1997**, *31*, 1255–1271. [CrossRef]
39. Ocaña, J.; Frutos, G.; Sánchez, P. Using the similarity factor f2 in practice: A critical revision and suggestions for its standard error estimation. *Chemom. Intell. Lab. Syst.* **2009**, *99*, 49–56. [CrossRef]
40. Mawazi, S.M.; Hadi, H.A.B.; Al-Mahmood, S.M.A.; Doolaanea, A. Development and Validation of UV-VIS Spectroscopic Method of Assay of Carbamazepine in Microparticles. *Int. J. Appl. Pharm.* **2019**, *11*, 34–37. [CrossRef]
41. Chan, E.-S.; Lim, T.-K.; Voo, W.-P.; Pogaku, R.; Tey, B.T.; Zhang, Z. Effect of formulation of alginate beads on their mechanical behavior and stiffness. *Particuology* **2011**, *9*, 228–234. [CrossRef]
42. Zhang, G.; Pinnamaraju, P.; Ali, M.A. Water Insoluble Polymer Based Sustained Release Formulation. U.S. Patent 6251430B1, 26 June 2001.
43. Follonier, N.; Doelker, E.; Cole, E.T. Evaluation of hot-melt extrusion as a new technique for the production of polymer-based pellets for sustained release capsules containing high loadings of freely soluble drugs. *Drug Dev. Ind. Pharm.* **1994**, *20*, 1323–1339. [CrossRef]
44. Li, X.-Y.; Zheng, Z.-B.; Yu, D.-G.; Liu, X.-K.; Qu, Y.-L.; Li, H.-L. Electrosprayed sperical ethylcellulose nanoparticles for an improved sustained-release profile of anticancer drug. *Cellulose* **2017**, *24*, 5551–5564. [CrossRef]
45. Parida, P.; Mishra, S.C.; Sahoo, S.; Behera, A.; Nayak, B.P. Development and characterization of ethylcellulose based microsphere for sustained release of nifedipine. *J. Pharm. Anal.* **2016**, *6*, 341–344. [CrossRef]
46. Maulvi, F.A.; Soni, T.G.; Shah, D.O. Extended release of timolol from ethyl cellulose microparticles laden hydrogel contact lenses. *Open Pharm. Sci. J.* **2015**, *2*. [CrossRef]
47. Sandoz Inc. *Carbamazepine Extended-Release Tablets, USP*; Sandoz Inc.: Princeton, NJ, USA, 2016; pp. 2917–2921.
48. Gefter, J.; Zaks, B.; Kirmayer, D.; Lavy, E.; Steinberg, D.; Friedman, M. Chlorhexidine sustained-release varnishes for catheter coating–Dissolution kinetics and antibiofilm properties. *Eur. J. Pharm. Sci.* **2018**, *112*, 1–7. [CrossRef]
49. Higuchi, T. Mechanism of sustained-action medication. Theoretical analysis of rate of release of solid drugs dispersed in solid matrices. *J. Pharm. Sci.* **1963**, *52*, 1145–1149. [CrossRef] [PubMed]
50. Barzegar-Jalali, M.; Adibkia, K.; Valizadeh, H.; Shadbad, M.R.S.; Nokhodchi, A.; Omidi, Y.; Mohammadi, G.; Nezhadi, S.H.; Hasan, M. Kinetic analysis of drug release from nanoparticles. *J. Pharm. Pharm. Sci.* **2008**, *11*, 167–177. [CrossRef] [PubMed]
51. BeMiller, J. *Carrageenans*, 3rd ed.; Elsevier: Amsterdam, The Netherlands, 2019; p. 12.

4

Development of a New Delivery System Based on Drug-Loadable Electrospun Nanofibers for Psoriasis Treatment

Leticia Martínez-Ortega †, Amalia Mira, Asia Fernandez-Carvajal, C. Reyes Mateo, Ricardo Mallavia * and Alberto Falco *,†

Institute of Research, Development and Innovation in Biotechnology of Elche (IDiBE) and Molecular and Cellular Biology Institute (IBMC), Miguel Hernández University (UMH), 03202 Elche, Spain; leticia.martinez@goumh.umh.es (L.M.-O.); a.mira@umh.es (A.M.); asia.fernandez@umh.es (A.F.-C.); rmateo@umh.es (C.R.M.)

* Correspondence: r.mallavia@umh.es (R.M.); alber.falco@umh.es (A.F.)

† These authors contributed equally to this work.

Abstract: Psoriasis is a chronic autoimmune systemic disease with an approximate incidence of 2% worldwide; it is commonly characterized by squamous lesions on the skin that present the typical pain, stinging, and bleeding associated with an inflammatory response. In this work, poly(methyl vinyl ether-*alt*-maleic ethyl monoester) (PMVEMA-ES) nanofibers have been designed as a delivery vehicle for three therapeutic agents with palliative properties for the symptoms of this disease (salicylic acid, methyl salicylate, and capsaicin). For such a task, the production of these nanofibers by means of the electrospinning technique has been optimized. Their morphology and size have been characterized by optical microscopy and scanning electron microscopy (SEM). By selecting the optimal conditions to achieve the smallest and most uniform nanofibers, approximate diameters of up to 800–900 nm were obtained. It was also determined that the therapeutic agents that were used were encapsulated with high efficiency. The analysis of their stability over time by GC-MS showed no significant losses of the encapsulated compounds 15 days after their preparation, except in the case of methyl salicylate. Likewise, it was demonstrated that the therapeutic compounds that were encapsulated conserved, and even improved, their capacity to activate the transient receptor potential cation channel 1 (TRPV1) channel, which has been associated with the formation of psoriatic lesions.

Keywords: PMVE/MA; electrospinning; nanofibers; capsaicin; psoriasis; TRPV1

---

1. Introduction

Psoriasis is a chronic immune-mediated disease that affects 2% of the population, comprising different clinical manifestations, which are mainly characterized by skin disorders such as erythematous papules or scaly teardrop-like lesions associated with the characteristic pain, stinging, and even bleeding of an inflammatory process. The most affected areas are usually the elbows, knees, scalp, and lower back [1,2].

The immune system plays a crucial role in the pathogenesis of the disease, and particularly, the deregulation of the crosstalk between the innate and adaptive immune system within the interleukin-23 (IL23)/T helper cell 17 (Th17) axis [1,3,4]. Thus, the therapeutic treatments focus on targeting the Th17 response, either as local or systemic non-specific immunosuppressors (conventional therapies) such as dermocorticoids and methotrexate. The side effects produced by these treatments have boosted the use of antibody-based systemic treatments that recognize, bind, and block the activity of those cytokines involved in the Th17 response (biological therapies), such as IL17A (Ixekizumab,

Taltz™; Secukinumab, Cosentyx™), IL23 (Guselkumab, Tremfya™), IL23 and IL12 (Ustekinumab, Stelara™), and TNF-α (Adalimumab, Humira™; Etanercept, Enbrel™; Infliximab, Remicade™) [1,5,6]. However, despite the promising results offered by this type of treatment, they also have limitations such as their high cost, some adverse effects, a loss of efficacy due to the development of anti-drug antibodies, and the inability to avoid occasional symptomatic outbreaks or to act on some poorly accessible locations [1,7–9]. Therefore, there is still a need to use therapeutic agents to alleviate the discomfort derived from the symptoms caused by the psoriatic lesions [1,6,10].

The main palliative agents for the dermal symptomatology of the disease are keratolytics, to reduce the generation of scales, and analgesics, to relieve the painful and itching sensation. Among the keratolytics, salicylic acid stands out, which acts by lowering the pH of the stratum corneum and thus preventing the adhesion of keratinocytes [11]. In turn, it also improves the absorption of other topical treatments by reducing the stiffness of the stratum, and also reduces the pruritus [12].

In terms of analgesic therapy, one of the most common targets in topical applications is the transient receptor potential cation channel 1 (TRPV1), commonly called the capsaicin receptor. This receptor is mainly found in the nociceptive neurons of the peripheral nervous system, although they have also been described in other non-neuronal tissues, including skin cells. TRPV1 is a non-selective tetrameric cation channel with high permeability to calcium (Ca^{2+}) that has been involved in the transmission and modulation of pain when triggered by different physical and chemical stimuli such as temperatures above 43 °C, acidic pH, capsaicin, and some endogenous mediators of inflammation [13–15]. Capsaicin, an alkaloid present in several species in the genus *Capsicum*, and some of its derivatives act as analgesic agents by producing TRPV1 desensitization [13,16]. Additionally, this family of compounds hold other biological properties such as cardiovascular stimulator, antioxidant, and anticancer, as well as anti-inflammatory, by for instance suppressing the inducement of TNF-α, which is also a psoriasis mediator [17–20]. Methyl salicylate, which is derived from salicylic acid, is another analgesic agent. This compound belongs to the family of non-steroidal anti-inflammatory drugs (NSAIDs), and has also been reported to activate TRPV1 [21,22]. In addition, it is easily absorbed through the skin, and is already used for the treatment of inflammation and pain [22].

However, for the maximization of the expected benefits of their combined delivery, it would be necessary to have a suitable system for their topical application, and desirably, an encapsulation procedure that allows combining all three compounds together without losing their activity, in addition to being simple and scalable to industrial production. In this sense, recent advances in nanotechnology applied to the field of medicine offer an alternative that meets all these requirements, i.e., polymer nanofibers produced by the electrospinning technique [23–25]. In addition, the correct choice of the integrating materials would allow the development of nanostructures with appropriate release properties according the particular dosage needs of their load, which in the specific case of capsaicin should be sustained in order to keep TRPV1 desensitized for a prolonged period.

In this work, based on the progress made in our previous study [26], the production process of electrospun nanofibers loaded with all three compounds described above is optimized using poly(methyl vinyl ether-*alt*-maleic ethyl monoester) (PMVEMA-ES) as the polymeric material. Such a biodegradable, biocompatible, bioadhesive, and low-toxic polymer is already commercialized, and used in other biomedical applications, and has already shown its suitability for the creation of these nanostructured systems with the appropriate release characteristics [26–30]. Additionally, this polymer not only allows the possibility of being used as the main building polymer for the creation of nanofibers, but also allows combining with other materials, such as fluorene-based copolymers [31,32], in order to combine functional properties within the same nanostructure [26,33,34]. The morphological characterization of these nanofibers, together with their encapsulation capacity, stability over time, and activity of the encapsulated compounds are also analyzed in this study.

2. Materials and Methods

2.1. Polymers, Solvents, Drugs, and Common Materials

The copolymer of poly(methyl vinyl ether-*alt*-maleic acid) monoethyl ester (PMVEMA-ES) (M_w: ~130 kg/mol) was supplied in a 50% *w/w* solution in ethanol (Sigma-Aldrich, Saint Louis, MO, USA).

The solvents used were dichloromethane, acetone, ethanol (Merck KGaA, Darmstadt, Germany), methanol (VWR International, Radnor, PA, USA), sulfuric acid, and anhydrous dimethyl sulfoxide (DMSO) (Sigma-Aldrich).

The reagents used were salicylic acid, capsaicin, ruthenium red (RR) (Sigma-Aldrich), magnesium sulfate anhydrous (Honeywell Fluka, Morris Plains, NJ, USA), sodium hydroxide (Panreac AppliChem—ITW Reagents, Cinisello Balsamo, Milan, Italy), and ferric chloride (Sigma-Aldrich). Although it is considered in the text as a unique therapeutic agent, according to the supplier's analysis certificate, the purity of the commercial capsaicin used in this work was 61.1%, and it contained 31.2% of dihydrocapsaicin, which is a derivative with very similar chemical and biological properties to capsaicin.

Methyl salicylate was synthesized from the esterification of salicylic acid in a solution of methanol and sulfuric acid by following the method proposed by Carrillo-Arcos *et al.* (2016) [35]. Briefly, the 2-hydroxybenzoic acid (28.96 mmol) was dissolved in 60 mL of methanol, and then sulfuric acid (98%, 2 mL) was added dropwise to the solution, and the mixture was stirred at reflux for 18 h. Next, the solvent of the reaction was removed by vacuum rotary-evaporation, and the crude product was neutralized to pH 5–6 with a solution of NaOH (1 M, 50 mL), which was extracted three times with dichloromethane (3 × 50 mL). The combined organic phases were dried (magnesium sulfate) and concentrated (rotavap). The crude oil was distilled in a Kugelrohr B-585 glass furnace (Büchi, Flawil, Switzerland) to finally obtain a colorless oil (yield of 75%).

2.2. Electrospinning

The preparation of nanofibers was performed by means of the methodology described before by Mira *et al.* (2017) [26]. After optimization, an electrospinnable solution containing 25% *w/w* of PMVE/MA-ES in ethanol was selected. As for the active agents, a combination of 1.5% salicylic acid, 1% capsaicin (2:1 together with dihydrocapsaicin), and 1% methyl salicylate, all *w/w* with respect to the polymer weight, was used.

The electrospinning process was performed on a device that included a two-mL Discardit II syringe (Becton Dickinson, Franklin Lakes, NJ, USA) through which the polymer solution was introduced, and from which it was pumped through a blunt-end stainless steel hypodermic needle 316 of 20 Gauge (101.6 mm in length, external diameter 0.902 mm, and internal diameter 0.584 mm) (Sigma-Aldrich) at a sustained flow controlled by a KDS 100 infusion pump (KD Scientific, Holliston, MA, USA). The needle and the aluminum foil collector, faced vertically, are connected to a Series FC high voltage source (Glassman High Voltage Inc., Whitehouse Station, NJ, USA), which provides the voltage responsible for the generation of the jet to be deposited on the collector located at a settled distance. Any material that is intended to be covered with a mat of electrospun nanofibers, as for example in this work, the adhesive dressings, would be placed on the aluminum collector. After the optimization of the operational parameters (see corresponding section for further details), values were selected for the elaboration of the batches of nanofibers for the following experiments.

2.3. Microscopy

For the observation in optical microscopy, the nanofibers were electropun on a microscope slide (Deltalab, Barcelona, Spain) arranged on top of the aluminum collector. The inverted fluorescence optical microscope that was used was a Microsystems DMI3000B (Leica, Bensheim, Germany) equipped with a Leica EL6000 compact light source and a Leica DFC 3000G digital camera. The images were taken with a 63× objective in phase contrast, and the image processing was done manually using the program Leica Application Suite AF 6000 Module Systems. By this methodology, an initial screening, and then a more exhaustive screening, were carried out.

After the optimization of the electrospinning parameters, selected nanofiber samples were also analyzed by scanning electron microscopy (SEM), without metal coating, in a JSM-6360 LV device (Jeol, Tokyo, Japan). In both cases, from the images obtained for each sample, a total of 100 measurements of nanofiber diameters were taken and analyzed by using the Image J software (National Institutes of Health, NIH, Bethesda, MD, USA).

2.4. Gas Chromatography and Mass Spectrometry (GC-MS)

The amount of the therapeutic agents contained in the nanofibers, which are necessary for analyzing the encapsulation efficiency and the stability of the encapsulation over time, was determined by means of a gas chromatograph coupled to a mass spectrometer, in particular, a GCMS-QP2010 SE equipment with quadrupole detector supplemented with a thermal TD-20 adsorption attachment and an AOC-20i/s automatic sample injector (Shimadzu, Kyoto, Japan). The employed GC column was an Agilent J&W capillary HP-5MS UI (5% diphenyl–95% dimethylpolysiloxane, 30 m $\times$ 0.25 mm id, film thickness 0.25 μm) (Agilent Technologies Inc., Santa Clara, CA, USA).

The procedure of this analytical methodology is based on a previous study [36]. Briefly, the temperatures of the injector and detector were 250 °C and 210 °C, respectively. Helium was used as a carrier gas at a flow rate of 1.5 mL/min. The chosen program was 40 °C for two minutes; then, the temperature was raised at a speed of 10 °C/min to 240 °C and, thereafter, at a rate of 5 °C/min up to 270 °C, which was finally maintained for five minutes.

In each experiment, a calibration curve was created for each of the analyzed compounds whose concentration ranges were between 0.018–1.420 mg/mL for capsaicin, 0.009–0.720 mg/mL for dihydrocapsaicin, 0.04–3.22 mg/mL for methyl salicylate, and 0.161–3.22 mg/mL for salicylic acid. All of the values that were provided for each curve corresponded to the area under the curve that was obtained for each concentration of the corresponding compound. In this way, the curves were preferably adjusted to a quadratic equation correlating area with concentration R^2 coefficients greater than 0.99 in all of the cases (see Figure S1 in supplementary information).

The analyzed samples corresponded to two independent productions of nanofibers loaded with the three therapeutic agents as described above. Each sample of nanofibers was analyzed when just prepared and at 5 and 15 days post-production. These samples were stored in a drawer, uncovered, protected from light, and at room temperature. Immediately prior to their analysis, the samples were dissolved in dichloromethane, filtered with 0.2-μm nylon membranes (Millipore, Bedford, OH, USA) and injected at a concentration of 10 mg/mL *w/v*. As controls, nanofibers without encapsulated compounds and fresh polymer solutions (made just prior to the electrospinning process) were used.

2.5. Cell Culture

For *in vitro* cell assays, human embryonic kidney cells stably expressing TRPV1 (HEK293-VR1) were used. The cells were maintained in Dulbecco's modified Eagle's medium (DMEM) supplemented with 10% *v/v* fetal bovine serum (FBS) (Sigma-Aldrich) and 50 μg/mL gentamicin (Thermo Fisher Scientific, Waltham, MA, USA). Cells were cultured in 25-cm^2 flasks at 37 °C in a humidified atmosphere with 5% CO_2, and for their harvest they were detached with 0.25% trypsin-EDTA solution. For the assays, cells were seeded in opaque 96-well plates with transparent bottoms (Corning Incorporated, Corning, NY, USA) at a cell density of 40,000 cells three days before treatment.

2.6. TRPV1 Channel Activity Assays

Since the TRPV1 channel allows the non-selective passage of cations such as Ca^{2+} when activated, a Ca^{2+} fluorescence probe has been used to indirectly quantify such activation, which might be induced by the experimental treatments. Thus, Ca^{2+} fluorography assays were performed by using the probe Fluo-4 NW (Molecular Probes-Thermo Fisher Scientific, Waltham, MA, USA) supplemented with

2.5 mM of probenecid, which improves the permeation of the probe in the cells and inhibits losses of fluorescence by avoiding its exit to the cellular exterior, as was recently reported by Serafini *et al.* (2018) [37].

Briefly, in cell plates prepared as described in the previous section, the culture medium was removed, and 100 μL/well of probe solution was added and incubated for 30 min at 37 °C followed by 30 min at 30 °C, always in the dark. Then, the fluorescence measurements were taken (excitation at 485 nm and emission at 535 nm) with a POLARstar Omega plate reader (BMG LABTECH GmbH, Offenburg, Germany) for 20 cycles (each one corresponding to a period of 156 s) and at a constant internal temperature of 30 °C. After the third cycle, one μL/well of each formulation that had been previously dissolved in DMSO at the corresponding concentration was added manually in order to reach the expected treatment doses in the well. In this sense, nanofibers were dissolved at 50 mg/mL in order to treat cells with 54 μM, 33 μM, and 10 μM of salicylic acid, methyl salicylate, and capsaicin, respectively. A solvent control (DMSO), capsaicin as agonist compound at 10 μM [38], and RR as a non-competitive inhibitor [39] at 10 μM were also included. Then, the measurements continued until cycle 20. After cycle 10, one μL of 10 μM capsaicin in DMSO was added to some wells that had been previously treated with RR in order to check the stability and selectivity of the system. Calibration curves for capsaicin and methyl salicylate were also included (range 0.1–30 μM and 15–120 μM, respectively). Each sample was analyzed in triplicate in each assay.

2.7. Preliminary In Vivo Test of Topical Application

An initial *in vivo* study was carried out with three healthy human volunteers to evaluate, when administered topically, the stability time of the experimental nanofibers, as well as to determine the functionality of the encapsulated TRPV1 agonists by analyzing the responsiveness to them. Each volunteer was given an adhesive dressing with electrospun nanofibers on each arm on the skin surface of the deltoid. This test was blind, since for each volunteer, one of the dressings contained empty nanofibers, and the other contained drug-loaded ones, but they were assigned randomly to each of their arms. Each dressing contained approximately 25 mg of nanofibers distributed over a surface area of 20 cm^2. The duration of the treatment was eight hours. The surface of the dressing was kept protected from light throughout the full period. Every two hours, photographs were taken of each dressing to determine the state of the nanofibers and treated skin. At the end of the trial, each volunteer was asked which dressing they thought contained the TRPV1 agonists. This study was approved by the Project Evaluation Board of Miguel Hernández University (approval no. 2018.12.05.FPRL).

2.8. Data Analysis and Graphics

Data were analyzed by either GraphPad Prism v6 and Microsoft Excel software. Both of them were used for creating the graphs. Statistical analysis was performed with GraphPad Prism v6 specifically. Applied statistical methods are stated together with the analyzed data in the Results section.

3. Results and Discussion

3.1. Optimization of PMVE/MA-ES Nanofibers Encapsulating Three Therapeutic Agents

Initially, we proceeded to the optimization of the morphology and size of the nanofibers without the encapsulated agent. For this, the operational values of the electrospinning procedure were modulated within a range that had been estimated from our previous study [26]. They included a concentration of PMVEMA-ES (20–28% *w*/*w*), pumping flow (0.25–1.35 mL/h), voltage (6–17.5 kV), and distance between the needle and collector (8–30 cm).

The concentration of polymer was shown to be determinant for the morphology and size of the final nanofibers. Independently of the other parameters, the values of greater uniformity and smaller fiber diameter were obtained with a concentration of 25% *w*/*w* of PMVE/MA-ES (as in our previous study [26]). Therefore, the concentration of polymer was fixed at this value for the analysis of the rest of the operational parameters, which were shown to be inversely proportional to the size of the nanofibers until reaching a critical value at which abrupt increases in size or the appearance of morphological aberrations could be observed. In short, the combination of values with which the smallest uniform fibers (810 ± 141 nm) were obtained were 15.5 kV, 12 cm, and 0.25 mL/h (Figure 1). However, when adding the therapeutic agents, nanofibers were significantly larger (about 200 nm more) by using these same parameters; the reason we proceeded to refine them again under these new circumstances was in order to reduce the size of the nanofibers below the micron. Thus, the optimal values to obtain uniform nanofibers of 878 ± 209 nm were 17 kV voltage, an eight cm needle–collector distance, and a flow of 0.25 mL/h (Figure 1).

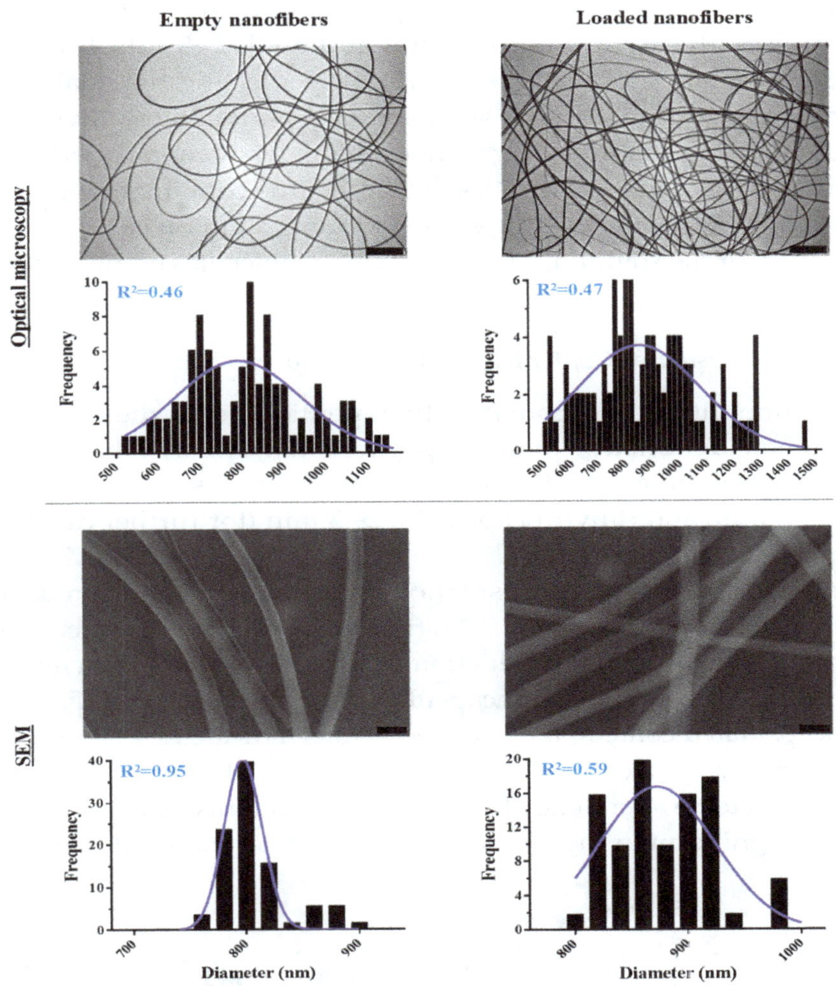

Figure 1. Optical microscopy and SEM analysis of optimized nanofibers. Representative optical microscopy and SEM images that include either empty or loaded nanofibers obtained by using optimized electrospinning parameters are shown (scale bars: 25 μm for optical microscopy, and 1 μm for SEM images). Corresponding frequency histograms of their diameters are also included. Each histogram was performed from the data obtained from several images until reaching 100 measurements. Best-fit adjustments (and their R^2) to a Gaussian distribution are indicated in blue.

So far, the analysis of the nanofibers had been done by optical microscopy; however, to analyze the morphology in more detail and with greater precision, the size of the optimized nanofibers was observed by SEM. The measurements obtained by electron microscopy are equivalent to those obtained by optical microscopy: 808 ± 31 nm for empty nanofibers, and 875 ± 49 nm for those with encapsulated therapeutic content (Figure 1).

The low amount of encapsulated drug that was used in this work (3.5% all together) does not explain the increase in size that was observed in the loaded nanofibers, even more considering that loading percentages are usually much higher for molecules that have a similar complexity, which even reduces nanofiber diameters [40,41]. Neither did an incompatibility in solubility, since all three compounds are soluble in the polymer-solvent system that was used. In fact, this aspect has been reported as critical, as well as the adequate selection of the solvent [42,43], for the morphology of fibers [44]. In this sense, from a broad perspective, the factors influencing fiber morphology are classified into two main groups: the processing and solution ones (briefly reviewed in [45]). Thus, while the processing factors are associated with the electrospinning mechanical set-up and environmental conditions, such as relative humidity, the solution factors refer to the physicochemical characteristics of the electrospinning solution, and, among them, some of the relevant ones are the conductivity and viscosity, according to several authors [41,45,46]. Therefore, if the addition of a compound, or a combination of them, is significantly affecting the final morphology of fibers, it might be as a consequence of modifying such solution parameters. Given that, as reported in studies, within moderate drug-loading ranges, fiber diameters generally increase with decreasing conductivity or increasing viscosity values [40,41,45,47,48], the combination of compounds that was used in the present work may be affecting the electrospinning solution either way, but most probably by increasing the viscosity of the solution, since none of the molecules employed was either a salt or a polyelectrolyte [40,41].

3.2. Determination of the Encapsulated Content and Its Stability over Time

To quantify the amount of encapsulated therapeutic agent, they were separated by gas chromatography, and then identified with mass spectrometry. In the calibration process, the elution times were precisely determined for the four compounds: methyl salicylate, 12.5 min; salicylic acid, 14.0 min; capsaicin, 29.0 min; and dihydrocapsaicin, 29.3 min (for further details in this regard, see Figure S1 in the supplementary information).

By following this procedure, the encapsulation efficiency was calculated for each therapeutic agent, which was found to be approximately 100% (in comparison to theoretical full encapsulation) in all cases when measuring right after the production of nanofibers ($t = 0$, data not shown). Such value was used as a reference for calculating the encapsulated content over time (Figure 2). Regarding the permanence of the encapsulated content, the obtained results indicate that methyl salicylate is lost over time; specifically, after 15 days, just 60.2 $\pm$ 7.8% of methyl salicylate remained in fibers. Regarding the other agents, there seemed to be a tendency to decrease the quantity of encapsulated compound, but these changes were not significant in the period of time that was analyzed (0–15 days).

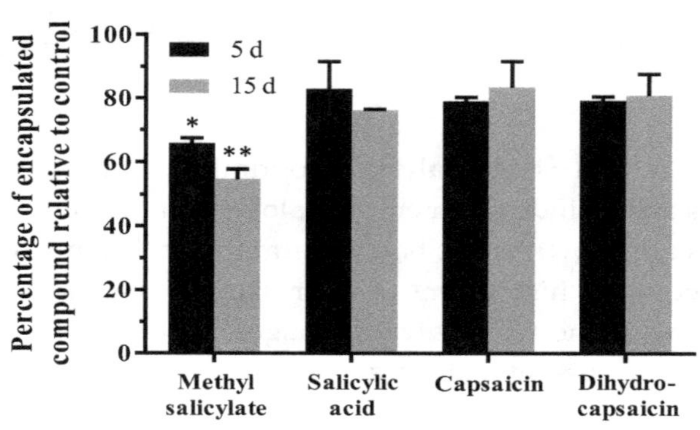

Figure 2. Stability of the loaded compounds over time. The graph indicates the percentage of compound that remained encapsulated in the nanofibers 5 and 15 days (d) after they were produced. Compound content was determined by GC-MS. Values are relative to the content measured right after the production of the nanofibers. Statistical analysis comprised multiple *t* test corrected for multiple comparisons by using the Holm–Sidak method. Significant changes in the content of each compound over time with respect to the corresponding initial values are indicated as: *, $p < 0.05$ and **, $p < 0.01$.

Thus, by adjusting the operational parameters, it is possible to load the nanofibers described here with approximately 100% efficiency by using a concentration of 3.5% *w*/*w* of the three compounds, all together. In addition, the absence of significant changes in size and shape suggests that their encapsulation capacity might be higher. In this sense, by using the same nanostructured system, they were loaded with up to 16.6% *w*/*w* of 5-aminolevulinic acid in PMVE/MA-ES and Ac nanofibers [26]. Other evidence of electrospun nanofibers made of a blend of other polymers and PMVE/MA were shown to be able to be loaded with even zinc oxide-containing nanoparticles [33] and silver nanoparticles [34]. Indeed, the electrospinning technique allows loadability concentrations of up to 60% *w*/*w* in some cases [49] and encapsulation yields close to full efficiency levels [26,50].

Regarding the concentration of each therapeutic agent proposed, salicylic acid is usually used at concentrations of 0.5–60% *w*/*w* for the treatment of psoriasis [51]. The concentration that was chosen in this work was 1.5% *w*/*w*, which is similar to the concentrations used in acne creams [52]. The use of methyl salicylate in nanostructures has not been described yet, but it is in other topical applications to treat pain in general, especially musculoskeletal pain [21]. The concentrations of this compound used in creams are usually 10–30% *w*/*w* (*Bengay* and *Icy Hot* creams) and even 45% in the case of the *Reflex* gel. In the case of capsaicin, it has been used at 1% *w*/*w*, as in the present study, with respect to the base polymer in nanofibers and nanoparticles for topical use in psoriasis [53,54]. In addition, there is a commercial patch of 8% capsaicin, *Qutenza Astellas*, which is used to treat neuropathic pain.

One of the most surprising results was the loss of product observed for methyl salicylate, which seems to be due to the increase in surface area with respect to the volume that occurs in one-dimensional materials when they are nanostructured, which increases the evaporation of the encapsulated substances [55]. This effect would also be increased in those more volatile molecules, such as in the case of methyl salicylate, which is liquid at room temperature (melting point (mp): −9 °C), while capsaicin and salicylic acid are solid (mp: 62 and 159 °C, respectively). In any case, this loss of compound could be avoided or delayed by packaging the nanofiber mats tightly and hermetically, as is done for other similar products with volatile compounds. On the contrary, this might be an advantage for topical applications because of the possibility of gradually alternating the release of different compounds. From the *in vitro* skin permeability studies performed in our previous work to evaluate the potential of this polymeric family for topical applications [26], it was concluded that nanofibers made with this same material can achieve both fast and high rates of transdermal release of a non-volatile compound (90% of 5-ALA release in two hours by following a Higuchi kinetic model). However, under these conditions that mimic those existing in the human dermal surface (high humidity and 32.5 °C), the diffusion of a more volatile compound, such as methyl salicylate, should be faster, anticipating its treatment with respect to the less volatile ones.

3.3. Assessment of the Activation Capacity of TRPV1 by the Encapsulated Agents

The activity of the TRPV1 agonist compounds encapsulated in the experimental nanofibers (only methyl salicylate and capsaicin, not salicylic acid), alone or in combination with the other two agents (i.e., all three compounds), was assessed by treating HEK293-VR1 cells. These results were represented in percentages relative to the highest value obtained for the activation induced by capsaicin at 10 μM and using the lowest one after inoculating RR as the baseline.

Firstly, in Figure 3A, records of values induced by control samples to check the validity of the system are shown. As can be observed, both methyl salicylate and capsaicin are able to activate TRPV1 by inducing an increase of fluorescence because of the internal increase of Ca^{2+} after being inoculated in cycle three. The graph also shows that TRPV1 is highly activated right after the inoculation of each agent and remains at high levels, which even increase in the case of capsaicin. The specificity of the system is checked by the blocking of the channel with RR, which is even able to desensitize it to a subsequent stimulation with capsaicin (cycle 10). Figure 3 also shows that the activation of TRPV1 is concentration-dependent for both compounds (Figure 3B and 3C for methyl salicylate and capsaicin, respectively), considering the highest value from each time-course analysis for the calculations. In the specific case of methyl salicylate, this curve seems to plateau within the range of concentrations used, from 60 μM in particular.

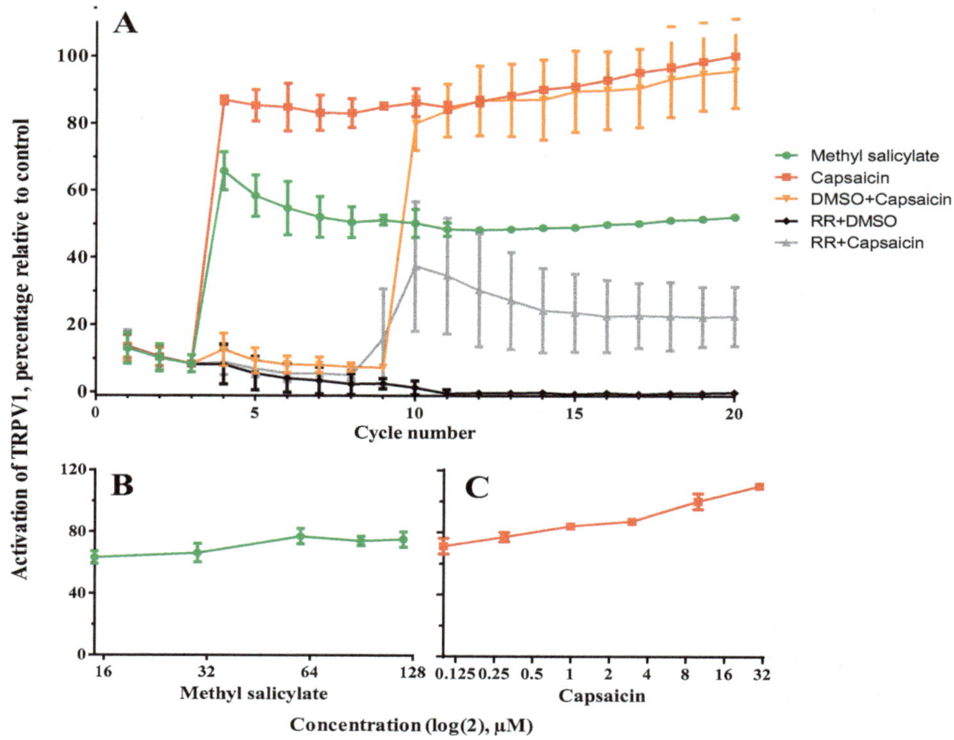

Figure 3. Functional analysis of transient receptor potential cation channel 1 (TRPV1) *in vitro* and calibration of its agonists. (**A**) TRPV1 activation dynamics were determined by performing fluorescence time-course assays in cells stably expressing TRPV1 after treatment with agonists (30 μM of methyl salicylate and 10 μM of capsaicin) and antagonist (ruthenium red, RR). TRPV1 activation was observed once agonists were added, while the inoculation of the antagonist attenuated this response. (**B**,**C**) Additionally, concentrations of agonists lower and higher than those to be tested from produced nanofibers under these experimental conditions were assayed in order to better assess the functionality of the compounds when they were encapsulated. For all analysis, the level of activation is calculated as the percentage relative to the highest value from the time-course in cells treated with 10 μM of capsaicin, and relative to the lowest value from RR treatment as the baseline.

For the comparison of the activity of the agonist compounds on TRPV1 when they are encapsulated in nanofibers, alone or together with the other therapeutic agents, the same above-described procedure was followed, but including experimental nanofibers that were previously dissolved in DMSO. In these *in vitro* cell assays (Figure 4), although the obtained values were moderately higher when the agent was encapsulated, no significant changes were found between the encapsulated and non-encapsulated compounds, and only significant variations were found, as expected, when comparing each compound among them (two-way ANOVA corrected with Tukey's test for multiple comparisons; F (3, 8) = 15.59; p = 0.0011), meaning that the encapsulation process did not affect the chemical properties of the encapsulated agents. Some activation of TRPV1 was also observed when treating with empty nanofibers.

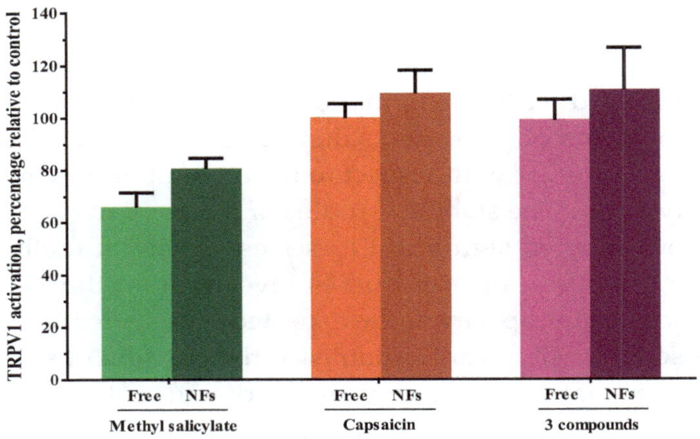

Figure 4. Effect of the encapsulation on the ability of the experimental compounds to activate TRPV1. Fluorescence time-course assays were performed on cells stably expressing TRPV1 and treated with the agonist compounds employed either alone or in combination, and also including salicylic acid (three compounds). These samples included compound-containing nanofibers (NFs) and non-encapsulated compounds (Free). The level of activation is calculated as the percentage relative to the highest value from the time-course in cells treated with 10 μM of capsaicin and the lowest value from RR treatment. Statistical analysis comprised two-way ANOVA corrected with Tukey's test for multiple comparisons (Free vs. NFs) and no significant differences were found between the experimental and control samples.

The combination of different compounds within the same formulation generally pursues a synergistic effect that could allow the reduction of the concentration of each one, and thus their potential adverse effects; however, other benefits from such an approach might be the combination of other functional properties such as, in this case, the ones introduced previously, which are also related to treating psoriasis and other factors such as their antimicrobial activities [56,57].

Finally, but also related to the assessment of the ability of the developed nanofibers to activate TRPV1, it has been possible to successfully electrospin the experimental nanofibers on adhesive dressings for topical application and preliminarily check their gradual degradation by visual observation, as well as their content release by assessing the typical reddening reaction of the capsaicin in the skin (Figure 5). Both effects were evident eight hours after the application of the patch covered with loaded nanofibers on the skin from volunteers' arms. In this sense, no effects were either observed or detected on skin when treating with control patches based on empty nanofibers. Future studies will be aimed at describing the release and dermal absorption of this system, as well as at revealing the possible effect of the polymers on TRPV1.

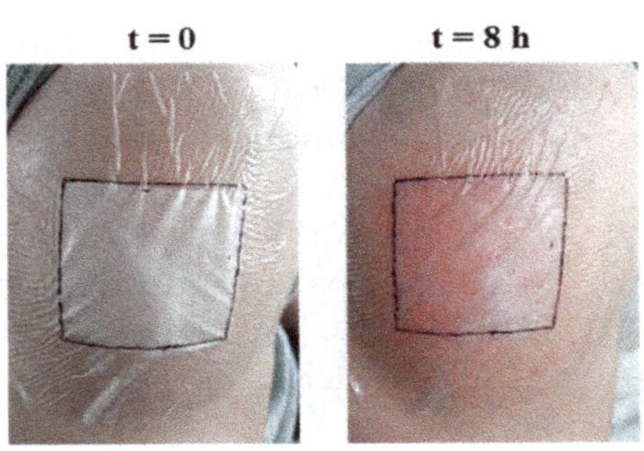

Figure 5. Preliminary assessment of the feasibility of transdermal patches based on experimental nanofibers. Dressings for topical applications produced by electrospinning experimental nanofibers onto adhesive patches were developed and tested for up to eight hours on volunteers' arms. Representative pictures of their application are shown at both the beginning and the end of the test. After eight hours of treatment, the degradation of the nanofibers and the typical reddening of the skin as a consequence of the action of capsaicin on the surface of the skin were observed.

4. Conclusions

In this work, it has been possible to optimize the electrospinning parameters to create PMVE/MA-ES nanofibers loaded with a combination of three compounds with therapeutic activity to alleviate the dermal symptoms of psoriasis (salicylic acid, methyl salicylate, and capsaicin at a concentration of 3.5% *w/w* all together with respect to the amount of polymer), with an encapsulation efficiency of approximately 100%. The stability studies of the content encapsulated over time (up to 15 days after its production) showed significant losses especially of methyl salicylate, which were probably due to its higher volatility. *In vitro* studies revealed that the TRPV1 agonist compounds maintained their channel-activating capacity at the expected levels after being encapsulated. Finally, it was found that the proposed nanofibers are suitable for the creation of skin adhesive dressings and allow the release of the encapsulated compounds by the disintegration of the nanostructure. In this study, the effect of those compounds with the capacity to activate TRPV1 was checked *in vivo*.

Author Contributions: Conceptualization, R.M. and A.F.; methodology, L.M.-O., A.M., A.F.-C. and A.F.; software, L.M.-O. and A.F.; validation, A.F.-C.; formal analysis, R.M. and A.F.; investigation, L.M.-O., A.M. and A.F.; resources, C.R.M. and R.M.; data curation, A.F.; writing—original draft preparation, A.F.; writing—review and editing, A.F.-C., C.R.M., R.M. and A.F.; visualization, A.F.; supervision, R.M. and A.F.; project administration, C.R.M. and R.M.; funding acquisition, C.R.M. and R.M.

Acknowledgments: We thank Elisa Pérez and Irene Mudarra-Fraguas for technical assistance. It is also appreciated the collaboration of the volunteers in the preliminary topical test.

References

1. Boehncke, W.H.; Schon, M.P. Psoriasis. *Lancet* **2015**, *386*, 983–994. [CrossRef]
2. Christophers, E. Psoriasis—Epidemiology and clinical spectrum. *Clin. Exp. Dermatol.* **2001**, *26*, 314–320. [CrossRef] [PubMed]
3. Nickoloff, B.J.; Qin, J.Z.; Nestle, F.O. Immunopathogenesis of psoriasis. *Clin. Rev. Allergy Immunol.* **2007**, *33*, 45–56. [CrossRef] [PubMed]
4. Nickoloff, B.J. Cracking the cytokine code in psoriasis. *Nat. Med.* **2007**, *13*, 242–244. [CrossRef] [PubMed]
5. Di Cesare, A.; Di Meglio, P.; Nestle, F.O. The IL-23/Th17 axis in the immunopathogenesis of psoriasis. *J. Investig. Dermatol.* **2009**, *129*, 1339–1350. [CrossRef] [PubMed]
6. MacDonald, A.; Burden, A.D. Psoriasis: Advances in pathophysiology and management. *Postgrad. Med. J.* **2007**, *83*, 690–697. [CrossRef]
7. Wozel, G. Psoriasis treatment in difficult locations: Scalp, nails, and intertriginous areas. *Clin. Dermatol.* **2008**, *26*, 448–459. [CrossRef]
8. Raut, A.S.; Prabhu, R.H.; Patravale, V.B. Psoriasis clinical implications and treatment: A review. *Crit. Rev. Ther. Drug Carrier Syst.* **2013**, *30*, 183–216. [CrossRef]
9. Hsu, L.; Snodgrass, B.T.; Armstrong, A.W. Antidrug antibodies in psoriasis: A systematic review. *Br. J. Dermatol.* **2014**, *170*, 261–273. [CrossRef]
10. Ryan, C.; Korman, N.J.; Gelfand, J.M.; Lim, H.W.; Elmets, C.A.; Feldman, S.R.; Gottlieb, A.B.; Koo, J.Y.; Lebwohl, M.; Leonardi, C.L.; et al. Research gaps in psoriasis: Opportunities for future studies. *J. Am. Acad. Dermatol.* **2014**, *70*, 146–167. [CrossRef]
11. Fluhr, J.W.; Cavallotti, C.; Berardesca, E. Emollients, moisturizers, and keratolytic agents in psoriasis. *Clin. Dermatol.* **2008**, *26*, 380–386. [CrossRef]
12. Dawn, A.; Yosipovitch, G. Treating itch in psoriasis. *Dermatol. Nurs.* **2006**, *18*, 227.
13. Caterina, M.J.; Schumacher, M.A.; Tominaga, M.; Rosen, T.A.; Levine, J.D.; Julius, D. The capsaicin receptor: A heat-activated ion channel in the pain pathway. *Nature* **1997**, *389*, 816–824. [PubMed]
14. Ferrer-Montiel, A.; García-Martínez, C.; Morenilla-Palao, C.; García-Sanz, N.; Fernández-Carvajal, A.; Fernández-Ballester, G.; Planells-Cases, R. Molecular architecture of the vanilloid receptor. *FEBS J.* **2004**, *271*, 1820–1826.

15. Baumann, T.K.; Martenson, M.E. Extracellular protons both increase the activity and reduce the conductance of capsaicin-gated channels. *J. Neurosci.* **2000**, *20*, RC80. [CrossRef] [PubMed]
16. Anand, P.; Bley, K. Topical capsaicin for pain management: Therapeutic potential and mechanisms of action of the new high-concentration capsaicin 8% patch. *Br. J. Anaesth.* **2011**, *107*, 490–502. [CrossRef] [PubMed]
17. Zhao, J.J.; Hu, Y.W.; Huang, C.; Ma, X.; Kang, C.M.; Zhang, Y.; Guo, F.X.; Lu, J.B.; Xiu, J.C.; Qiu, Y.R.; et al. Dihydrocapsaicin suppresses proinflammatory cytokines expression by enhancing nuclear factor ia in a nf-kappab-dependent manner. *Arch. Biochem. Biophys.* **2016**, *604*, 27–35. [CrossRef]
18. Tang, J.; Luo, K.; Li, Y.; Chen, Q.; Tang, D.; Wang, D.; Xiao, J. Capsaicin attenuates LPS-induced inflammatory cytokine production by upregulation of LXR alpha. *Int. Immunopharmacol.* **2015**, *28*, 264–269. [CrossRef]
19. Reyes-Escogido, M.d.L.; Gonzalez-Mondragon, E.G.; Vazquez-Tzompantzi, E. Chemical and pharmacological aspects of capsaicin. *Molecules* **2011**, *16*, 1253–1270. [CrossRef]
20. Bode, A.M.; Dong, Z. The two faces of capsaicin. *Cancer Res.* **2011**, *71*, 2809–2814. [CrossRef]
21. Ohta, T.; Imagawa, T.; Ito, S. Involvement of transient receptor potential vanilloid subtype 1 in analgesic action of methylsalicylate. *Mol. Pharmacol.* **2009**, *75*, 307–317. [CrossRef] [PubMed]
22. Wu, K.K.-Y. Biochemical pharmacology of nonsteroidal anti-inflammatory drugs. *Biochem. Pharmacol.* **1998**, *55*, 543–547. [PubMed]
23. Xie, J.; Li, X.; Xia, Y. Putting electrospun nanofibers to work for biomedical research. *Macromol. Rapid Commun.* **2008**, *29*, 1775–1792. [CrossRef] [PubMed]
24. Ji, W.; Sun, Y.; Yang, F.; van den Beucken, J.J.; Fan, M.; Chen, Z.; Jansen, J.A. Bioactive electrospun scaffolds delivering growth factors and genes for tissue engineering applications. *Pharm. Res.* **2011**, *28*, 1259–1272. [CrossRef] [PubMed]
25. Bhardwaj, N.; Kundu, S.C. Electrospinning: A fascinating fiber fabrication technique. *Biotechnol. Adv.* **2010**, *28*, 325–347. [CrossRef] [PubMed]
26. Mira, A.; Mateo, C.R.; Mallavia, R.; Falco, A. Poly (methyl vinyl ether-alt-maleic acid) and ethyl monoester as building polymers for drug-loadable electrospun nanofibers. *Sci. Rep.* **2017**, *7*, 17205. [CrossRef] [PubMed]
27. Iglesias, T.; de Cerain, A.L.; Irache, J.; Martín-Arbella, N.; Wilcox, M.; Pearson, J.; Azqueta, A. Evaluation of the cytotoxicity, genotoxicity and mucus permeation capacity of several surface modified poly (anhydride) nanoparticles designed for oral drug delivery. *Int. J. Pharm.* **2017**, *517*, 67–79. [CrossRef]
28. Iglesias, T.; Dusinska, M.; El Yamani, N.; Irache, J.M.; Azqueta, A.; Lopez de Cerain, A. In vitro evaluation of the genotoxicity of poly(anhydride) nanoparticles designed for oral drug delivery. *Int. J. Pharm.* **2017**, *523*, 418–426. [CrossRef]
29. Prieto, E.; Puente, B.; Uixera, A.; Garcia de Jalon, J.A.; Perez, S.; Pablo, L.; Irache, J.M.; Garcia, M.A.; Bregante, M.A. Gantrez an nanoparticles for ocular delivery of memantine: In vitro release evaluation in albino rabbits. *Ophthalmic Res.* **2012**, *48*, 109–117. [CrossRef]
30. Gardner, C.M.; Burke, N.A.; Chu, T.; Shen, F.; Potter, M.A.; Stover, H.D. Poly(methyl vinyl ether-alt-maleic acid) polymers for cell encapsulation. *J. Biomater. Sci. Polym. Ed.* **2011**, *22*, 2127–2145. [CrossRef]
31. Kahveci, Z.; Vazquez-Guillo, R.; Mira, A.; Martinez, L.; Falco, A.; Mallavia, R.; Mateo, C.R. Selective recognition and imaging of bacterial model membranes over mammalian ones by using cationic conjugated polyelectrolytes. *Analyst* **2016**, *141*, 6287–6296. [CrossRef] [PubMed]
32. Vázquez-Guilló, R.; Falco, A.; Martínez-Tomé, M.J.; Mateo, C.R.; Herrero, M.A.; Vázquez, E.; Mallavia, R. Advantageous microwave-assisted suzuki polycondensation for the synthesis of aniline-fluorene alternate copolymers as molecular model with solvent sensing properties. *Polymers* **2018**, *10*, 215. [CrossRef]
33. Chhabra, H.; Deshpande, R.; Kanitkar, M.; Jaiswal, A.; Kale, V.P.; Bellare, J.R. A nano zinc oxide doped electrospun scaffold improves wound healing in a rodent model. *RSC Adv.* **2016**, *6*, 1428–1439. [CrossRef]
34. Xavier, P.; Jain, S.; Chatterjee, K.; Bose, S. Designer porous antibacterial membranes derived from thermally induced phase separation of PS/PVME blends decorated with an electrospun nanofiber scaffold. *RSC Adv.* **2016**, *6*, 10865–10872. [CrossRef]
35. Carrillo-Arcos, U.A.; Rojas-Ocampo, J.; Porcel, S. Oxidative cyclization of alkenoic acids promoted by agoac. *Dalton Trans.* **2016**, *45*, 479–483. [CrossRef] [PubMed]
36. Gonzalez-Penas, E.; Lopez-Alvarez, M.; de Narvajas, F.M.; Ursua, A. Simultaneous gc determination of turpentine, camphor, menthol and methyl salicylate in a topical analgesic formulation (dologex®). *Chromatographia* **2000**, *52*, 245–248. [CrossRef]

37. Serafini, M.; Griglio, A.; Aprile, S.; Seiti, F.; Travelli, C.; Pattarino, F.; Grosa, G.; Sorba, G.; Genazzani, A.A.; Gonzalez-Rodriguez, S.; et al. Targeting transient receptor potential vanilloid 1 (TRPV1) channel softly: The discovery of passerini adducts as a topical treatment for inflammatory skin disorders. *J. Med. Chem.* **2018**, *61*, 4436–4455. [CrossRef]
38. Kim, S.; Kang, C.; Shin, C.Y.; Hwang, S.W.; Yang, Y.D.; Shim, W.S.; Park, M.-Y.; Kim, E.; Kim, M.; Kim, B.-M. TRPV1 recapitulates native capsaicin receptor in sensory neurons in association with Fas-associated factor 1. *J. Neurosci.* **2006**, *26*, 2403–2412. [CrossRef]
39. Dray, A.; Forbes, C.; Burgess, G. Ruthenium red blocks the capsaicin-induced increase in intracellular calcium and activation of membrane currents in sensory neurones as well as the activation of peripheral nociceptors in vitro. *Neurosci. Lett.* **1990**, *110*, 52–59. [CrossRef]
40. Shen, X.; Yu, D.; Zhu, L.; Branford-White, C.; White, K.; Chatterton, N.P. Electrospun diclofenac sodium loaded Eudragit® L 100-55 nanofibers for colon-targeted drug delivery. *Int. J. Pharm.* **2011**, *408*, 200–207. [CrossRef]
41. Samprasit, W.; Akkaramongkolporn, P.; Ngawhirunpat, T.; Rojanarata, T.; Kaomongkolgit, R.; Opanasopit, P. Fast releasing oral electrospun PVP/CD nanofiber mats of taste-masked meloxicam. *Int. J. Pharm.* **2015**, *487*, 213–222. [CrossRef] [PubMed]
42. Moghe, A.; Gupta, B. Co-axial electrospinning for nanofiber structures: Preparation and applications. *Polym. Rev.* **2008**, *48*, 353–377. [CrossRef]
43. Liu, Y.; Ma, G.; Fang, D.; Xu, J.; Zhang, H.; Nie, J. Effects of solution properties and electric field on the electrospinning of hyaluronic acid. *Carbohydr. Polym.* **2011**, *83*, 1011–1015. [CrossRef]
44. Zeng, J.; Xu, X.; Chen, X.; Liang, Q.; Bian, X.; Yang, L.; Jing, X. Biodegradable electrospun fibers for drug delivery. *J. Control. Release* **2003**, *92*, 227–231. [CrossRef]
45. Nezarati, R.M.; Eifert, M.B.; Cosgriff-Hernandez, E. Effects of humidity and solution viscosity on electrospun fiber morphology. *Tissue Eng. Part C Methods* **2013**, *19*, 810–819. [CrossRef] [PubMed]
46. Fong, H.; Chun, I.; Reneker, D. Beaded nanofibers formed during electrospinning. *Polymer* **1999**, *40*, 4585–4592. [CrossRef]
47. Reda, R.I.; Wen, M.M.; El-Kamel, A.H. Ketoprofen-loaded eudragit electrospun nanofibers for the treatment of oral mucositis. *Int. J. Nanomed.* **2017**, *12*, 2335–2351. [CrossRef] [PubMed]
48. Canbolat, M.F.; Celebioglu, A.; Uyar, T. Drug delivery system based on cyclodextrin-naproxen inclusion complex incorporated in electrospun polycaprolactone nanofibers. *Colloids Surf. B* **2014**, *115*, 15–21. [CrossRef]
49. Krogstad, E.A.; Woodrow, K.A. Manufacturing scale-up of electrospun poly (vinyl alcohol) fibers containing tenofovir for vaginal drug delivery. *Int. J. Pharm.* **2014**, *475*, 282–291. [CrossRef]
50. Ball, C.; Woodrow, K.A. Electrospun solid dispersions of maraviroc for rapid intravaginal preexposure prophylaxis of hiv. *Antimicrob. Agents Chemother.* **2014**, *58*, 4855–4865. [CrossRef]
51. Lebwohl, M. The role of salicylic acid in the treatment of psoriasis. *Int. J. Dermatol.* **1999**, *38*, 16–24. [CrossRef] [PubMed]
52. Zheng, Y.; Wan, M.; Chen, H.; Ye, C.; Zhao, Y.; Yi, J.; Xia, Y.; Lai, W. Clinical evidence on the efficacy and safety of an antioxidant optimized 1.5% salicylic acid (SA) cream in the treatment of facial acne: An open, baseline-controlled clinical study. *Skin Res. Technol.* **2013**, *19*, 125–130. [CrossRef] [PubMed]
53. Opanasopit, P.; Sila-on, W.; Rojanarata, T.; Ngawhirunpat, T. Fabrication and properties of capsicum extract-loaded PVA and CA nanofiber patches. *Pharm. Dev. Technol.* **2013**, *18*, 1140–1147. [CrossRef] [PubMed]
54. Gupta, R.; Gupta, M.; Mangal, S.; Agrawal, U.; Vyas, S.P. Capsaicin-loaded vesicular systems designed for enhancing localized delivery for psoriasis therapy. *Artif. Cells Nanomed. Biotechnol.* **2016**, *44*, 825–834. [CrossRef]
55. Sánchez, L.M.D.; Rodríguez, L.; López, M. Electrospinning: La era de las nanofibras. *Rev. Iberoam. Polím.* **2013**, *14*, 10–27.
56. Özçelik, B.; Kartal, M.; Orhan, I. Cytotoxicity, antiviral and antimicrobial activities of alkaloids, flavonoids, and phenolic acids. *Pharm. Biol.* **2011**, *49*, 396–402. [CrossRef]
57. Kantouch, A.; El-Sayed, A.A.; Salama, M.; El-Kheir, A.A.; Mowafi, S. Salicylic acid and some of its derivatives as antibacterial agents for viscose fabric. *Int. J. Biol. Macromol.* **2013**, *62*, 603–607. [CrossRef]

5

Drug Bioavailability Enhancing Agents of Natural Origin (Bioenhancers) that Modulate Drug Membrane Permeation and Pre-Systemic Metabolism

Bianca Peterson, Morné Weyers, Jan H. Steenekamp, Johan D. Steyn, Chrisna Gouws and Josias H. Hamman *

Centre of Excellence for Pharmaceutical Sciences (Pharmacen™), North-West University, Potchefstroom 2520, South Africa; bianca.peterson@nwu.ac.za (B.P.); weyers.morne@gmail.com (M.W.); jan.steenekamp@nwu.ac.za (J.H.S.); dewald.steyn@nwu.ac.za (J.D.S.); chrisna.gouws@nwu.ac.za (C.G.)

* Correspondence: sias.hamman@nwu.ac.za

Abstract: Many new chemical entities are discovered with high therapeutic potential, however, many of these compounds exhibit unfavorable pharmacokinetic properties due to poor solubility and/or poor membrane permeation characteristics. The latter is mainly due to the lipid-like barrier imposed by epithelial mucosal layers, which have to be crossed by drug molecules in order to exert a therapeutic effect. Another barrier is the pre-systemic metabolic degradation of drug molecules, mainly by cytochrome P450 enzymes located in the intestinal enterocytes and liver hepatocytes. Although the nasal, buccal and pulmonary routes of administration avoid the first-pass effect, they are still dependent on absorption of drug molecules across the mucosal surfaces to achieve systemic drug delivery. Bioenhancers (drug absorption enhancers of natural origin) have been identified that can increase the quantity of unchanged drug that appears in the systemic blood circulation by means of modulating membrane permeation and/or pre-systemic metabolism. The aim of this paper is to provide an overview of natural bioenhancers and their main mechanisms of action for the nasal, buccal, pulmonary and oral routes of drug administration. Poorly bioavailable drugs such as large, hydrophilic therapeutics are often administered by injections. Bioenhancers may potentially be used to benefit patients by making systemic delivery of these poorly bioavailable drugs possible via alternative routes of administration (i.e., oral, nasal, buccal or pulmonary routes of administration) and may also reduce dosages of small molecular drugs and thereby reduce treatment costs.

Keywords: bioenhancer; cytochrome P450; drug absorption enhancer; efflux; metabolism; P-glycoprotein; pharmacokinetic interaction; tight junction

---

1. Introduction

Drug absorption is the process whereby drug molecules are transferred from the site of administration across biological membranes into the systemic blood circulation to produce a systemic pharmacological effect. Biological cell membranes have a lipophilic nature due to their phospholipid bilayer structures. Molecules should therefore have sufficient hydrophilic properties to dissolve in the aqueous environments surrounding the biological membranes, but should also have sufficient lipophilic properties to partition into the membranes in order to achieve passive absorption via the transcellular pathway [1]. Adjacent epithelial/endothelial cells are connected by tight junctions, which are traversed by aqueous channels/fenestrae through which only small water-soluble molecules (<600 Da) can pass to get absorbed via the paracellular pathway [2].

A number of active transporter molecules (including both uptake transporters and efflux transporters) are present in various cell types in different organs. Drug efflux transporters found in the plasma membranes of intestinal epithelial cells can pump structurally diverse compounds from within the intestinal epithelial cells back to the gastro-intestinal lumen and thereby reduce drug bioavailability [3]. Efflux of compounds occurs by active transporters that need energy and this process is adenosine triphosphate (ATP)-dependent [4]. The ATP-binding cassette (ABC) transporter superfamily is among the largest and most broadly expressed efflux transporters discovered so far, consisting of P-glycoprotein (P-gp), the multidrug resistant protein (MRP) and the breast cancer resistance protein (BCRP) [5–7]. Another major determinant of oral drug bioavailability besides drug permeation across the epithelial cells is pre-systemic metabolism or first-pass metabolism, which is the metabolism that takes place during uptake before the drug molecules reach the systemic circulation, as observed for olanzapine treatment [8]. Pre-systemic metabolism occurs mainly in the enterocytes of the gastrointestinal epithelium and the hepatocytes of the liver. The cytochrome P450 (CYP) family of enzymes account for the majority of oxidative metabolic reactions of xenobiotics during pre-systemic and systemic metabolism. More than 30 different human CYP enzymes have been identified, of which CYP3A4 appears to be one of the most important drug-metabolizing enzymes in humans [9].

For the purpose of this paper, the term bioenhancer is reserved for molecules of natural origin that are capable of increasing the rate and/or extent at which co-administered drug molecules reach the systemic circulation unchanged (i.e., increased bioavailability). The main mechanisms that have been identified through which bioenhancers can improve the bioavailability of drug molecules include alteration of the plasma membrane fluidity to increase passive transcellular drug permeation; modulation of tight junctions to allow for increased paracellular diffusion; and active efflux transporter modulation, such as P-gp-related efflux inhibition. Inhibition of CYP enzymes in the intestinal epithelium and liver can significantly impact upon the bioavailability of drugs that are substrates of these enzymes by means of reducing pre-systemic metabolism [10–12].

The most popular route of drug administration remains the oral route [2]. As mentioned before, the oral bioavailability of a drug molecule is determined by its ability to penetrate the gastrointestinal epithelial membrane, which is mainly determined by its physico-chemical properties (e.g., pKa, lipophilicity, molecular size, charge, dissolution and solubility) [13], together with the extent of enzymatic metabolism during its movement to the systemic circulation (known as pre-systemic metabolism or the first-pass effect). Some other factors that may affect the oral bioavailability of a drug include the gastric emptying rate, pH of the gastrointestinal fluid, interactions with other compounds (e.g., other drugs, food or herbs) and its affinity for active transporters [2,14].

Drug administration via the nasal route can easily be accomplished by patients for both local and systemic drug delivery, which is non-invasive and painless. A relatively large epithelial surface is available that is highly permeable and offers a rapid onset of therapeutic effect. For drugs that target the central nervous system, direct nose-to-brain drug delivery is possible [13,15,16]. Additionally, intranasal drug administration bypasses hepatic first-pass metabolism [13,17,18]. However, the protective mucous layer and ciliary clearance may potentially have a negative impact on intranasal absorption [13,15].

The buccal route of administration is a good alternative for drugs that are unstable in gastric fluids and those that are severely affected by first-pass metabolism. However, absorption across the buccal mucosa is relatively slow due to the limited surface area, poor permeability of buccal epithelial tissue, removal of drug by saliva and the presence of peptidases within the buccal mucosa [15]. Hence this route of drug administration is mostly suited for highly potent, low dose drugs [15].

The buccal route of administration is a good alternative for drugs that are unstable in gastric fluids and those that are severely affected by first-pass metabolism. However, absorption across the buccal mucosa is relatively slow due to the limited surface area, poor permeability of buccal epithelial tissue, removal of drug by saliva and the presence of peptidases within the buccal mucosa [15]. Hence this route of drug administration is mostly suited for highly potent, low dose drugs [15].

The pulmonary route of drug administration (i.e., administration via the lungs) is associated with rapid drug delivery due to the large surface area and abundant blood supply [2,15]. Pulmonary drug delivery can occur through different dosage forms, such as aerosol or nebulizer, for both local treatment (e.g., bronchodilators) or systemic drug delivery [2]. In the case of volatile anesthetics or for voluptuary drugs, the inhalation route is the preferred way of administration [2,19].

In this paper, discussions regarding drug absorption enhancing agents are restricted to bioenhancers of natural origin (therefore purely synthetic chemical permeation enhancers are excluded). The selected bioenhancers are discussed in terms of their main effects on drug bioavailability as well as their mechanisms of action as elucidated by in vitro and in vivo studies. Furthermore, a comprehensive list of bioenhancers is included in Table 1 for each of the four selected routes of administration including the buccal, nasal, pulmonary and oral routes of drug administration.

2. Buccal Route of Administration

Figure 1 illustrates the main mechanisms of action of selected bioenhancers for improved drug delivery via the buccal route of administration.

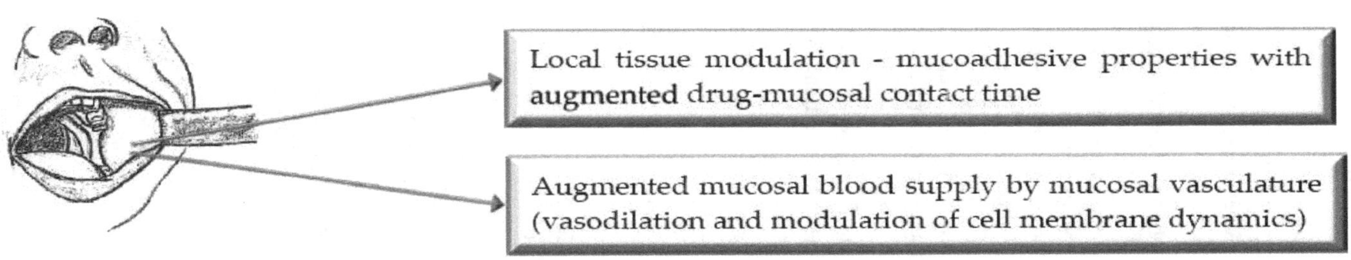

Figure 1. Illustration of the main mechanisms of action of bioenhancers for enhanced buccal drug delivery.

2.1. Aloe Vera

The effect of *Aloe vera* gel on the permeability of didanosine (ddI) across porcine buccal mucosae was investigated using Franz diffusion cells. The control solution contained ddI in phosphate buffer saline (PBS) at pH 7.4 alone (5, 10, 15, 20 mg/mL), and the test solutions contained ddI (20 mg/mL) in the presence of *A. vera* gel (0.25, 0.5, 1, 2, 4, and 6% *w/v*) [20].

At concentrations of 0.25 to 2% *w/v*, *A. vera* gel significantly enhanced the buccal permeability of ddI with enhancement ratios ranging from 5.09 (0.25% *w/v*) to 11.78 (2% *w/v*). However, at higher concentrations (4 and 6% *w/v*) of *A. vera* gel, decreased ddI permeability across the buccal tissue was observed. This may be attributed to the high viscosity of the *A. vera* gel at these high concentrations, which caused resistance to drug diffusion. *A. vera* gel may be used as a potential buccal permeation enhancer for ddI in the treatment of HIV and AIDS [20].

Table 1. Summary of selected natural bioenhancers and their main mechanisms of action on various drugs for enhanced nasal, oral, buccal and pulmonary drug delivery.

Route of Administration	Bioenhancer (Class)	Biological Source	Mechanism(s) of Action	Study Design Model	Research Compound	Reference(s)
Buccal	*Aloe vera* (gel, whole leaf)	Plant (*Aloe vera*)	Intercellular modulation	In vitro (Franz diffusion cells)	Didanosine: Antiviral reverse transcriptase inhibitor	[20]
Buccal	Chitosan (Biopolymer)	Deacetylated chitin from crustaceans and fungi	Mucoadhesion; changes in lipid organization and loosening of intercellular filaments	In vitro (T146 cells [1])	FITC–dextran: Hydrophilic polysaccharide	[21]
Buccal	Chitosan (Biopolymer)	Deacetylated chitin from crustaceans and fungi	Mucoadhesion; mucosal membrane modulation	Ex vivo (porcine buccal mucosa)	Hydrocortisone: Corticosteroid TGF-beta: Cytokine polypeptide	[22]
Buccal	Chitosan–TBA (Thiolated polymer)	Deacetylated chitin from crustaceans and fungi	Mucoadhesion; mucosal membrane modulation	Ex vivo (porcine buccal mucosa); in vivo (pig)	PACAP: Pituitary Adenylate Cyclase-activating Peptide	[23,24]
Buccal	Cod-liver oil extract (Fatty acid)	Animal (Cod fish)	No mechanism specified	Ex vivo (hamster cheek pouch)	Ergotamine tartrate: Ergopeptine alkaloid	[25]
Buccal	Menthol (Alcohol)	Plant (Corn mint, peppermint, or other mint oils)	No mechanism specified	Ex vivo (porcine buccal mucosa)	Dideoxycytidine: Nucleoside analog reverse transcriptase inhibitor (NRTI)	[26]
Buccal	Oleic acid, eicosapentaenoic acid, docosahexaenoic acid (Fatty acids)	Animal (Cod fish)	No mechanism specified	In vitro (membraneless dissolution test), in vivo (rat)	Insulin: Peptide hormone	[27]
Buccal	Sodium glycodeoxycholate (Bile salt)	Intestinal bacterial by-product	No mechanism specified	Ex vivo (porcine buccal mucosa)	Dideoxycytidine: Nucleoside analog reverse transcriptase inhibitor (NRTI)	[28]
Buccal	TMC (Cationic polymers)	Chemically modified chitosan (crustaceans, fungi)	Mucoadhesion; mucosal membrane modulation	Ex vivo (porcine buccal mucosa)	FD4: Hydrophilic polysaccharide	[29]
Nasal	Chitosan (Biopolymer)	Chemically modified chitosan (crustaceans, fungi)	Tight junction modulation	In vivo (sheep)	sCT: Endogenous polypeptide hormone	[30]
Nasal	Chitosan (Biopolymer)	Deacetylated chitin from crustaceans and fungi	Increased mucoadhesion; tight junction modulation	In vivo (sheep, human)	Morphine: Opium alkaloid	[31]
Nasal	Chitosan–TBA (Thiolated polymer)	Deacetylated chitin from crustaceans and fungi	Increased mucoadhesion; tight junction modulation	In vivo (rat)	Insulin: Peptide hormone	[32]

Table 1. *Cont.*

Route of Administration	Bioenhancer (Class)	Biological Source	Mechanism(s) of Action	Study Design Model	Research Compound	Reference(s)
Nasal	TMC (Cationic polymers)	Chemically modified chitosan (crustaceans and fungi)	Increased mucoadhesion; tight junction modulation	In vivo (rat)	Mannitol: Sugar alcohol	[33]
Oral	(-)-Epicatechin (Flavonoid)	Plant (woody plants)	Metabolism (glucuronidation) inhibition	Ex vivo (rat small intestine)	Alpha-naphtol: Organic fluorescent compound	[34]
Oral	*Aloe vera* (gel and whole leaf)	Plant (*Aloe vera*)	Tight junction modulation	Ex vivo (rat intestinal tissue)	Atenolol: Beta-receptor activity compound	[35]
Oral	Aloe vera (gel and whole leaf)	Plant (*Aloe vera*)	Tight junction modulation	In vitro (Caco-2 cells [2])	Insulin: Peptide hormone	[36]
Oral	Aloe vera (juice)	Plant (*Aloe vera*)	Local mucosal tissue modulation	In vivo (human)	Vitamin C and E: Ascorbic acid, tocopherols, tocotrienols.	[37]
Oral	Aloe vera (gel polysaccharides)	Plant (*Aloe vera*)	Metabolism inhibition; tight junction modulation	In vitro (Caco-2, LS180 cells [3]), In vivo (rat)	Indinavir: Antiviral protease inhibitor	[38]
Oral	BHCl (Flavonoid)	Acidification of betaine Plant (beetroot: *Beta vulgaris*)	Metabolism enhancement (transient re-acidification of gastric pH)	In vivo (human)	Dasatinib: Protein kinase inhibitor	[39]
Oral	Caraway (Flavonoid)	Plant (meridian fennel/Persian cumin: *Carum carvi*)	Local mucosal tissue modulation	In vivo (human)	Rifampicin: Semisynthetic rifamycin derivative, Isoniazid: Isonicotinic acid derivative, pyrazinamide: nicotinamide pyrazine analogue	[40]
Oral	Chitosan (Biopolymer)	Deacetylated chitin from crustaceans and fungi	Tight junction modulation	In vitro (HT-29 clone B6 cells [4])	Heparin: Anticoagulant	[41]
Oral	Chitosan (Biopolymer)	Deacetylated chitin from crustaceans and fungi	Tight junction modulation	In vitro (Caco-2 cells [2])	Chitosan–(Lissamine–rhodamine labelled)	[42]
Oral	Chitosan–TBA (Thiolated polymer)	Deacetylated chitin from crustaceans and fungi	Mucoadhesion; tight junction modulation	Ex vivo (guinea pig small intestinal mucosa)	Cefadroxil: Cephalosporin	[43]
Oral	Chitosan–TBA (Thiolated polymer)	Deacetylated chitin from crustaceans and fungi	Mucoadhesion; tight junction modulation	In vivo (rat)	Insulin: Peptide hormone	[44]
Oral	Curcumin (Flavonoid)	Plant (turmeric: *Curcuma longa*)	Metabolism (UDP-glucuronyl transferase) inhibition	In vitro (rat microsomes)	Mycohenolic acid: Immunosuppressant	[45]
Oral	Curcumin (Flavonoid)	Plant (turmeric: *Curcuma longa*)	Efflux transporter inhibition; metabolism inhibition	In vivo (rabbit)	Norfloxacin: Fluoroquinolone	[46]
Oral	Curcumin (Flavonoid)	Plant (turmeric: *Curcuma longa*)	Metabolism (CYP3A4) inhibition	In vitro (human liver microsomes)	Midazolam: Benzodiazepine	[47]

Table 1. *Cont.*

Route of Administration	Bioenhancer (Class)	Biological Source	Mechanism(s) of Action	Study Design Model	Research Compound	Reference(s)
Oral	Curcumin (Flavonoid)	Plant (turmeric: *Curcuma longa*)	Efflux transporter (P-gp) inhibition; metabolism (CYP3A4) inhibition	In vivo (rat)	Midazolam: Benzodiazepine	[48]
Oral	Cyclosporine A (Immunosuppressant)	Fungi (*Tolypocladium inflatum Gams*)	Efflux transporter (P-gp) inhibition	In vivo (rat, dog)	Clopidogrel: Platelet aggregation inhibitor	[49]
Oral	Diosmin (Flavonoid)	Plant (citrus fruits)	Efflux transporter (P-gp) inhibition	In vitro (Caco-2 cells [2])	Digoxin: Digitalis glycoside	[50]
Oral	Emodin (Anthraquinone derivative)	Plant (senna: *Cassia angustifolia*, *Aloe vera* (syn *Aloe barbadensis*), rhubarb: *Rheum officinale*)	Efflux transporter (P-gp) inhibition	In vitro (MDR1-MDCKII cells [6], Caco-2 cells[2])	Digoxin: Digitalis glycoside	[51]
Oral	Fulvic acid (Organic acid)	Plant (decomposed material)	Metabolism enhancement (enhanced drug water solubility)	In vivo (rat)	Glibenclamide: Sulfonylurea antidiabetic Insulin: Peptide hormone Pentazocin: Opioid analgesic	[52]
Oral	Gallic acid ester (Organic acid)	Plant (gallnuts, sumac, witch hazel, tea leaves, oak bark)	Metabolism (CYP3A) inhibition	In vitro (human liver microsomes)	Nifedipine: Calcium channel blocker	[53]
Oral	Genistein (Flavonoid)	Plant (soyabean: *Glycine max, kudzu: Pueraria lobata*)	Efflux transporter (MRP) inhibition	In vitro (HT-29 cells[4]), In vivo (rat)	Epigalllocatechin-3-gallate (EGCG): Phenolic antioxidant	[54]
Oral	Genistein (Flavonoid)	Plant (soyabean: *Glycine max, kudzu: Pueraria lobata*)	Efflux transporter (P-gp, BCRP, MRP2) inhibition; metabolism (CYP3A4) inhibition	In vivo (rat)	Paclitaxel: Tetracyclic diterpenoid	[55]
Oral	Gokhru extract (Herbal)	Plant (Tribulus: *Tribulus terrestris*)	Local mucosal tissue modulation	In vitro (goat everted sac)	Metformin: Biguanide	[56]
Oral	Gokhru extract (Herbal)	Plant (Tribulus: *Tribulus terrestris*)	Local mucosal tissue modulation	In vitro (chicken everted intestine)	Metformin: Biguanide	[57]
Oral	Grapefruit juice (Citrus fruit)	Plant (grapefruit: *Citrus paradisi*)	Efflux transporter (P-gp, MRP2); metabolism (CYP3A4) inhibition; renal uptake transporter (OATP) inhibition	Various	Various	[58]
Oral	LSC (Chitosan derivative)	Modified chitosan (crustaceans and fungi)	Increased mucoadhesion; tight junction modulation	In vitro (Caco-2 cells [2]), In vivo (rat), Ex vivo (rat intestine)	Insulin: Peptide hormone	[59]
Oral	Lycopene (Carotenoid)	Plant (red fruits and vegetables)	Dual carotenoid/LDL receptor mechanism for targeted hepatic delivery	In vivo (human)	Simvastatin: HMG–CoA reductase inhibitor	[60]

Table 1. *Cont.*

Route of Administration	Bioenhancer (Class)	Biological Source	Mechanism(s) of Action	Study Design Model	Research Compound	Reference(s)
Oral	Lysergol (Alkaloid)	Plant (morning glory plant: *Ipomoea* spp.)	Metabolism inhibition	In vivo (rat)	Berberine: Benzylisoquinoline alkaloid	[61]
Oral	Lysergol (Alkaloid)	Plant (morning glory plant: *Ipomoea* spp.)	Efflux transporter (BCRP) inhibition; metabolism inhibition	In vitro (rat liver microsomes)	Curcumin: Zingiberaceae Sulfasalazine: Aminosalicylic agent	[62]
Oral	Moringa oleifera pods (Traditional herbal medicine)	Plant (*Moringa oleifera*)	Metabolism (CYP450) inhibition	In vivo (mice)	Rifampicin: Semisynthetic rifamycin derivative	[63]
Oral	Naringin (Flavonoid glycoside)	Plant (grapefruit, apple, onion, tea)	Efflux transporter (P-gp) inhibition; metabolism inhibition	In vivo (rat)	Diltiazem: Benzothiazepine derivates	[64]
Oral	Naringin (Flavonoid glycoside)	Plant (grapefruit, apple, onion, tea)	Metabolism (CYP3A4) inhibition	In vivo (rat)	Tamoxifen: selective estrogen receptor modulator (SERM)	[65]
Oral	Naringin (Flavonoid glycoside)	Plant (grapefruit, apple, onion, tea)	Efflux transporter (P-gp) inhibition; metabolism (CYP3A4) inhibition	In vivo (rat)	Paclitaxel: Tetracyclic diterpenoid	[66]
Oral	Naringin (Flavonoid glycoside)	Plant (grapefruit, apple, onion, tea)	Efflux transporter (P-gp) inhibition; metabolism (CYP3A4) inhibition	Ex vivo (rat everted gut sac)	Clopidogrel: Platelet aggregation inhibitor	[67]
Oral	Naringin (Flavonoid glycoside)	Plant (grapefruit, apple, onion, tea)	Metabolism (CYP3A4) inhibition	In vivo (rabbit)	Verapamil: Calcium channel blocker	[68]
Oral	Palmitoyl carnitine chloride (Chelating agents)	Esterification of carnitinePlant/animal (various)	Tight junction modulation	In vitro (Caco-2 cells [2])	Clodronate: Bisphosphonate	[69]
Oral	Peppermint oil (Herbal)	Plant (peppermint: *Mentha pipertita*)	Metabolism (CYP3A) inhibition	Ex vivo (rat intestinal tissue)	Cyclosporine: Immunosuppressant	[70]
Oral	Piperine (Alkaloid)	Plant (*Piper longum* and *Piper nigrum*)	Local mucosal tissue modulation; thermogenic activity	In vivo (human)	B-carotene: Terpenoid	[71]
Oral	Piperine (Alkaloid)	Plant (*Piper longum* and *Piper nigrum*)	Local mucosal tissue modulation; thermogenic activity	In vivo (human)	Coenzyme Q10: benzoquinone	[72]
Oral	Piperine (Alkaloid)	Plant (*Piper longum* and *Piper nigrum*)	Decreased elimination (gastrointestinal transit inhibition; gastric emptying inhibition)	In vivo (rat, mice)	Phenol red: Spheroid	[73]
Oral	Piperine (Alkaloid)	Plant (*Piper longum* and *Piper nigrum*)	Metabolism inhibition	In vivo (human)	Propanol: Beta-receptor activity compound, theophylline: methylxanthine	[74]

Table 1. *Cont.*

Route of Administration	Bioenhancer (Class)	Biological Source	Mechanism(s) of Action	Study Design Model	Research Compound	Reference(s)
Oral	Piperine (Alkaloid)	Plant (*Piper longum* and *Piper nigrum*)	Metabolism (CYP450) inhibition	In vivo (rat)	Nimesulide: Non-steroidal anti-inflammatory	[75]
Oral	Piperine (Alkaloid)	Plant (*Piper longum* and *Piper nigrum*)	Efflux transporter (P-gp) inhibition	In vivo (rat)	Fexofenadine: Terfenadine metabolite	[76]
Oral	Piperine (Alkaloid)	Plant (*Piper longum* and *Piper nigrum*)	Metabolism inhibition	In vivo (mice)	Resveratrol: Phytoalexin	[77]
Oral	Piperine (Alkaloid)	Plant (*Piper longum* and *Piper nigrum*)	Metabolism inhibition	In vivo (human)	Nevirapine: Non-nucleoside reverse transcriptase inhibitor	[78]
Oral	Piperine (Alkaloid)	Plant (*Piper longum* and *Piper nigrum*)	Metabolism inhibition	In vivo (mice)	Epigalllocatechin-3-gallate (EGCG): Phenolic antioxidant	[79]
Oral	Piperine (Alkaloid)	Plant (*Piper longum* and *Piper nigrum*)	Metabolism inhibition	In vivo (rat)	Pentobarbitone: Barbiturate.	[80]
Oral	Piperine (Alkaloid)	Plant (*Piper longum* and *Piper nigrum*)	Metabolism (CYP3A4) inhibition	In vivo (human)	Carbamazepine: Carboxamide derivative	[81]
Oral	Piperine (Alkaloid)	Plant (*Piper longum* and *Piper nigrum*)	Metabolism (CYP450) inhibition	In vivo (rat)	Nateglinide: Meglitinide	[82]
Oral	Piperine (Alkaloid)	Plant (*Piper longum* and *Piper nigrum*)	Metabolism (hepatic and intestinal glucuronidation) inhibition	In vivo (rat, human)	Curcumin: Zingiberaceae agent	[83]
Oral	Piperine (Alkaloid)	Plant (*Piper longum* and *Piper nigrum*)	Metabolism inhibition	In vivo (hen)	Oxytetracycline: Bacterial protein synthesis inhibitor	[84]
Oral	Quercetin (Flavonoid)	Plant (citrus fruits, vegetables, leaves, grains)	Efflux transporter (P-gp) inhibition	In vivo (rat), Ex vivo (rat and chick everted intestinal sac)	Ranolazine: Piperazine derivative	[85]
Oral	Quercetin (Flavonoid)	Plant (citrus fruits, vegetables, leaves, grains)	Efflux transporter (P-gp) inhibition	In vivo (rat), In vitro (Caco-2 cells [2])	Irinotecan: Cytotoxic alkaloid	[86]
Oral	Quercetin (Flavonoid)	Plant (citrus fruits, vegetables, leaves, grains)	Efflux transporter (P-gp) inhibition	In vivo (rats), Ex vivo (rat intestinal everted sac)	Valsartan: Angiotensin II receptor antagonist	[87]
Oral	Quercetin (Flavonoid)	Plant (citrus fruits, vegetables, leaves, grains)	Metabolism (CYP3A) inhibition	In vivo (rabbit)	Verapamil: Calcium channel blocker	[88]
Oral	Quercetin (Flavonoid)	Plant (citrus fruits, vegetables, leaves, grains)	Efflux transporter (P-gp) inhibition; metabolism (CYP3A) inhibition	In vivo (rabbit)	Dilitiazem: Nondihydropyridine calcium channel blocker	[89]
Oral	Quercetin (Flavonoid)	Plant (citrus fruits, vegetables, leaves, grains)	Efflux transporter (P-gp) inhibition; metabolism (CYP3A) inhibition	In vivo (rat)	Doxorubicin: Daunorubicin precursor	[90]

Table 1. *Cont.*

Route of Administration	Bioenhancer (Class)	Biological Source	Mechanism(s) of Action	Study Design Model	Research Compound	Reference(s)
Oral	Quercetin (Flavonoid)	Plant (citrus fruits, vegetables, leaves, grains)	Efflux transporter (P-gp) inhibition	In vivo (human)	Fexofenadine: Terfenadine metabolite	[91]
Oral	Quercetin (Flavonoid)	Plant (citrus fruits, vegetables, leaves, grains)	Efflux transporter (P-gp) inhibition	In vivo (rat, dog)	Clopidogrel: Platelet aggregation inhibitor	[49]
Oral	Quercetin (Flavonoid)	Plant (citrus fruits, vegetables, leaves, grains)	Efflux transporter (P-gp) inhibition; metabolism (CYP3A) inhibition	In vivo (rat)	Etoposide: Podophyllotoxin derivative	[92]
Oral	Quercetin (Flavonoid)	Plant (citrus fruits, vegetables, leaves, grains)	Efflux transporter (P-gp) inhibition; metabolism (CYP3A) inhibition	Various	Epigalllocatechin-3-gallate (EGCG): Phenolic antioxidant	[93]
Oral	Quercetin (Flavonoid)	Plant (citrus fruits, vegetables, leaves, grains)	Efflux transporter (P-gp) inhibition	In vitro (human MCF-7 ADRr cells [7])	Doxorubicin: Daunorubicin precursor	[94]
Oral	Quercetin (Flavonoid)	Plant (citrus fruits, vegetables, leaves, grains)	Efflux transporter (MRP) inhibition; metabolism (CYP3A) inhibition	In vivo (rat)	Tamoxifen: selective estrogen receptor modulator (SERM)	[95]
Oral	Quercetin (Flavonoid)	Plant (citrus fruits, vegetables, leaves, grains)	Metabolism (CYP3A) inhibition	In vivo (rat)	Pioglitazone: Thiazolidinedione	[96]
Oral	Quinidine (Class I antiarrhythmic agent)	Chemically modified: stereoisomer of quinine Plant (cinchona tree: *Cinchona* sp.)	Efflux transporter (P-gp) inhibition	Ex vivo (everted rat gut sac)	Paeoniflorin: *Paeonia lactiflora* derivative	[97]
Oral	Resveratrol (Polyphenolic phytoalexin)	Plant (berries, grape skins, red wine)	Metabolism (CYP2C9, CYP2E1) inhibition	In vivo (human)	Diclofenac: NSAID	[98]
Oral	Resveratrol (Polyphenolic phytoalexin)	Plant (berries, grape skins, red wine)	Efflux transporter (P-gp, MRP-2) inhibition; reduced elimination; renal uptake transporter (OAT1, OAT3) inhibition	In vitro (Caco-2 cells [2], mock-MDCK, MDR1-MDCK [6], MRP2-MDCK [6], mock-HEK293, hOAT1-HEK293 [8], hOAT3-HEK293 [8] cells), Ex vivo (rat everted intestine, rat kidney slices), In vivo (rat)	Methotrexate: Immunosuppressant	[99]
Oral	Sinomenine (Alkaloid)	Plant (*Sinomenium acutum*)	Efflux transporter (P-gp) inhibition	Ex vivo (everted rat gut sac)	Paeoniflorin: *Paeonia lactiflora* derivative	[97]
Oral	Sinomenine (Alkaloid)	Plant (*Sinomenium acutum*)	Efflux transporter (P-gp) inhibition	In vivo (rat)	Paeoniflorin: *Paeonia lactiflora* derivative	[100]

Table 1. *Cont.*

Route of Administration	Bioenhancer (Class)	Biological Source	Mechanism(s) of Action	Study Design Model	Research Compound	Reference(s)
Oral	Sodium caprate (Fatty acid)	Chemically modified: salification of caproic acid Animal (fats and oils)	Tight junction modulation	In situ (recirculating intestinal perfusion), ex vivo (everted rat gut sacs), in vivo (rat)	Berberine: Antidiabetic plant alkaloid	[101]
Oral	Sodium cholate/phospholipid-mixed micelles (Bile salts)	Intestinal bacterial by-product	Mucosal membrane modulation	In vivo (dog)	Silybin, the major active component of silymarin (antihepatotoxic polyphenolic substance isolated from milk thistle plant, Silybum marianum)	[102]
Oral	Soybean phosphotidylcholine/ sodium deoxycholate (SPC/SDC) (Bile salts)	SPC: plant (soya bean: *Glycine max*) SDC: chemically modified: salification of deoxycholic acid (metabolic byproduct of intestinal bacteria)	Mucosal membrane modulation	In vivo (dog)	Fenofibrate	[103]
Oral	Tamarixetin (metabolite of quercetin) (Flavonoid)	Plant (hogweed/cow parsnip: *Heracleum stenopterum*)	Metabolism (CYP2C isozyme) inhibition	In vitro (rat liver microsomes), In vivo (rat)	Fluvastatin: HMG CoA reductase inhibitor	[104]
Oral	TMC (Cationic polymers)	Modified chitosan (crustaceans, fungi)	Mucoadhesion; tight junction modulation	In vitro (Caco-2 cells [2])	Mannitol: Sugar alcohol PEG 4000: Polyethylene glycol	[105]
Oral	TMC (Cationic polymers)	Modified chitosan (crustaceans, fungi)	Tight junction modulation	In vitro (Caco-2 cells [2])	Mannitol: Sugar alcohol FITC–dextran: Hydrophilic polysaccharide Buserelin: Gonadotropin-releasing hormone agonist	[106]
Oral	TMC (Cationic polymers)	Modified chitosan (crustaceans, fungi)	Tight junction modulation	In vitro (Caco-2 cells [2])	Clodronate: Bisphosphonate	[69]
Oral	ZOT (Toxins and venom extracts)	Bacteria (*Vibrio cholerae*)	Tight junction modulation	In vitro (Caco-2 cells [2])	PEG 4000: Polyethylene glycol FITC–dextran: Hydrophilic polysaccharide Inulin: Naturally occurring polysaccharide Paclitaxel: Tetracyclic diterpenoid Acyclovir: HSV-specified DNA polymerases inhibitor Cyclosporine: Immunosuppressant Doxorubicin: Daunorubicin precursor	[107]

Table 1. *Cont.*

Route of Administration	Bioenhancer (Class)	Biological Source	Mechanism(s) of Action	Study Design Model	Research Compound	Reference(s)
Pulmonary	Aprotinin, bestatin (Protease inhibitors)	Animal (bovine lung tissue), bacteria (*Streptomyces olivoreticuli*)	Metabolism inhibition	In vivo (rat)	rhG-CSF: Granulocyte-colony stimulating factor	[108]
Pulmonary	Chitosan (Biopolymer)	Chemically modified: deacetylation of chitin Animal (crustaceans), fungi	Tight junction modulation	In vitro (Calu-3 cells [5]); in vivo (rat)	Octreotide: Somatostatin analog	[109]
Pulmonary	Citric acid (Chelating agents)	Plant (citrus fruits and vegetables), fungi (*Aspergillus niger*)	Local mucosal tissue modulation; metabolism inhibition	In vivo (rat)	Insulin: Peptide hormone	[110]
Pulmonary	HPBCD, Crysmeb (Cyclodextrin derivatives)	Plant (starch)	Tight junction modulation	In vitro (Calu-3 cells [5])	Mannitol: Sugar alcohol	[111]
Pulmonary	Lanthanum, cerium, gadolinium (Lanthanides)	Natural elements	Drug targeting	In vivo (rat)	Insulin: Peptide hormone	[112]
Pulmonary	Sodium glycocholate (Bile salt)	Intestinal bacterial by-product	Tight junction modulation	Ex vivo (rabbit trachea and jejunum)	Thyrotropin-releasing hormone (TRH): Tripeptidal hypothalamus hormone Insulin: Peptide hormone	[113]
Pulmonary	Sodium taurocholate (Bile salt)	Intestinal bacterial by-product	Metabolism enhancement (dissociation of insulin hexamers); tight junction modulation; metabolism (enzymatic degradation) inhibition	In vitro (Caco-2 cells [2]), In vivo (dog)	Insulin: Peptide hormone	[114]
Pulmonary	Dideoxycytidine: Nucleoside analog reverse transcriptase inhibitor (NRTI)	Plant (Starch)	Tight junction modulation	In vitro (Calu-3 cells [5]), in vivo (rat)	Enoxaparin: Anticoagulant	[115]
Pulmonary	TMC (Cationic polymers)	Chemically modified: deacetylation of chitin Animal (crustaceans), fungi	Tight junction modulation	In vitro (Calu-3 cells [5]); in vivo (rat)	Octreotide: Octapeptide	[109]

[1] T146 cells: buccal epithelium cells. [2] Caco-2 cells: human epithelial colorectal adenocarcinoma cells. [3] LS180 cells: intestinal human colon adenocarcinoma cells. [4] HT-29 clone B6: human colon carcinoma cells. [5] Calu-3 cells: mammalian airway epithelium cells. [6] MDR1-MDCKII/MRP2-MDCK cells: Madin–Darby Canine Kidney cells with multidrug resistance 1 (MDR1) or multidrug resistance-associated protein 2 (MRP2) gene. [7] MCF-7 ADRr (re-designated NCI-ADR-RES) cells: ovarian tumor cells. [8] hOATP1/3-HEK293 cells: human embryonic kidney cells transfected with human organic anion-transporting polypeptide 1 or 3.

2.2. Bile Salts

The in vitro permeation of 2′,3′-dideoxycytidine (ddC) across porcine buccal mucosae was studied in the absence and presence of sodium glycocholate using in-line flow-through diffusion cells [28]. Fresh isotonic McIlvaine buffer solution (IMB, pH 7.4), which simulated gingival fluid without enzyme, with 10 mg/mL ddC, 0.01% (*w/v*) gentamicin and sodium glycocholate in concentrations varying from 0.6 to 50 mM, were added to the donor chambers. A flow rate of 0.8 mL/h was maintained, and samples were collected every 90 min for 22.5 h. Results demonstrated a concentration-dependent increase in ddC permeation across buccal mucosa as donor concentrations of ddC was increased from 1 to 20 mg/mL. This is indicative of passive diffusion [28]. In the presence of sodium glycocholate (4 mM), the permeability of ddC was significantly increased (~32-fold) to an apparent permeability coefficient (P_{app}) value of $5.11 \pm 1.46 \times 10^{-6}$ cm/s. At lower sodium glycocholate concentrations (<4 mM), a limited enhancement effect was observed, while the P_{app} value was only increased to $5.61 \pm 1.06 \times 10^{-6}$ cm/s at higher concentrations of sodium glycocholate (10 and 50 mM). Earlier studies indicated that 4 mM sodium glycocholate was close to the critical micelle concentration (CMC) of sodium glycocholate [116,117]. Since sodium glycocholate can solubilize the membrane lipids by incorporating them into sodium glycocholate micelles, a low enhancement effect was expected at sodium glycocholate concentrations below the CMC of 4 mM. On the other hand, interfacial saturation between sodium glycocholate micelles and lipid could explain the restricted enhancement effect observed with sodium glycocholate at concentrations beyond the CMC [28].

2.3. Chitosan and Derivatives

It was shown that chitosan could enhance the absorption of the transforming growth factor-β (TGF-β), a large bioactive peptide, across buccal mucosal tissue. A gel was prepared that consisted of 2% chitosan-H (MW: 1 400,000; degree of deacetylation: 80%) in dilute lactic acid solution. I125-labelled TGF-b (MW: ~25 Kda) was incorporated into the chitosan gel, as well as in a control solution of PBS. Continuous-flow perfusion chambers were used to study the permeability of TGF-β across porcine buccal mucosa dermatomed to a thickness of approximately 700 μm. Additionally, horizontal sectioning and counting was performed to determine the localization of TGF-β within the buccal mucosa [22]. Results demonstrated that chitosan enhanced the permeability of the TGF-β bioactive peptide in buccal mucosa six- to seven-fold, even though oral mucosa is relatively impermeable to TGF-β due to its large size [22].

Furthermore, compared to the control PBS solution, an increased amount of TGF-β was found in the superficial layers of the epithelium [22]. Enhanced penetration of TGF-β into buccal mucosa may be the result of increased retention of the drug at the application site due to the mucoadhesive nature of chitosan [22]. Another potential mechanism whereby chitosan improved drug transport across the buccal epithelium, is interference with the lipid organization in the intercellular regions of the epithelium [22].

Another in vitro study demonstrated decreased trans-epithelial electrical resistance (TEER) of the buccal epithelial TR146 cell culture model when chitosan was used as a bioenhancer for peptide and protein absorption. In this study, chitosan glutamate concentrations of 20 μg/mL and higher showed enhanced transport of large hydrophilic compounds, ^{3}H-mannitol and fluorescein isothiocyanate labeled dextrans (FITC–dextrans), at pH 6. ^{3}H-mannitol demonstrated the highest cellular permeability, and decreasing permeability was observed for FITC–dextran with molecular weight (MW) of 4000 Da (FD4), FD10 (MW of 10,000 Da), and FD20 (MW of 20,000 Da) as their molecular weights increased [21]. Enhanced permeability caused by chitosan of all the test substances, except FD20, was statistically significant. Compared to untreated cells, the TEER of the TR146 cell culture model was drastically reduced to ~30% in the presence of chitosan glutamate at concentrations of 20 μg/mL and higher [21]. Contrary to nasal and intestinal mucosal membranes, the buccal mucosal intercellular barrier is not based on tight junctions [22], therefore tight junction modulation cannot be the mechanism by which permeability enhancement proceeded. It was thus suggested that interference with the lipid organization in the buccal mucosa was responsible for improved drug transport in the presence of chitosan glutamate or also potential loosening of intercellular filaments [21].

Thiolated chitosans have shown the ability to significantly improve mucoadhesion and drug permeation [118]. A mucoadhesive buccal peptide drug delivery system with thiolated chitosan was designed and evaluated in vitro and in vivo as an approach for the buccal delivery of pituitary adenylate cyclase-activating polypeptide (PACAP) [23,24]. Chitosan-4-thiobutylamidine (chitosan–TBA) was synthesized and homogenized with enzyme inhibitor and permeation mediator glutathione (GSH), lyophilized and compressed into flat-faced discs. Two experimental formulations were prepared for in vivo evaluation, namely, formulation A that comprised chitosan–TBA (69.5 mg), GSH (3.75 mg), Brij 35 (0.75 mg), and PACAP (1 mg); whereas formulation B contained an innermost layer of chitosan–TBA (50 mg), GSH (2.5 mg), Brij 35 (2.5 mg), PACAP (1 mg) and an outermost layer of chitosan–TBA (50 mg). Additionally, formulation B contained a palm wax coating on one side to ensure unidirectional release of the drug toward buccal mucosa, whilst avoiding losses in the oral cavity [23]. Control formulations contained unmodified chitosan and PACAP (formulation C) or unmodified chitosan, Brij 35, and PACAP (formulation D). These test formulations were given to pigs via buccal administration for 6 h. An absolute bioavailability of 1% was obtained with formulations A and B, whereas the controls (formulations C and D) did not allow PACAP to even reach the systemic circulation [23].

In another study, trimethyl chitosan (TMC) with different quaternization degrees (QDs of 4%, 35% and 90%) showed increased mucoadhesive properties and enhanced permeation of FD4 (FITC–dextran with a molecular weight (MW) of 4000 Da) across porcine cheek mucosa [29]. The epithelium of the porcine cheek mucosa was peeled from the underlying tissues and mounted in Franz diffusion cells. TMC polymer solutions were prepared at 4% (*w/w*) concentration by gentle stirring at room temperature, followed by addition of FD4 at 0.2% (*w/w*) concentration [29]. A tensile stress tester was used to evaluate the mucoadhesive properties of the polymer solutions on cheek buccal mucosa and submaxillary bovine mucin. Results from the in vitro permeation studies demonstrated that permeation of FD4 across the excised cheek mucosal tissue was poor and difficult in the absence of a penetration enhancer. Mucoadhesive performance increased with increasing QD, regardless of media or biological substrate used. However, increased permeation of FD4 was only observed with pH 6.4 buffer, which can be attributed to increased polymer solubility. The best permeation enhancement results were obtained with low molecular weight TMCs with high QD [29].

2.4. Fatty Acids

A study investigated the effect of unsaturated fatty acids (including oleic acid, eicosapentaenoic acid (EPA), and docosahexaenoic acid (DHA)) when concomitantly administered with insulin in a Pluronic F-127 (PF-127) gel formulation [27]. PF-127 (MW: 12,500 Da) was used to prepare insulin gel formulations with or without unsaturated fatty acids. The final concentrations of PF-127 and unsaturated fatty acids were 20 and 5%, respectively. The control formulation consisted of a 20% PF-127 gel containing only insulin [27]. In vitro release studies were performed using membrane-less dissolution tests. In vivo studies were performed by buccally administering a volume of 0.2 mL of a formulation (insulin dose, 25 IU/kg) to anesthetized rats. Blood samples were taken before and after buccal dosing to determine the serum glucose levels [27].

A decreased rate of insulin release together with a remarkable and continuous hypoglycemic effect was observed with PF-127 gels (insulin dose, 25 IU/kg) containing unsaturated fatty acids. The reduced release rate may be partly due to reductions in the numbers and dimensions of the aqueous channels through which the hydrophilic solutes diffuse, or it may be due to the viscosity of the formulations [27]. The serum glucose levels were significantly reduced with all formulations containing unsaturated fatty acids. Results demonstrated that PF-127 gels containing oleic acid yielded the highest bioavailability (15.9 ± 7.9%) of insulin relative to subcutaneous administration. In comparison, EPA and DHA yielded bioavailabilities of 3.4 ± 1.2% and 4.1 ± 3.4%, respectively. However, increased bioavailability observed in the presence of DHA was not statistically significant [27].

Similarly, a study investigated the effect of cod-liver oil extract (CLOE) and hydrogenated castor oil (HCO) on the buccal permeation of ergotamine tartrate (ET) [25]. Hamster cheek pouch was used as a model membrane for the in vitro permeation study using a two-chamber diffusion cell (37 °C). The buccal membrane was pre-treated for 1 or 3 h with a solution of phosphate buffer (PB, pH 7.4) and propylene glycol (PG) (PB:PG, 1:1) containing 5% of each of the permeation enhancers which was each added to the donor cell. After pre-treatment, the solutions in both cells were removed and the cells were rinsed multiple times using a fresh PG/PB mixture. This was immediately followed by the permeation experiment where the donor cell was filled with a suspension of ET in PG/PB, and the receiver cell was filled with the PG/PB mixture only [25]. Results from the permeation study demonstrated that the permeation rate of ET was markedly increased in the presence of each of the permeation enhancers (5%). In the presence of HCO, the solubility of ET was noticeably increased, which resulted in a relatively low flux of ET due to a decrease in the partitioning of ET to the mucosa [25]. On the other hand, the solubility of ET increased ~2-fold in the presence of CLOE, which produced a ~8-fold increase in the flux of ET. These results suggest that CLOE has a direct action on the mucosa in addition to the solubilizing effect it has on ET [25]. Increasing concentrations of CLOE did not enhance the permeation of ET greatly, and 3% concentration of CLOE was considered to be sufficient to exhibit the enhancing action. Furthermore, the flux of ET was almost constant with or without pre-treatment, and an extended period of pre-treatment had no effect on the flux of ET. These findings suggest that CLOE exhibits a transient enhancing effect [25].

The permeation study was repeated on four of the major fatty acids in CLOE, namely palmitic acid, oleic acid, eicosapentaenoic acid (EPA), and docosahexaenoic acid (DHA). However, the concentration of each fatty acid in the donor solution was calculated according to its composition ratios in CLOE. Results from this permeation study revealed that the individual fatty acids had a significantly lower effect on the flux of ET than that of 5% CLOE, of which oleic acid showed the greatest enhancing action. This suggests that the synergistic action of the individual fatty acids in CLOE likely contributes to the greater enhancing action of CLOE [25].

2.5. Menthol

A study of the trans-buccal permeation of dideoxycytidine (ddC) using menthol as an enhancer demonstrated a significant increase in ddC permeability. Porcine buccal tissue was used for the permeation experiments using side-bi-side flow-through diffusion cells at 37 °C. The P_{app} of ddC across the buccal mucosa increased 2.02 times at a menthol concentration of 0.3 mg/mL. However, no significant difference was observed between the permeation enhancement of ddC in the presence of lower concentrations (0.1 and 0.2 mg/mL) of l-menthol. This may be due to the limited effect of menthol on the intercellular lipid extraction over the range of concentrations studied [26]. It was suggested that the observed enhancement in ddC permeation may be partly due to the partition coefficient enhancing effects of l-menthol [26].

3. Nasal Route of Administration

Figure 2 illustrates the main mechanisms of action of selected bioenhancers for improved drug delivery via the nasal route of administration.

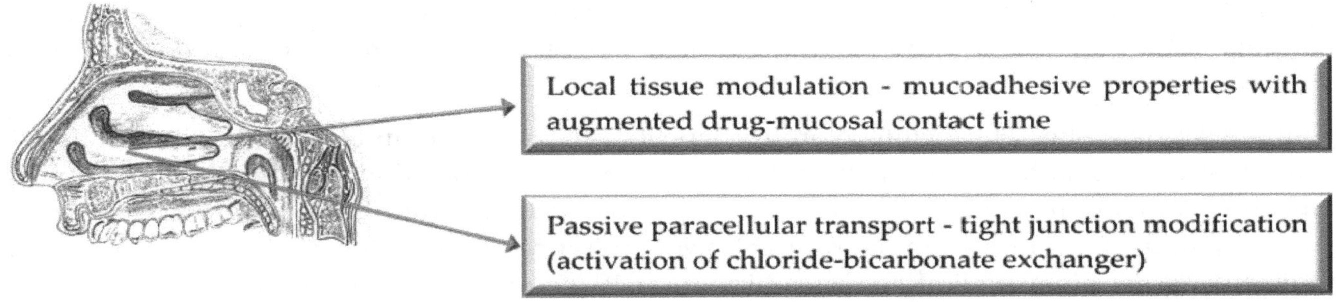

Figure 2. Illustration of the main mechanisms of action of bioenhancers for enhanced nasal drug delivery.

3.1. *Bile Salts*

The bioavailability of insulin from a nasal formulation with 5% glycofurol (GF) was studied in rabbits [119]. Zinc-free human insulin, Novolin® Nasal (Novo Nordisc) and glycofurol 75 (Hoffman La-Roche) were used in this study. Preparation of intranasal formulations consisted of 6.6 mg insulin dissolved in 1 mL phosphate buffer (12.5 mM, pH 7.4) containing 5% glycofurol. The dosage administered was 50 μL of the nasal solution within each nostril equivalent to 0.66 mg insulin (15.8 IU). Blood glucose was determined in blood collected at pre-determined time intervals. The frog palate model described by Gizurarson, et al. [120] was used to test local toxicity on mucocilliary clearance with phosphate buffer (12.5 mM) at pH 7.4 and 5% glycofurol. The results demonstrated greater decreased plasma glucose levels when glycofurol was included in the nasal formulation, which were comparable with previously published results [121]. Although the absorption enhancing mechanism of glycofurol is not known, the results demonstrated rapid insulin absorption with 90% reduction in the initial glucose blood concentration after 15 min. Furthermore, the plasma glucose was still suppressed with 85% of the initial value at a time interval of 120 min. The results are indicative of glycofurol having the ability to enhance insulin absorption in rats with enduring suppression of blood glucose levels.

Bagger, et al. [122] investigated the absolute nasal bioavailability of peptide T in rabbits when administered with sodium glycocholate and glycofurol. Previous nasal absorption studies with the bile salt sodium glycocholate as a drug absorption enhancer of peptide and peptide-like compounds has shown apparent bioenhancing effects [123–127]. In this study, the absorption enhancing action of sodium glycocholate and glycofurol was investigated by using T_{max}, C_{max} and time-dependent concentration profiles of peptide T. The bioavailability of peptide T administered with the selected bioenhancers was compared to a control formulation consisting of peptide T in water, which gave a bioavailability of 5.9%. Sodium glycocholate showed the highest increase in the bioavailability of peptide T (59%), while glycofurol also increased its bioavailability (22%). On the other hand, when the two bioenhancers were combined (i.e., glycoferol and sodium glycocholate), a bioavailability of 29% was obtained for peptide T. Furthermore, when peptide T was co-administered with sodium glycocholate, the bioenhancing effect was characterized by rapid absorption but relatively short duration of action. The glycofurol showed a lower absorption enhancement effect, but with a longer duration of action [122].

3.2. *Chitosan and Derivatives*

Chitosan is a polysaccharide obtained from deacetylation of chitin, the second most abundant natural polymer that is contained in the exoskeletons of insects and crustaceans. Illum and co-workers were the first to demonstrate the nasal drug absorption enhancement effects of chitosan. Chitosan showed, for example, the ability to increase the C_{max} of insulin in sheep from 34 mIU/L to 191 mIU/L, while the AUC was elevated 7-fold [128]. The use of chitosan as a novel absorption enhancer for peptide drugs has been described previously [129], while its use in nasal delivery systems for a range of therapeutics has recently been comprehensively reviewed [130]. Selected studies will briefly be discussed below as illustration of the nasal drug delivery enhancement potential of the natural polymer, chitosan.

Illum, Watts, Fisher, Hinchcliffe, Norbury, Jabbal–Gill, Nankervis and Davis [31] showed that the co-administration of either chitosan in solution or chitosan formulated in microspheres can improve the bioavailability of morphine hydrochloride after nasal administration in sheep. Chitosan caused an increase in the C_{max} of morphine from 151 nM in the control group (morphine alone) to 657 nM, and improved the bioavailability of morphine from 10.0% (control group) to 26.6%. Furthermore, the rate of absorption was increased as indicated by the T_{max} of 14 min as opposed to 20 min in the control group. Chitosan formulated into microspheres even further improved the bioavailability parameters of morphine with a C_{max} of 1,010 nM and bioavailability of 54.65%. The rate of absorption was also improved with a T_{max} of 8 min, which was statistically significantly different from that of the control [128].

Hinchcliffe, Jabbal–Gill and Smith [30] investigated the pharmacokinetic effects of a chitosan-based intranasal delivery system on salmon calcitonin within a sheep model. A control nasal solution containing salmon calcitonin (2200 IU/mL) only was compared to a salmon calcitonin solution containing chitosan glutamate (5 mg/mL) as well as to Miacalcin®, a commercially available salmon calcitonin containing nasal spray. A C_{max} value of 99 pg/mL (range 50–107 pg/mL) was obtained for the salmon calcitonin solution containing chitosan compared to 33 pg/mL (range 13–49 pg/mL) for the salmon calcitonin control solution and 42 pg/mL (range 15–79 pg/mL) for the Miacalcin® nasal spray. Furthermore, the average AUC value of the chitosan-containing solution of 3220 pg/mL/min (range 1606–4972 pg/mL/min) demonstrated a 3.5-fold increase compared to that of the control salmon calcitonin solution (943 pg/mL/min, range 198–2519 pg/mL/min) and 2-fold increase towards that of the Miacalcin® nasal spray (1636 pg/mL/min, range 87–3792 pg/mL/min) [30].

Since chitosan is only soluble at acidic pH values below its pKa value, chemically modified derivatives, such as N-trimethyl chitosan chloride (TMC), have been synthesized to improve solubility at more neutral pH values [131]. In a study where TMC polymers with different quaternisation degrees (QD) was nasally administered with ^{14}C-mannitol to rats, it was shown that the QD of TMC played an important role at a neutral environment (pH 7.4) in terms of its nasal absorption enhancement effects. The nasal delivery of ^{14}C-mannitol increased with an increase in QD until a threshold value was reached at 45% [33].

3.3. Starch Microspheres

In vivo studies in sheep found augmented nasal drug absorption for bioadhesive starch microsphere delivery systems, which could be improved synergistically by combination with other absorption enhancing agents. The comparison of control solutions with starch microspheres containing insulin and gentamicin showed 5-fold and 10-fold increases in absorption efficiency, respectively [132–134]. Similar starch microsphere formulations and drug compounds demonstrated approximately 30-fold increases in the bioavailability of the drugs when administered nasally to rats [135].

4. Oral Route of Administration

Figure 3 illustrates the main mechanisms of action of selected bioenhancers for improved drug delivery via the oral route of administration.

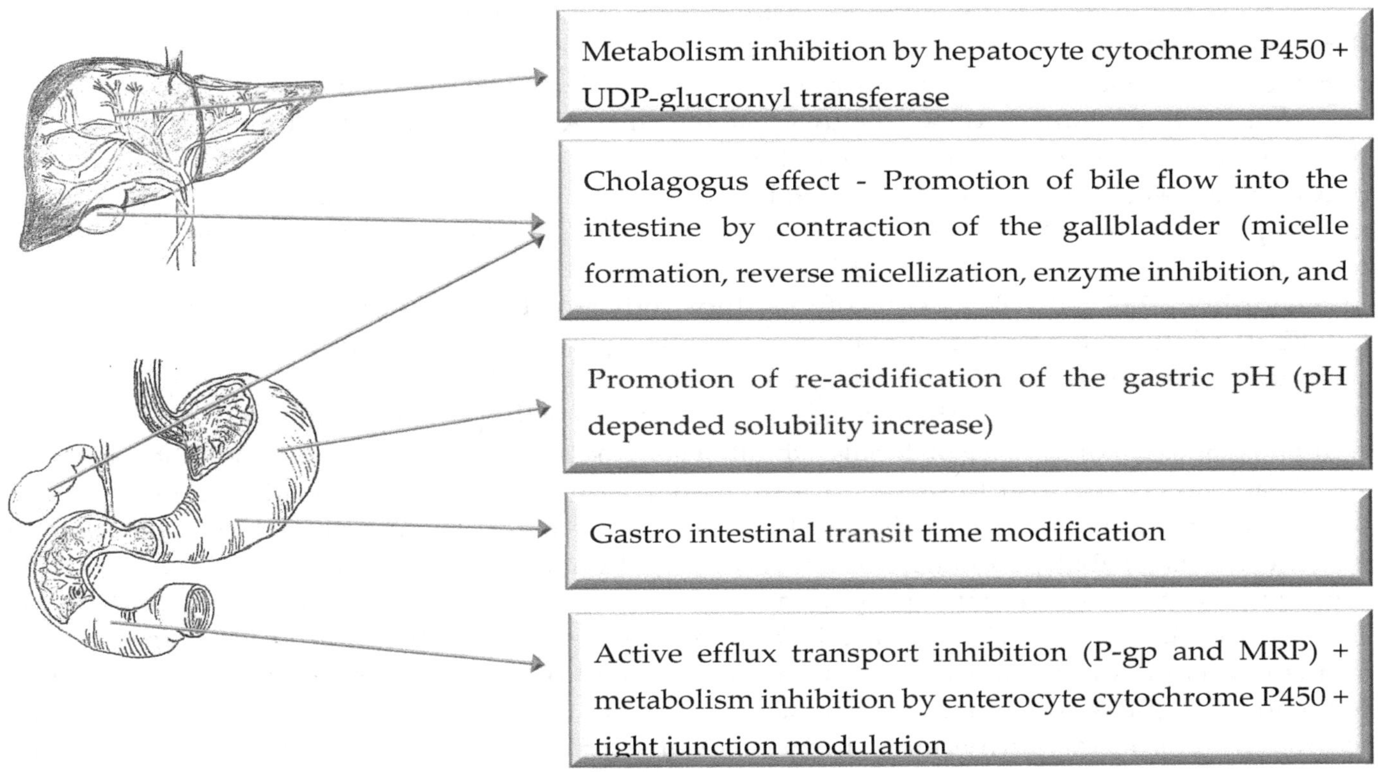

Figure 3. Illustration of the main mechanisms of action of bioenhancers for enhanced oral drug delivery.

4.1. Aloe Vera

Aloe vera leaf materials and extracts have been found to modify in vitro drug transport and in vivo drug bioavailability. In a double-blind, cross-over clinical study investigating the effect of *A. vera* liquid products on the absorption of vitamins C and E in human subjects, both *A. vera* gel product (AVG) and *A. vera* whole leaf product (AVWL) were investigated. AVG caused a 3.7-fold and AVWL a 2-fold increase in the bioavailability of vitamin C in comparison to the control (i.e., vitamin C administered with water). With respect to the influence on the bioavailability of vitamin E, both *Aloe* products caused a statistically significant increase in the baseline levels of vitamin E at 6 and 8 h post administration. However, due to large inter-individual variation, the AUC values between the different treatments were not statistically significant. The authors attributed the improvement in the bioavailability of vitamins C and E by the *A. vera* products to a protective action against degradation in the gastrointestinal tract, however, this was not proven in the study [37].

Both *A. vera* gel and whole leaf materials increased insulin transport extensively across Caco-2 cell monolayers over a concentration range of 0.1 to 5% *w/v* at two different pH values of 5.8 and 7.4. The *Aloe* materials decreased the TEER of the Caco-2 cell monolayers markedly at concentrations higher than 0.5% *w/v*, which was reversible [36]. A study was conducted using *A. ferox* and *A. vera* gel material, whole leaf material as well as precipitated polysaccharides (from these materials) in a concentration of 2% *w/v* in combination with atenolol as model drug across excised rat intestinal tissues in diffusion chambers. All the *Aloe* materials lowered the TEER of the excised rat intestinal tissues statistically significantly ($p < 0.05$) in comparison to the control (atenolol alone) and to a larger extent than the positive control (0.2% *w/v* sodium lauryl sulfate). In this study, it was also shown that some precipitated polysaccharides resulted in a higher decrease in TEER than their corresponding gel and whole leaf material counterparts. This reduction in TEER was indicative of the ability of the *Aloe* leaf materials to open tight junctions and consequently enhance paracellular transport of hydrophilic drug molecules such as atenolol. Only the precipitated polysaccharide fraction from dehydrated *A. vera* gel (Daltonmax 700®) material could enhance the transport of atenolol across intestinal rat tissue statistically significantly in comparison to the control. Although not statistically significant in comparison to the control, the polysaccharide fraction obtained from the *A. vera* whole leaf extract (Daltonmax 700®) caused a substantial increase in atenolol transport. The *A. ferox* materials were, however, not able to enhance the transport of atenolol across the excised rat intestinal tissues [35].

In a study by Wallis, Malan, Gouws, Steyn, Ellis, Abay, Wiesner, P Otto and Hamman [38], the effect of *A. vera* gel and polysaccharides (i.e., crude polysaccharides as well as fractionated polysaccharides based on molecular weight) on the bioavailability of indinavir was investigated in Sprague–Dawley rats. As part of this study, the effect of the selected *Aloe* materials was also investigated on the TEER of Caco-2 cell monolayers as well as their influence on the metabolism of indinavir in LS 180 cells. The results of this study indicated that all of the *Aloe* materials decreased the TEER of the Caco-2 cell monolayers indicating opening of tight junctions. The precipitated polysaccharides decreased the TEER to a larger extent than the gel material. However, no clear correlation between the different molecular weight fractions of the polysaccharides and TEER reduction could be made. All of the *Aloe* materials exhibited enzyme inhibitory effects, although not statistically significant, in comparison to the control (indinavir alone). With respect to the influence on the bioavailability of indinavir as indicated by AUC, all the investigated *Aloe* materials rendered an increase in bioavailability although not statistically significant. The increase in indinavir bioavailability caused by the crude precipitated polysaccharide and polysaccharide fractions were higher than that seen for the *A. vera* gel. The increase in bioavailability of indinavir in this study was attributed to a combination of mechanisms including the opening of the tight junctions (as indicated by a reduction in TEER) and an inhibition in the metabolism of indinavir (as indicated by the metabolite plasma concentration). Furthermore, from the results of this study, it is evident that the biologically active components responsible for the modulation of drug pharmacokinetics and absorption are most probably concentrated in the polysaccharide component of the *A. vera* gel material although it cannot be directly correlated with the molecular size of the polysaccharide component [38].

4.2. Bile Salts

The ability of bile salts to enhance the oral bioavailability of compounds, especially poorly water-soluble drugs, has been discovered many years ago [136–138].

The study by Yu, Zhu, Wang, Peng, Tong, Cao, Qiu and Xu [102] investigated the bioavailability of silybin when mixed with bile salt micelles compared with silybin-*N*-methylglucamine alone after oral administration in dogs. The prepared mixed bile salt micelles showed a mean particle size of 75.9 ± 4.2 nm. Silybin-sodium cholate/phospholipid-mixed micelles revealed a very slow release of the silybin, only 17.5% (*w/w*) over 72 h in phosphate buffer (pH 7.4) and 15.6% (*w/w*) in HCl solution (pH 1.2). In spite of this slow release, the relative bioavailability of silybin in the mixed micelles versus silybin-*N*-methylglucamine in dogs was 252% [102].

An in vivo study in diabetic rats was used to investigate the regional-specific intestinal delivery of insulin by co-administration of sodium glycocholate [139]. Insulin (10 UI/kg) was administered intestinally (duodenum, jejunum and ileum) to rats by surgical technique without (control) and with 5% sodium glycocholate. Insulin absorbed from the gastrointestinal tract was investigated by measuring the hypoglycemic effect in the rats at 45 and 60 min post administration. The hypoglycemic effect (100%) of the positive control was specified at 77.9 mg/100 mL glucose at 45 min and 70.5 mg/100 mL glucose at 60 min. For the duodenum region, the insulin control showed a hypoglycemic effect of 71% at 45 min and 84% at 60 min, while the insulin with sodium glycocholate showed hypoglycemic effects of 90% and 95% at 45 and 60 min post administration, respectively. For the jejunum region, the insulin control showed 34% and 54% hypoglycemic effects, while the insulin with sodium glycocholate showed 39% and 60% hypoglycemic effects at 45 and 60 min post administration, respectively. However, administration within the ileum of rats did not demonstrate a significant decrease in blood glucose concentration profiles compared to control. For the ileum, the insulin control showed 9% and 5%, while insulin with sodium glycocholate showed 5% and 8% at 45 and 60 min post administration, respectively [139].

These effects could be contributed to the increased insulin absorption in the presence of the bile salt, potentially by mechanisms of mucus layer modification as well as tight junction modulation [140,141]. Finally, the effects of sodium glycocholate on the intestinal absorption enhancement of insulin demonstrated site-dependent effects with duodenum being the optimal site for insulin oral delivery [139].

4.3. Black Cumin

Nigella sativa, commonly known as black cumin/caraway, was previously evaluated as a bioenhancer for amoxicillin [142]. *N. sativa* extracts were prepared by cleaning, milling and sieving seeds, followed by extractions with methanol and hexane for 6 h [142]. Everted rat intestinal sacs were used to study the transfer of amoxicillin (6 mg/mL) in PBS (pH 7.4) with or without methanol (3 mg) and hexane (6 mg) extract of *N. sativa* seeds. The amount of amoxicillin transported across the gut was quantified spectrophotometrically at 273 nm [142]. For in vivo studies, amoxicillin (25 mg/kg) was orally co-administered with *N. sativa* hexane extract (25 mg/kg) to rats. Blood samples were collected at 0, 0.25, 0.5, 0.75, 1, 1.5, 2, 4, 6 and 8 h post-dosing, after which UPLC-MS/MS was used to quantify the amount of amoxicillin in rat plasma [142].

Results from the in vitro study demonstrated that both the methanol and hexane extracts of *N. sativa* significantly increased the permeation of amoxicillin, with the latter showing the greatest increase [142]. Hence, hexane extract was selected for in vivo evaluation. Results from the in vivo study also demonstrated a significant increase in amoxicillin plasma concentration in rats. *N. sativa* extract increased the rate and extent of amoxicillin absorption, increasing the C_{max} from 4138.251 $\pm$ 156.93 to 5995.045 $\pm$ 196.28 ng/mL, while $AUC_{0\rightarrow t}$ increased from 8890.40 $\pm$ 143.33 to 13483.46 $\pm$ 152.45 ng/mL·h. It was suggested that this permeation enhancing effect of *N. sativa* might be attributed to the presence of fatty acids [142]. It has previously been demonstrated that fatty acids are able to enhance permeation of low permeable drugs by increasing the fluidity of the apical and basolateral membranes [143]. A similar in vivo study performed on rabbits yielded opposite results. In that study, the C_{max} and $AUC_{0-\infty}$ of cyclosporine (30 mg/kg) significantly decreased by 35.5% and 55.9%, respectively, after pretreatment with *Nigella* (200 mg/kg). However, a significant increase in cyclosporine clearance (~2-fold) was observed, thus suggesting that intestinal P-gp and/or CYP3A4 are activated in the presence of *N. sativa* [144].

4.4. Capsaicin

In vitro, in situ and in vivo evaluations of the effect of capsaicin pre-treatment on fexofenadine showed significantly enhanced intestinal absorption of fexofenadine [145]. Non-everted intestinal sacs of rats were employed in the in vitro study, while an in situ single-pass intestinal perfusion study was conducted on rats where the ileal segment (~8–12 cm) was isolated and cannulated. For the in vivo study, the same pre-treatment was applied for 7 days in rats. Results from the non-everted sac study indicated a significant increase in the intestinal transport and P_{app} of fexofenadine in the presence of capsaicin. It was suggested that P-gp efflux inhibition in intestine of rats was the action mechanism, since the results obtained with capsaicin pre-treatment and verapamil, a standard P-gp inhibitor, were comparable [145]. In situ single-pass intestinal perfusion results demonstrated a significant increase in the absorption rate constant, fraction absorbed, and effective permeability of fexofenadine in rats pre-treated with capsaicin and verapamil in comparison with control group [145]. In vivo results showed a significant increase in the AUC and C_{max} of fexofenadine orally administered to rats pretreated with capsaicin. Additionally, the apparent oral clearance of fexofenadine was significantly decreased, while t_{max} and $t_{1/2}$ were unchanged. Findings from this study thus provide in vivo evidence that capsaicin might increase the bioavailability of fexofenadine via the inhibition of P-gp-mediated drug efflux [145].

4.5. *Caraway*

Caraway is obtained from the dried ripe fruit of the plant *Carum carvi*. In an open-label, cross-over in vivo study, the bioenhancing effect of *C. carvi* (Caraway) extract (100 mg) on the pharmacokinetics of rifampicin, isoniazid and pyrazinamide administered as a fixed-dose combination (FDC) was investigated. The Caraway extract increased both C_{max} and AUC as indicators of bioavailability for all three drugs, statistically significantly. The increase in C_{max} was 32.22%, 36.01% and 33.22% for rifampicin, isoniazid and pyrazinamide, respectively, while the increase in $AUC_{0-24\,h}$ was 32.16%, 29.06% and 27.92% for rifampicin, isoniazid and pyrazinamide, respectively. According to the authors, the improvement in bioavailability caused by Caraway extract may be attributed to an enhancement of mucosal to serosal permeation as well as its influence on P-gp efflux [40]. Caraway was shown to act as an inhibitor of P-gp efflux and the main active components were found to be carvone and limonene [146].

4.6. *Cylcosporine A*

Cyclosporine A is a polypeptide consisting of 11 amino acids and was initially derived from a fungus, *Tolypocladium inflatum Gams* [147]. Cyclosporine A is used amongst other indications as an immunosuppresive agent during organ transplantation, to treat autoimmune diseases and in the treatment of certain viral diseases such as Hepatitis C, to name but a few uses. Cyclosporine A has been shown to act as an inhibitor of the efflux transporter, P-gp and as a result may increase the bioavailability of drugs that are substrates for this active efflux transporter [51]. Cyclosporine A has been shown to improve the bioavailability of clopidogrel, an antiplatelet drug, in rats. Co-administration of a dose of 10 mg/kg of cyclosporine A and 30 mg/kg of clopidogrel resulted in a 3.48-fold and 2.83-fold increase in the AUC and C_{max} of clopidogrel, respectively. The authors attributed this increase in bioavailability to the inhibition of P-gp-mediated efflux [49].

4.7. *Chitosan and Derivatives*

The oral drug absorption enhancing effects of chitosan and its derivatives have previously been reviewed extensively [148,149]. In brief, several studies have shown that chitosan (including chitosan salts such as chitosan hydrochloride and chitosan glutamate) is an effective oral drug absorption enhancer across in vitro cell models as well as in vivo animal models [42,150–152]. The major mechanism of drug absorption enhancement has been shown to involve tight junction modulation to allow for enhanced paracellular uptake of hydrophilic and macromolecular drug compounds. Although a number of studies indicated interactions of chitosan with epithelial cells to open tight junctions [153] through redistribution of F-actin and ZO-1 [148,154], it was shown on HT-29/B6 cells with two-path impedance spectroscopy that the tight junction opening effect of chitosan was due to changes in intracellular pH caused by the activation of a chloride-bicarbonate exchanger [155].

To improve some of the characteristics of chitosan, several derivatives and chemically modified chitosans have been investigated for their drug delivery potential including trimethyl-chitosans, thiolated chitosans, carboxymethyl chitosan and derivatives, hydrophobic chitosans, chitosan succinate and phthalate, PEGylated chitosans and chitosan-enzyme inhibitor conjugates, which have been published in a review previously [156].

4.8. *Curcumin*

Curcumin (diferuloylmethane) is the major curcuminoid contained in the rhizome of *Curcuma longa* L. (turmeric) that has been shown to have several biological and pharmacological activities [157]. A previously published review on pharmacokinetic interactions of curcuminoids with conventional drugs revealed potential interactions via modulation of CYP450 and phase II enzymes as well as P-gp efflux inhibition and potential effects on organic anion transporting polypeptides (OATP).

Unfortunately, contrasting results were obtained by different studies ranging from drug absorption enhancement to drug absorption reduction by curcumin [158].

An example of a study where curcumin was found to significantly increase drug bioavailability is an in vivo study in Sprague–Dawley rats that received curcumin (60 mg/kg) for four days prior to drug administration (pre-treatment group), while another group received curcumin (60 mg/kg) once only concomitantly with the drug and the control group received no curcumin. The bioavailability of celiprolol increased statistically significantly in the curcumin pre-treated rats, but not in rats where it was co-administered once only with curcumin. Although the bioavailability of midazolam increased in both the pre-treatment group as well as the co-administered group, it was only statistically significant in the pre-treatment group. Western blot analyses revealed that intestinal P-gp protein expression reduced by 49%, while CYP3A protein content reduced by 42% after 4 days of pre-treatment with curcumin. On the other hand, the hepatic P-gp protein expression increased by 144% and the CYP3A protein content was increased by 91%. Renal P-gp protein levels remained unchanged, but renal CYP3A was enhanced by 41%. Since celiprolol is a P-gp substrate and midazolam is extensively metabolized by CYP3A enzymes, it was deduced from this study that the pharmacokinetics of these two drugs have been changed by curcumin due to down regulation of P-gp and CYP3A in the small intestine [48]. Furthermore, when curcumin was administered at a dose of 10 mg/kg with tamoxifen to rats, the AUC and C_{max} values of tamoxifen were significantly increased (i.e., by 64% and 71%, respectively) [159]. Pre-treatment of broiler chickens with 100 mg/kg curcumin for ten days enhanced the absolute and relative bioavailabilities of marbofloxacin in these animals [160]. The P-gp inhibiting effects of curcumin was confirmed in an in vitro study on a human P-gp overexpressing cell line (LLC-GA5-COL300) where the uptake of calcein-AM was increased [161].

4.9. Diosmin

Certain flavones (e.g., tangeretin, nobiletin and bergamottin) from citrus fruits have shown P-gp inhibitory effects, which caused pharmacokinetic interactions with drugs that are substrates for this efflux transporter. Diosmin, a flavonoid contained in citrus fruit, was investigated in the Caco-2 cell model for P-gp inhibitory effects using rhodamine 123 and digoxin as model compounds. Rhodomine 123 accumulation in the Caco-2 cells was investigated in the absence and presence of diosmin. At a concentration of 50 μM, diosmin caused a 494 ± 8.4% increase in the cellular accumulation of rhodamine 123 in reference to the control. To further investigate the initial observation of P-gp-mediated efflux inhibition by diosmin, bi-directional transport (i.e., in the apical-to-basolateral [A-B] and basolateral-to-apical [B-A] direction) of digoxin across Caco-2 cell monolayers was conducted in the absence and presence of diosmin. At a concentration of 50 μM diosmin, the $P_{app\ (A–B)}$ was significantly increased from $2.8 \pm 0.07 \times 10^{-6}$ cm/s to $9.5 \pm 0.06 \times 10^{-6}$ cm/s, while the $P_{app\ (B–A)}$ was significantly decreased from $41.1 \pm 1.20 \times 10^{-6}$ cm/s to $17.1 \pm 0.10 \times 10^{-6}$ cm/s. These P_{app} values corresponded to transport ratio values of 15.2 in the absence and 2.3 in the presence of diosmin. Based on the results of this study, it is clear that diosmin act as a P-gp efflux transport inhibitor and as such has the potential to improve the bioavailability of drugs that are substrates for P-gp [50].

In a more recent study, the effect of diosmin on the in vivo pharmacokinetics of fexofenadine in rats was investigated. In this study, rats were pre-treated for 7 days with diosmin (50 mg/kg) where after fexofenadine (10 mg/kg) was administered on day 8. Pre-treatment with diosmin resulted in a 2.5- and 2.2-fold increase in C_{max} and $AUC_{0\text{-}\infty}$, respectively. The enhanced bioavailability of fexofenadine in this study was attributed to the fact that diosmin is a potent P-gp inhibitor [162].

4.10. Emodin

Anthraquinones such as emodin (1,3,8-trihydroxy-6-methyl-anthraquinone) occur naturally in a wide variety of plants and herbs such as *Rheum palmatum* [163], *Polygonum multiflorum* [164], *Polygonum cuspidatum* [165], *Cassia obtusifolia* [166] and *Aloe vera* [167]. Administration of emodin may lead to synergistic and/or inhibitory effects on P-gp-related efflux and/or modulation of multidrug-resistance associated protein 1, 2 and 3 (MRP1, MRP2 and MRP3) and these effects may have a profound effect on the bioavailability of co-administered substrate molecules [163,168–171].

In an extensive study conducted by Min, et al. [172], potential interactions between emodin and rhodamine 123 were investigated in various in vitro models. In this study, human myelogenous myeloid leukemia cells (K562), the P-gp over-expressing adriamycin resistant K562 cells (K562/ADM) and Caco-2 cells were used as in vitro models to investigate if the co-administration of emodin at various concentrations had any significant effect on the intracellular accumulation of rhodamine 123 (1 μM). The results showed that addition of emodin increased the intracellular accumulation of rhodamine 123 in a concentration-dependent manner in both the Caco-2 and K562/ADM cell models. The extent of the accumulation of rhodamine 123 in Caco-2 cells by emodin (20 μM) was comparable to that of a much higher verapamil concentration (200 μM). Binding site competition between emodin and rhodamine 123 on P-gp was also investigated. The results showed that the calculated K_i values increased consistently in conjunction with increasing rhodamine 123 concentrations (0 to 20 μM), which indicated that a competitive interaction occurred between emodin and rhodamine 123. It was concluded that emodin and rhodamine 123 shared the same R-binding site on P-gp [172].

An MTT method was also used in conjunction with the K562/ADM cell line to investigate if the addition of emodin could potentially reverse P-gp-mediated MDR. The results showed that the addition of emodin (20 μM), alone or in combination with 10 μM adriamycin, exerted down regulation of P-gp expression in comparison to the control group. The authors concluded that emodin could potentially reverse P-gp-mediated MDR due to inhibition of P-gp expression in K562/ADM cells and also by competitive interactions between emodin and rhodamine 123 at the R-binding site of P-gp. The results confirmed that emodin is an effective inhibitor of P-gp and its effects are mediated either by direct binding to P-gp and subsequent weakening of the P-gp-mediated efflux function or by indirect mechanisms related to a reduction in P-gp expression [172].

In another study, it was also shown that the addition of emodin to the Caco-2 cell model had the ability to decrease P-gp-mediated efflux, but additionally it was also reported that P-gp expression was mediated via the MAPK/AP-1 pathway by means of COX-2 inhibition [173]. An in vitro transport study across rat intestinal tissues using an Ussing-chamber technique showed that the transport of digoxin was decreased in the presence of emodin while the transport of teniposide was increased in the presence of emodin. The authors concluded that emodin was an inducer of P-gp-related efflux and also an inhibitor of MRP3 [174].

4.11. Gallic Acid Ester

Gallic acid is a water soluble phenolic acid which is found in grapes and in the leaves of various plants and forms part of a larger group of plant polyphenols known as gallotannins [175]. Gallotannins are transformed in the gastrointestinal tract by hydrolysis to form free gallic acid [176]. Various health benefits are associated with the intake of gallic acid and it is reported in the literature to exert anti-cancer, anti-inflammatory, cardio-protective and anti-diabetic properties [175]. Gallic acid has been reported to exhibit inhibitory effects on P-gp-mediated drug efflux and also on CYP450-related isozymes such as CYP3A4 [177–179].

In vitro and in situ transport studies were conducted to investigate the effects of gallic acid on the transport of diltiazem. The in vitro studies entailed the use of non-everted gut sacs from Wistar rat intestinal tissue. The results from the in vitro study showed that the apparent permeability of diltiazem had increased in the presence of gallic acid by 4.4-, 5.1- and 4.9-fold in the respective segments of the duodenum, jejunum and ileum of non-everted intestinal gut sacs when compared with the control group [180].

For the in situ single-pass intestinal perfusion study, rats were randomly divided into four groups ($n = 5$) (control, standard inhibitor, and pre-treated with either gallic acid or ellagic acid). Perfusion of the cannulated intestinal segment was performed using phosphate buffered saline (pH = 7.2) containing diltiazem (100 μg/mL) and phenol red (50 mg/mL). A constant flow rate of 0.2 mL/min was maintained for a period of 90 min and samples were collected at 10 min intervals. The results from the in situ study showed that pre-treatment with gallic acid (50 mg/kg) for 7 days resulted in a significant ($p < 0.05$) increase in diltiazem transport in rats when compared to the control group (diltiazem alone) following pre-treatments with gallic acid for 7 days. The C_{max}, AUC_{0-t}, and $AUC_{0-\infty}$ of diltiazem were increased by 1.90-, 2.06- and 2.08-fold, respectively (Athukuri and Neerati., 2018). Based on these results, it was suggested that gallic acid was most likely a dual inhibitor of both P-gp and CYP3A4 and that this dualistic effect may have resulted in the significant enhancement in the bioavailability of diltiazem [180].

The transport of metoprolol was assessed in a similar in situ single-pass intestinal perfusion study to evaluate the pharmacokinetic parameters of orally administered metoprolol in Wistar rats. The rats were pre-treated with gallic acid (50 mg/kg) for 7 days before the start of the study. A significant increase in the C_{max} and AUC values of metoprolol were evident. It was concluded that gallic acid had enhanced the oral bioavailability by inhibiting CYP2D6 activity in the liver, which caused reduced metabolism of metoprolol [181].

4.12. Genistein

The flavonoid genistein (5,7-Dihydroxy-3-(4-hydroxyphenyl)chromen-4-one) is a plant-derived (*Glycine max* and *Pueraria lobata*) isoflavone and a phytoestrogen, frequently ingested by humans [54,55,182]. Genistein has very poor bioavailability in itself and although some studies have suggested that genistein may have anticancer effects, these effects could not be obtained in clinical studies because of its low bioavailability [183]. Genistein is purported to be an enhancer of bioavailability of drugs, since it has been shown to inhibit efflux of P-gp, BCRP and MRP2 transporters. These properties were investigated in a Caco-2 antiparasitic agent transport study, where taxol (a P-gp substrate) was applied in combination with 33 or 100 μM genistein [184]. Although no inhibition of transport could be measured for 33 μM genistein, 100 μM genistein resulted in 20% inhibition. It was subsequently determined that although genistein inhibited P-gp, it did not appear to be a substrate of P-gp. Another study showed 10–30 μM genistein increased sensitivity of a P-gp hyper-expressing drug resistant human cervical carcinoma cell line (KB-V1) to vinblastine and paclitaxel, while reducing efflux of Rhodamine 123 and vinblastine in a dose-dependent manner (10–200 μM) [185]. However, no correlating change in P-gp expression was observed following exposure to genistein, indicating only P-gp activity was modulated. Li and Choi [55] later demonstrated that a single oral dose of 30 mg/kg paclitaxel 30 min after ingesting 3.3 mg/kg or 10 mg/kg genistein, significantly increased the AUC by 54.7% in male Sprague–Dawley rats. This was as a result of decreased plasma clearance (35.2%), thereby increasing systemic exposure. The same effect was seen when the paclitaxel was administered intravenously (3.3 mg/kg). It was proposed that the genistein inhibited the efflux transporters and metabolic enzymes for which paclitaxel is known to be a substrate, probably being P-gp and CYP3A [55,182].

Genistein also inhibited efflux of 2′,7′-bis-(carboxypropyl)-5(6)-carboxyfluorescein (BCPCF), an MRP1 substrate, from human erythrocytes. Genistein displayed an IC_{50} concentration of 50–70 μM for BCPCF efflux. It was reported that genistein inhibited MRP1 efflux transporters, but that this modulation was substrate sensitive [186].

Genistein has been shown to inhibit the biotransformation and intestinal efflux of (-)-epigallocatechin-3-gallate (EGCG) in more recent studies. EGCG is a flavonoid in various foods and beverages, but especially in *Camellia sinensis* (green tea), and has been shown to have several therapeutic effects such as anti-cancer, anti-viral and anti-inflammatory effects, but it has very poor oral systemic absorption [187]. Lambert, Kwon, Ju, Bose, Lee, Hong, Hao and Yang [54] demonstrated an increase in cytosolic EGCG of 2- to 5-fold in the presence of genistein (20 μM), in HT-29 human colon cancer cells. They also treated CF-1 mice with 200 mg/kg genistein and 75 mg/kg EGCG, resulting in increased plasma half-life and maximal concentration of the EGCG. However, in a male adenomatous polyposis coli (APC) min/+ mouse model, this combination also enhanced tumor genesis.

An in vitro and in vivo study treated Mardin-Darby canine kidney (MDCK-II) cells and Assaf sheep with the antibacterial fluoroquinolone, danofloxacin, concomitantly with genistein [188]. Danofloxasin is exclusive for animal use and is actively secreted into milk. The in vitro transport study showed that genistein inhibited BCRP transport of danofloxasin efficiently, while the in vivo study indicated no change in danofloxasin plasma levels following isoflavone supplementation. A prolonged diet of soy, however, did reduce antimicrobial concentrations in the milk.

Important to note are the findings of Chen, et al. [189], which indicated that genistein can induce the phase II drug-metabolizing enzyme, sulfotransferase. Enzymatic activity, protein levels and mRNA expression were evaluated in a transformed human liver cell line (HepG2) and a colon carcinoma cell line (Caco-2). It was concluded that gene expression (SULT1A1 and SULT2A1) was induced by genistein in a time and dose-dependent (0–25 μM) manner. Contrary, approximately 0.1 μM genistein inhibited human liver phenol sulfotransferase by 50% in a competitive manner [190].

4.13. Gokhru Extract

Gokhru extract, a popular plant extract used in Ayurvedic medicines, is derived from *Tribulus terrestris* Linn (Zygophyllaceae) [56,191]. Some of the phytochemicals previously identified in *T. terrestris* include saponins, steroids, flavonoids and carboline alkaloids. Gokhru extract is traditionally used as a diuretic, anti-inflammatory, anabolic, spasmolytic, muscle relaxant, hypotensive, and hypoglycemic agent, but it has been reported to influence bioavailability of co-administered drugs.

One study investigated the effect of Gokhru extract on the absorption of metformin hydrochloride (HCl) in an everted sac model [56]. Metformin is an anti-diabetic drug that is known to be highly soluble, but poorly membrane permeable (BCS class III). In this study, the extract was prepared from dried plant material (fresh fruits, leaves and stems) with hot ethanol. The results showed increased absorption of metformin in the presence of the Gokhru extract, and the authors suggested the major saponin component in the extract may have contributed largely to this increase in drug transport. Saponins consist of one or more sugar chains, connected to a steroid or triterpenoid aglycon. It can solubilize cholesterol, while maintaining most of the structure of the cell membranes, thereby permeabilizing it to increase membrane permeability [57].

A similar study formulated metformin HCl tablets (175–500 mg) with varying concentrations Gokhru extract (0–100 mg), which were then investigated using a chicken intestine everted sac model. In this study, the drug absorption enhancement properties of Gokhru extract was confirmed with increased metformin permeation across the chicken intestinal membranes from 29% to 54% [57].

A methanol extract was prepared from dried *T. terrestris* leaves and applied together with salicylic acid (aspirin) to the mucosal side of the goat intestinal tissues used in an everted sac technique. The Gokhru extract increased aspirin transport and it was proposed that the permeability enhancing action was a result of the saponins effects on the membranes [191].

4.14. Grapefruit Juice

The pharmacokinetic interaction between grapefruit (*Citrus paradisi*) juice and the calcium channel antagonist, felodipine, was discovered serendipitously during an in vivo clinical study in 1989 that was designed to evaluate the potential interaction between ethanol and felodipine. Grapefruit juice was used to mask the taste of ethanol in this study. Concomitant intake of felodipine with grapefruit juice caused higher anti-hypertensive effects as well as higher felodipine plasma concentrations. This observation led to a follow-up pilot study in a single volunteer where felodipine plasma concentrations were found to be more than 5-fold higher when it was taken with grapefruit juice than with water [192]. Since this initial discovery, more than 85 drugs have shown to interact with grapefruit juice in terms of pharmacokinetics of which most experienced increased plasma concentrations [193].

In a study on borderline hypertensive patients where the effect of different fruit juices was evaluated on felodipine pharmacokinetics, it was shown that grapefruit juice, but not orange juice, could markedly increase felodipine's bioavailability parameters (both C_{max} and AUC were increased).

In addition, grapefruit juice reduced the ratio of dehydrofelodipin (the primary metabolite of felodipine produced by CYP3A4) to felodipine. This effect was not observed for intravenous administration of felodipine with grapefruit juice, which indicated selective inhibition of pre-systemic metabolism involving CYP3A4 [194].

Several studies showed that three groups could be distinguished with respect to the effect of grapefruit juice on the pharmacokinetic parameters of drugs, namely "increase", "decrease" and "no change" [195]. The uptake and bioavailability enhancement effect of grapefruit juice was shown in a study where both in vitro and in vivo models were used. Lyophilized freshly-prepared grapefruit juice significantly increased the uptake of doxorubicin into human uterine sarcoma (MES-SA/DX5) cells and significantly increased the bioavailability of timolol maleate in rabbits [196]. However, it was shown that both regular strength and double strength grapefruit juice did not have a significant effect on the pharmacokinetic parameters of simvastatin when administered concomitantly to Sprague–Dawley rats in a dose of 20 mg/kg over 28 days. On the other hand, simvastatin plasma concentrations were elevated by double strength grapefruit juice when the drug was administered at a dose of 80 mg/kg [197], indicating a dose-dependent pharmacokinetic interaction. In another in vivo study, grapefruit juice decreased the oral bioavailability of fexofenadine [58].

Results from different studies revealed, over time, that the pharmacokinetic effect of several forms of grapefruit (i.e., whole fruit, fresh fruit juice or frozen concentrate) is drug-specific and it may in some cases be concentration-dependent. It was also shown that the lower the inherent bioavailability of the drug due to pre-systemic metabolism, the higher the chance is that the interaction with grapefruit can be dangerous [193].

One of the main mechanisms of action of grapefruit juice by which the bioavailability of drugs (e.g., felodipine) is increased, is by mechanism-based inhibition of CYP3A4 in the enterocytes of the small intestine and hepatocytes of the liver [58,198]. It was also shown that grapefruit juice could inhibit the P-gp efflux transporter and thereby increase the bioavailability of drugs that are substrates for this efflux transporter (e.g., talinolol) [199,200]. Furthermore, a study on 10 volunteers that received grapefruit juice three times a day for 6 days revealed that their small intestinal CYP3A4 protein expression reduced by 62%, but not their liver CYP3A4 protein expression. This selective down regulation of CYP3A4 correlated well with the C_{max} increase of felodipine after grapefruit juice consumption relative to that taken with water [201]. On the other hand, it was found that grapefruit juice has the ability to inhibit uptake transporters such as OATP, specifically OATP1A2 and OATP2B1, and thereby it can decrease the absorption of certain drugs (e.g., fexofenadine) [202,203].

4.15. Lycopene

The effect of a lycopene-containing nano-formulation containing simvastatin on low density lipoprotein (LDL) was investigated in mildly hypercholesterolemic patients [60]. The aim of this study was to evaluate lycopene as a vector of intrahepatic transport to specifically enhance the hepatic bioavailability of simvastatin. This is important, since hepatic cholesterologenesis is the main site of statin action. Furthermore, the plasma lipid profile is not affected by extrahepatic inhibition of HMG-CoA reductase, and extrahepatic toxicity is observed with increasing statin concentrations [60]. A total of 10 patients with moderately increased plasma LDL levels (150 to 200 mg/dL) received 20 mg of either unmodified simvastatin or lycosome-formulated statin (Lyco–Simvastatin) daily. Plasma samples were obtained after 30-day treatment and analyzed for lipids. The results demonstrated that the solubilized lycosome nanoparticles increased the intestinal absorption rate in comparison with unmodified simvastatin and were able to bind hepatocyte membranes. The lycopene-containing simvastatin formulation significantly ($p = 0.0049$) reduced LDL levels in the hypercholesterolemic patients as compared to unmodified simvastatin [60].

The mechanism of action of lycopene is enhanced hepatic uptake via a dual carotenoid/LDL receptor-mediated mechanism [60]. It was shown that lycopene crystals and/or lycopene-containing nanoparticles (lycosomes) became incorporated into chylomicrons upon absorption. The chylomicrons are then distributed by lymph and likely undergo a dual receptor-mediated uptake associated with the lycopene core. The latter is a powerful ligand for carotenoid receptors that are expressed by hepatocytes and therefore promoted intrahepatic delivery of lycosome-formulated statins [60]. Enhanced hepatic uptake of lycostatin is also possible due to a second pathway of intrahepatic uptake involving an LDL-receptor mechanism. Chylomicrons and their enzymatically degraded products, LDL and very low density lipoprotein (VLDL), contain ApoB that mediates their transport inside hepatocytes using the LDL receptor [60]. Although further research related to the pharmacology of Lyco-Simvastatin is needed, lycopene seems to a promising bioenhancer for targeted hepatic delivery of simvastatin [60].

4.16. Lysergol

Lysergol (9,10-Didehydro-6-methylergoline-8-*O*-methanol) is a compound present in several higher plants (e.g., *Ipomoea violacea*, *I. muricata* and *Rivea corymbosa*) and lower fungi (e.g., *Claviceps*, *Penicillium* and *Rhizopus*) [182,204]. Lysergol is traditionally used as a psychotropic, analgesic, analeptic, hypotensive and immuno-stimulant. It usually maintains normal blood flow through its vaso-activity and can promote drug absorption from the gastrointestinal tract [205]. An in vivo study by Shukla, Malik, Jaiswal, Sharma, Tanpula, Goyani and Lal [62] indicated that lysergol increased the bioavailability and decreased the clearance of curcumin significantly. This was followed by in vitro mechanistic studies using rat liver microsomes and probe substrates for P-gp and BCRP transporter proteins. The results suggested that BCRP, rather than P-gp, was inhibited by lysergol. In situ single-pass intestinal perfusion studies of the P-gp substrate, digoxin, and the BCRP substrate, sulfasalazine, were then performed in Sprague–Dawley rats following pre-treatment with 20 mg/kg lysergol. These studies supported the conclusion that P-gp was not involved in the permeation-enhancing effect of lysergol, but that BCRP was inhibited [62].

Lysergol (2–10 μg/mL) isolated from *I. muricata* seeds with methyl alcohol has been shown to act as a bioenhancer of antibiotics. The authors showed that rifampicin and tetracycline intestinal transport could be enhanced (2.96–8.53 fold) by lysergol in vitro [204]. Lysergol also increased the oral bioavailability of the quaternary protoberberine alkaloid, berberine, in male Sprague–Dawley rats. Berberine is used for numerous ailments, including bacterial infection, intestinal parasitic infection and diarrhea, but it is very poorly absorbed in the intestines and extensively metabolized. The study indicated that 20 mg/kg lysergol could increase the bioavailability of the berberine [61].

4.17. Naringin and Bergamottin

Certain phytochemicals such as naringin (a flavonoid) and bergamottin (a furanocoumarin) contained in grapefruit have been associated with the pharmacokinetic interactions observed for grapefruit juice co-administered with certain drugs [195]. When paclitaxel has been orally co-administered with naringin to Sprague–Dawley rats, the paclitaxel plasma concentrations increased statistically significantly. Since naringin affected the bioavailability of paclitaxel similar to that of quercetin, a known inhibitor of CYP3A and P-gp, it was deduced that naringin enhanced the bioavailability of paclitaxel by means of inhibition of CYP3A metabolism and P-gp efflux transporters [66]. Similarly, the pharmacokinetic parameters of diltiazem (AUC and C_{max}) were increased by 2-fold when the rats were pre-treated with naringin (administered 30 min prior to diltiazem) compared to the control group. In addition, the AUC metabolite-to-parent ratio decreased by 30% in the presence of naringin compared to the control. This confirmed the ability of naringin to inhibit metabolism of diltiazem [64].

The CYP3A4 inhibition activities of bergamottin and 6′,7′-dihydroxybergamottin were investigated in a human intestinal microsome study on two model compounds namely testosterone and midazolam. Bergamottin was identified as a substrate-dependent reversible inhibitor, but a substrate-independent mechanism-based inhibitor of CYP3A4. On the other hand, 6′,7′-dihydroxybergamottin was found to be a substrate-independent reversible and mechanism-based CYP3A4 inhibitor [206].

4.18. *Palmitoyl Carnitine Chloride*

Initial drug absorption enhancement studies on palmitoyl carnitine, a fatty acid ester of carnitine, showed that it is capable of intestinal drug absorption enhancement by means of tight junction opening (paracellular transport) and disruption of brush-border membrane lipids (transcellular transport) [207,208]. An in depth study on Caco-2 cell monolayers indicated that lytic effects and reduction in cell viability accompanied transport enhancement of hydrophilic macromolecules at all concentrations of palmitoyl carnitine that were investigated. It was concluded that the alteration of the tight junctional network, which was shown by TEER reduction and confocal laser scanning microscopic localization of ZO-1, occurred secondary to the interaction of palmitoyl carnitine with the membrane. Since complete recovery of TEER could not be obtained, the use of palmitoyl carnitine for drug absorption enhancement should be considered with caution [209].

4.19. *Piperine*

Piperine is an alkaloid contained in black pepper (*Piper nigrum*) and long pepper (*Piper longum*) [11]. Piperine can probably be considered as one of the world's first bioenhancers since its use dates as far back as the 7th century BC [205,210]. Piperine is traditionally used for its anti-inflammatory, anti-pyretic, anti-fungal, anti-diarrheal and anti-cancer effects [211]. Possible mechanisms by which piperine caused bioenhancing effects include alteration of membrane dynamics, inhibition of P-gp efflux, and inhibition of gastrointestinal and hepatic metabolism [11,83,210].

A study that investigated the effects of piperine on the serum levels of resveratrol (3,5,4′-trihydroxystilbene) when orally co-administered to C57BL mice, showed that AUC and C_{max} were increased by 229% and 1,544%, respectively [77]. Jin and Han [76] investigated the bioavailability changing effects of orally administered piperine in rats when co-administering fexofenadine either orally (10 mg/kg) or intravenously (5 mg/kg). The results suggested that there were no significant variations in the C_{max} of fexofenadine or its half-life, but the oral exposure (AUC) of fexofenadine was almost doubled. It was deduced from this study that the effects of piperine are more prominent after oral administration (likely due to the P-gp-mediated efflux inhibition and metabolism inhibition in the gastrointestinal epithelium) than after intravenous administration (due to hepatic metabolism inhibition) [76].

4.20. *Quercetin*

Quercetin, which is a CYP3A4 and P-gp inhibitor, has shown the ability to significantly enhance the bioavailability of orally administered tamoxifen and 4-hydroxytamoxifen in rats [95]. In that study, tamoxifen (10 mg/kg) was orally administered with or without quercetin (2.5, 7.5 and 15 mg/kg) in rats. Tamoxifen (10 mg/kg) was added to 1.5 mL distilled water for the control solution, whereas the required quercetin dose was dissolved in 1 mL distilled water to prepare quercetin suspensions for oral administration. Plasma concentrations of tamoxifen were measured in blood samples (0.5 mL) collected at 0, 0.5, 1, 2, 3, 4, 5, 6, 8, 12, 24 and 36 h after tamoxifen administration using HPLC [95].

The relative bioavailability of tamoxifen was 1.35- and 1.61-fold higher, with an absolute bioavailability of 20.2% and 24.1% with 2.5 and 7.5 mg/kg quercetin, respectively. These changes in bioavailability were significant ($p < 0.05$). Interestingly, higher concentrations of quercetin (15 mg/kg) did not induce any significant changes. No significant changes in the terminal half-life ($t_{1/2}$) and the time to reach the peak concentration (T_{max}) of tamoxifen was observed when co–administered with quercetin. When 4-hydroxytamoxifen, one of tamoxifen's metabolites, were co-administered with quercetin (7.5 mg/kg), a significant increase in the AUC of 4-hydroxytamoxifen was observed. These results suggested that MDR efflux and first-pass metabolism of tamoxifen was inhibited by quercetin [95].

Another in vivo study demonstrated an inhibitory effect on P-gp efflux of fexofenadine when it was co-administered with quercetin [91]. Twelve healthy subjects received an oral dose of quercetin

(500 mg) or placebo 3 times daily for 7 days. On the 7th day, a single dose of 60 mg fexofenadine was administered orally with 240 mL water under fasting conditions of more than 10 h. The healthy volunteers received the oral administration of fexofenadine while in the sitting position, and remained seated for 4 h [91]. Four and 10 h after dosing, subjects received standardized meals with only minor amounts of flavonoids, so as not to influence the absorption of fexofenadine or quercetin. Subsequently, blood samples were drawn immediately before, as well as 0.25, 0.5, 1, 1.5, 2, 2.5, 3, 4, 6, 8, 12, and 24 h after fexofenadine administration. Urine samples were collected during time intervals of 0–2, 2–4, 4–8, 8–12, and 12–24 h after dosing. Plasma and urinary fexofenadine concentrations were quantified using HPLC [91].

Results indicated that quercetin significantly enhanced the mean plasma concentrations of fexofenadine. The AUC of plasma fexofenadine increased by 55% from 2,005.3 to 3,098.6 ng.h/nL ($p < 0.001$) in the presence of quercetin. The C_{max} was similarly increased by 68% from 295.3 to 480.3 ng/mL ($p = 0.006$) when co-administered with quercetin. After quercetin treatment, the oral clearance of fexofenadine was significantly decreased by 37% from 61.4 to 38.7 L/h ($p < 0.001$). However, no differences in the renal clearance and half-life were observed between the groups receiving placebo versus quercetin [91].

In summary, quercetin can be used as a bioenhancer for enhanced intestinal absorption, and hence bioavailability, of tamoxifen [95] and fexofenadine [91]. The action mechanisms employed by quercetin are MDR transporter efflux inhibition, as well as first-pass metabolism inhibition [95]. If the results obtained with tamoxifen from the rats' model is confirmed in the clinical trials, the dose of tamoxifen should be adjusted for potential drug interactions when quercetin or the quercetin-containing dietary supplements are simultaneously consumed with this drug [95]. Although the inhibitory effect of quercetin on P-gp-mediated efflux of fexofenadine was demonstrated in the short-term (7 days), it is uncertain whether long-term use of quercetin will yield the same results [91].

4.21. *Quinidine*

A research study using everted gut sacs demonstrated that quinidine could significantly enhance the absorption of paeoniflorin (20 μM) [97]. Increased absorption of paeoniflorin was observed with an increase of incubation time, indicating that the absorption of this compound was time-dependent. In addition, the absorptive profiles with different concentrations of paeoniflorin indicated that absorption increased with increasing concentrations, but saturation of the in vitro gut sac system was observed at a concentration of ~80 μM. This saturation indicates that transport of paeoniflorin might be facilitated by an active transporter or carrier [97]. Co-administration of quinidine (1.3 mM) and paeoniflorin (20 μM) yielded a 1.5-fold increase in the absorption of paeoniflorin after 45 min of incubation. Absorption of paeoniflorin in the intestine could thus be significantly enhanced by co-administration of quinidine [97].

4.22. *Resveratrol*

A recent study demonstrated that resveratrol could significantly increase rat intestinal absorption of methotrexate in vivo and in vitro [99]. Furthermore, resveratrol was also able to inhibit efflux transport and decrease renal clearance of methotrexate. The bidirectional transport of methotrexate across mock-MDCK, MDR1-MDCK, and MRP2-MDCK cell monolayers were evaluated using an experimental buffer solution containing methotrexate (10 μM) and/or resveratrol (10 μM). This experimental buffer solution was added to the donor chamber, either 400 μL apical or 600 μL basolateral chamber, respectively. At time intervals of 0.5, 1, 2, and 3 h, 50 μL samples were removed from the opposite (receiver) chamber and replenished with 50 μL fresh Hanks' balanced salt solution (HBSS, pH 7.4) [99].

Additionally, the in vitro uptake of methotrexate in the absence and presence of resveratrol in kidney slices and Caco-2 cells were determined by liquid chromatography-tandem mass spectrometry (LC-MS/MS). To clarify the action mechanism of resveratrol, transporter uptake assays were similarly performed using mock-human embryonic kidney (HEK) 293 cells, human organic anion transport 1 (hOAT1)-HEK293 cells and hOAT3-HEK293 cells. The transport buffer contained 10 μM methotrexate, *p*-amino hippuric acid (PAH), Penicillin G (PCG) or resveratrol. PAH and PCG are specific substrates of OAT1 and OAT3, respectively [99].

The in vivo absorption experiment in rats entailed an oral administration of 5 mg/kg methotrexate dissolved in 2% sodium bicarbonate with or without resveratrol (100 mg/kg, dissolved in 0.5% sodium carboxymethyl cellulose) and brought up to volume with normal saline. Blood samples were collected at 5, 10, 20, 30, 60, 120, 240, 360, 480, and 600 min to determine plasma concentrations of methotrexate. In order to establish the renal excretion of methotrexate, a solution of methotrexate (5 mg/kg) and/or resveratrol (10 mg/kg) dissolved in normal saline solution of hydroxypropyl-β-cyclodextrin was intravenously administered to rats. Again, blood samples were collected at the specified times to determine the plasma concentration of methotrexate. Furthermore, urine was collected at 2, 4, 6, 8, 10, 12, 16, and 24 h after dosing to determine the concentration of methotrexate excreted through urine [99].

In vivo results indicated that a significant increase in the plasma exposure of methotrexate was observed when methotrexate was orally or intravenously co-administered. In vitro results using the rat everted gut sac model demonstrated that serosal concentrations of methotrexate increased significantly in the presence of resveratrol, as well as verapamil and/ or CDF, inhibitors of P-gp and MRP2, respectively. These results thus suggest that resveratrol can enhance methotrexate intestinal absorption by inhibiting P-gp or MRP2. Furthermore, co-administration of methotrexate and resveratrol resulted in a 37.3% decreased cumulative urinary excretion of methotrexate, indicating that resveratrol could inhibit renal excretion of methotrexate. To clarify the action mechanism of the latter, methotrexate uptake experiments were conducted using rat kidney slices. Results from this experiment showed significantly decreased uptake of methotrexate in the presence of resveratrol and probenecid, a well-known inhibitor of OATs. Furthermore, PAH and PCG (substrates of OAT1 and OAT3, respectively), as well as methotrexate uptake was significantly inhibited by resveratrol in hOAT1-HEK293 or hOAT3-HEK293 cells. These results indicated that resveratrol was able to inhibit OAT1/3, which were target transporters involved in drug-drug interactions between methotrexate and resveratrol in the kidney. The rate of basal-to-apical transepithelial methotrexate transport in MDR1-MDCK and MRP2-MDCK cells increased 32.5- and 20.8-fold, respectively, in the presence of resveratrol. These results thus indicated that P-gp and MRP2 are also target transporters of methotrexate, which is inhibited by resveratrol [99].

In vivo and in vitro results indicated that resveratrol could significantly increase the absorption of methotrexate in the intestine, and also decreased methotrexate renal clearance. Uptake, transport and renal clearance studies confirmed that the mechanisms of action of resveratrol entailed inhibition of P-gp, MRP2, OAT1 and OAT3. This corresponds with previous studies demonstrating that methotrexate is mainly eliminated rapidly by OAT1 and OAT3 in the unchanged form into urine [212,213].

A recent study demonstrated contradictory results where resveratrol stimulated P-gp efflux of saquinavir in MDR1-expressing Madin–Darby canine kidney (MDCKII-MDR1) cells [214]. In this study, MDCKII-MDR1 cells were incubated with 50 μM saquinavir and/or resveratrol (1, 10, 33, and 100 μM) or verapamil (50 μM) at 37 °C for 4 h. Verapamil, a P-gp inhibitor, served as the positive control. Additionally, an in vitro metabolism experiment in microsomes assessed the effect of resveratrol on the intestinal CYP3A-mediated metabolism of saquinavir. In order to assess the effects of resveratrol on the pharmacokinetic profiles of saquinavir, 30 mg/kg saquinavir was orally administered, with or without resveratrol (20 mg/kg), to rats. Saquinavir was suspended in solvent (20% ethanol, 30% propylene glycol, and 50% saline) at a concentration of 6 mg/mL, whereas resveratrol was suspended in saline with 30% polyethylene glycol 400 at 20 mg/mL concentration. Subsequently, blood samples were collected at 0, 0.25, 0.5, 1, 2, 4, 8, 12, and 24 h after drug administration, and analyzed with LC-MS/MS [214].

Results demonstrated significantly decreased saquinavir intracellular concentrations in the presence of resveratrol in a concentration-dependent manner, which indicated that resveratrol stimulated P-gp-mediated efflux of saquinavir. Results from the metabolism experiment demonstrated a significant increase in residual saquinavir in the presence of resveratrol in a dose-dependent manner. This suggests that resveratrol has a concentration-dependent inhibitory effect on the intestinal CYP3A-mediated metabolism of saquinavir. Oral co-administration of resveratrol (20 mg/kg) decreased the mean $AUC_{0-\infty}$ of saquinavir by ~31%, while the mean apparent systemic clearance (CL/F) was increased by ~51%. However, both these changes were not statistically significant ($p > 0.05$) [214].

4.23. Sinomenine

Previous research using everted gut sacs demonstrated that sinomenine at 16 and 136 μM concentrations could significantly enhance the absorption of paeoniflorin (20 μM) by 1.5- and 2.5-fold, respectively [97]. Similarly, the absorption of digoxin (13 μM) could significantly be enhanced by 2.5-fold in the presence of sinomenine (136 μM). Increased absorption of paeoniflorin was observed with increase of incubation time, indicating that the absorption of this compound was time-dependent. In contrast, absorptive profiles with different concentrations of paeoniflorin indicated that absorption increased with increasing concentrations, but saturation of the in vitro gut sac system was observed at a concentration of ~80 μM [97]. This saturation indicated that transport of paeoniflorin might be facilitated by an energy-dependent carrier. Enhanced bioavailability of paeoniflorin (150 mg/kg) in the presence of sinomenine (90 mg/kg) has also previously been demonstrated in vivo in rats, yielding a 12-fold increase [100].

In order to investigate the potential mechanism underlying the observed enhanced absorption of paeoniflorin, two Pg-inhibitors (verapamil or quinidine) and a P-gp substrate (digoxin) was employed. Co-administration of verapamil (20 μM) and paeoniflorin (20 μM) yielded a 2.1-fold increase in the absorption of paeniflorin after 45 min of incubation. Similarly, when quinidine (1.3 mM) was co-administered, a 1.5-fold increase in the absorption of paeoniflorin was observed. Transportation and absorption of paeoniflorin in the intestine could thus be significantly enhanced by inhibition of P-gp by verapamil and quinidine [97]. Sinomenine (136 μM) was also able to significantly enhance the absorption of 13 μM digoxin, which is a well-known P-gp substrate-like drug, by 2.5-fold after 45 min of incubation.

4.24. Sodium Caprate (Fatty Acid)

Enhancement of sodium caprate on the intestinal absorption of berberine has been studied by in situ, in vitro and in vivo experiments [101]. Results from the recirculating perfusion model demonstrated an increased absorption rate of berberine (50 μmol/L) at 4 h from 9.3% to 18.5% in the presence of sodium caprate. In comparison, 100 μmol/L and 200 μmol/L berberine with sodium caprate (0.2% *w/v*) showed increased absorption rates of 13.1% and 20.1%, respectively. The in vitro everted rat gut sac experimental results showed that small amounts of berberine is absorbed in the intestine, with the highest and lowest amounts being absorbed in the jejunum and ileum, respectively. In the presence of sodium caprate, absorption of berberine was rapidly and significantly increased after 90 min incubation. Sodium caprate also resulted in an enhanced P_{app}. The greatest absorption of berberine in the presence of sodium caprate, was in the ileum (ER = 3.49), which showed the weakest absorption in the absence of sodium caprate. The duodenum and jejunum showed enhancement ratios (ERs) of 2.08 and 1.49, respectively. In vivo studies demonstrated that the bioavailability of berberine could be improved by co-administration of sodium caprate. A significant increase in the peak plasma concentration (from 721.39 ± 53.46 to 988.84 ± 135.56 ng/mL) of berberine in rats was observed, together with delayed peak time (from 30 to 60 min) and increased $AUC_{0\text{-}6\,h}$ (28%). Compared with the berberine treatment group, berberine with sodium caprate remarkably decreased the blood glucose levels and the areas under the glucose curves, thus enhancing the antidiabetic activity of insulin [101].

It is suggested that the low bioavailability of berberine is due to P-gp efflux. It has previously been demonstrated that sodium caprate can inhibit P-gp efflux [215].

4.25. Zonula Occludens Toxin (Zot)

Research demonstrated that the permeability of high molecular weight markers and poorly bioavailable compounds can be increased across Caco-2 cell monolayers by co-administration of the absorption enhancer Zonula occludens toxin (Zot, MW: 45 kDa), a toxin produced by the *Vibrio cholerae* bacteria [107]. During this study, the transport of hydrophilic high molecular weight markers (i.e., PEG4000, FITC–dextran 10,000, and inulin) and hydrophobic therapeutic agents (i.e., acyclovir, cyclopsorin, paclitaxel, and doxorubicin) were evaluated with Zot using Caco-2 cell monolayers. It has previously been established that Zot can reversibly open tight junctions between intestinal epithelial cells by binding to a specific receptor on the luminal surface of the intestine [216]. After cell monolayers were pre-incubated with Zot (0, 1, 2, and 4 μg/mL) for 30 min, markers or therapeutic agents were added to inserts at time 0 and samples were collected over 120 min from the basolateral chamber. Radio-graphic or HPLC methods were used for transport analysis, and TEER values were monitored over a 3 h period. Results indicated that 4 μg/mL Zot significantly enhanced the transport of markers with MW < 5 kDa by 6.2-fold. Similarly, Zot significantly increased transport of therapeutic agents at a concentration of 4 μg/mL, yielding enhancement ratios of 1.8 and 3.13 for acyclovir and paclitaxel, respectively. Significantly lower TEER values were observed between 0.5 and 2 h, although this effect of Zot on TEER across Caco-2 cell monolayers was reversible.

Caco-2 transport studies with the transcellular marker propranolol indicated that Zot does not significantly modulate the transcellular pathway [107]. Furthermore, a lactate dehydrogenase (LDH) assay demonstrated no significant difference in LDH activity in the presence of Zot, thus suggesting Zot is non-cytotoxic at the effective concentration level after a 3 h incubation period [107]. The permeation of FITC was not significantly enhanced, whereas a significant increase (6.3-fold) in permeability of inulin from 7×10^{-7} cm/s (control) to 4.37×10^{-6} cm/s (4 μg/mL) was observed. It was suggested that the compact cylindrical configuration of inulin results in higher permeability of inulin vs. PEG4000, even though inulin has a higher molecular weight [107]. The in vitro results with the therapeutic agents displayed a range of permeation increase by Zot from 20–300%. The rank order of permeability enhancement observed with the therapeutic agents in the presence of Zot was paclitaxel $>$ doxorubicin $>$ acyclovir $>$ cyclosporine A. Paclitaxel and cyclosporine A demonstrated P_{app} enhancement ratios of 3.13 and 1.2, respectively [107].

5. Pulmonary Route of Administration

Figure 4 illustrates the main mechanisms of action of selected bioenhancers for improved drug delivery via the pulmonary route of administration.

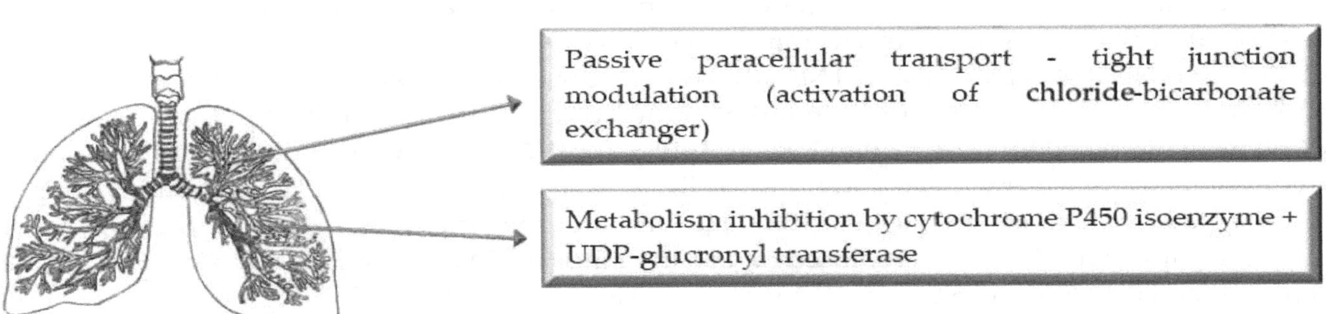

Figure 4. Illustration of the main mechanisms of action of bioenhancers for enhanced pulmonary drug delivery.

5.1. Bile Salts

A research study demonstrated that the tracheal permeability of thyrotropin-releasing hormone (TRH, MW: 362 Da) and insulin (MW: 5814 Da) was significantly increased by sodium glycocholate [113]. Non-everted sac segments of excised rabbit trachea were used. In addition to the transport study, the peptidase activities in the trachea and jejunum were measured and compared to examine the enzymatic barrier for TRH and insulin permeation across rabbit tracheal epithelium [113]. Results demonstrated that the permeability of both TRH (5 mM) and insulin (10 IU/mL) significantly increased in the presence of 10 mM glycocholate. The P_{app} values for TRH (5 and 10 mM) were $2.51 \pm 0.31 \times 10^{-7}$ and $3.54 \pm 0.87 \times 10^{-7}$ cm/s, respectively. Sodium glycocholate (10 mM) increased the tracheal permeability of TRH ~3-fold [113]. The P_{app} value for insulin (10 IU/mL) was $6.66 \pm 0.11 \times 10^{-9}$ cm/s. However, the half-life of insulin was about 14 h, and only showed slight degradation by luminal secreted enzymes for the duration (150 min) of the experiment. The tracheal and jejunal peptidases showed the following decreasing order of activity: DPP IV > Leu-aminopeptidase > cathepsin-B > trypsin [113]. These four peptidases had significantly lower activities in the tracheal epithelial cells compared to jejunal epithelial cells. Since TRH had no metabolites during tracheal permeation, a potential action mechanism of tight junction modulation and therefore enhanced paracellular permeability is suggested for sodium glycocholate [113]. Glycocholate is known to be a Leu-aminopeptidase inhibitor. However, insulin was slightly degraded during tracheal permeation. It is therefore suggested that insulin (MW: 5814 Da) is mainly transported via paracellular diffusion with slight metabolism by proteolytic enzymes such as trypsin-like and aminopeptidase-like enzymes through isolated rabbit tracheal epithelium [113].

Similarly, previous in vitro and in vivo research indicated that absorption of inhaled insulin could be enhanced by the bile salt sodium taurocholate [114]. For the in vivo study, beagle dogs were starved for at least 16 h, after which they were intubated and exposed to insulin or insulin-sodium taurocholate aerosols for differing times. As an intravenous reference, insulin in 0.9% NaCl was infused for 5 min (0.2 U/kg, 0.5 U/mL, 0.08 mL/kg per min) in the right foreleg vein. The insulin–sodium taurocholate solutions were aerosolized by a PARI LC jet nebulizer. The flow from the nebulizer was 3.2 L/min (1 Bar) and the target inhaled dose of insulin was 1 U/kg. Blood samples were collected before dosing and at 5, 10, 15, 25, 35, 50, 65, 95, 125 and 245 min after start ($t = 0$) of inhalation [114]. The bioavailability of pure insulin was $2.6 \pm 3\%$, while the bioavailability of nebulized insulin solutions increased to $23.2 \pm 4.4\%$ with addition of 32 mM sodium taurocholate. In comparison, a $3.81 \pm 1.12\%$ bioavailability of insulin was obtained when aerosolized powder was administered to the lungs. In vitro results indicated increased insulin transport, accompanied by reduced TEER, at sodium taurocholate concentrations between 25 and 30 mM. Unfortunately, the viability of cell layers was approximately zero at sodium taurocholate concentrations exceeding 32 mM [114].

5.2. Chitosan and Derivatives

The enhancement of bronchial octreotide absorption by chitosan and N-trimethyl chitosan (TMC) was evaluated with an integral in vitro/in vivo correlation approach [109]. The TMC derivatives with 20% and 60% QD (TMC20 and TMC60) were synthesized by alkaline methylation of chitosan. Chitosan was dissolved at 1.5% (*w/v*) in HBSS, buffered with 30 mM HEPES at pH 5.5. TMC20 and TMC60 were dissolved at 1.5% (*w/v*) in HBSS/HEPES at pH 7.4. Two hours prior to the TEER studies, the culture medium was removed and Calu-3 cells were equilibrated in 1 ml HBSS/HEPES at pH 7.4 in the basolateral chamber and 200 μL HBSS/HEPES, at pH 5.5 or pH 7.4, in the apical compartment. At $t = 0$, the apical medium was replaced by 200 μL chitosan, TMC20 or TMC60 formulations or by 200 μL HBSS/HEPES at pH 5.5 or pH 7.4 that served as controls. The TEER was measured at $t = 120$ and 60 before administration and $t = 0$, 30, 60, 90, 120, 150, 210 and 240 min after administration.

Octreotide was dissolved to an end concentration of 0.97 mM in 0.9% saline containing 1.5% chitosan (pH 5.5), TMC20 (pH 7.4) or TMC60 (pH 7.4). Control solutions contained octreotide in 0.9% saline of pH 5.5 and 7.4. From these solutions, 200 μL were instilled into the trachea of rats.

Intratracheal instillation was employed to ensure dose deposition in bronchial region of rats. Blood samples of 200 μL were collected initially, and every 30 min thereafter for 4 h. A group of 6 rats received a 200 μL intravenous bolus containing 190 μM octreotide in 0.9% saline in order to determine the absolute bioavailability of octreotide [109].

A significant, but reversible, reduction in TEER was observed in the presence of chitosan, TMC20 and TMC60, accompanied by 21-, 16- and 30-fold enhanced octreotide permeation, respectively. The bioavailability was enhanced by 2.4-, 2.5- and 3.9-fold, respectively. TMC60 induced a strong decrease in TEER, which suggested that pH, solubility and cationic charge density are important factors for paracellular barrier modulation [109]. A linear in vitro/in vivo correlation was observed between calculated absorption rates (R^2 = 0.93), which suggested that an analogous mechanism causes permeation enhancement by the polymers, both in vitro and in vivo. The permeation studies showed zero order kinetic profiles, suggesting that the polymers altered the structural integrity of tight junctions to facilitate passive paracellular diffusion of octreotide [109].

5.3. Citric Acid (Chelating Agent)

The effect of additives on the pulmonary absorption of insulin from solutions and dry powders was examined in male Sprague–Dawley rats [110]. Results from this study demonstrated a slight hypoglycemic effect in the absence of citric acid [110]. In the presence of citric acid, a significant and extended dose-dependent hypoglycemic effect was observed after insulin administration. Bioavailabilities of 43% and 57% were obtained with the citrate buffer solutions (0.19 mg/dose of citric acid in 0.1 mL) at pH 5 and 3, respectively. However, a greater hypoglycemic effect was achieved with citrate in dry powder than in solution. For the 0.2% (0.036 mg/dose) citric acid formulation, the blood glucose level rapidly decreased after insulin dry powder administration and the effect continued for the duration of the experiment [110]. An absolute bioavailability greater than 50% was achieved. LDH activity, which is a sensitive indicator of acute toxicity to lung cells, was as low for 0.2% citric acid as it was for PBS administration. This suggested that citric acid is a safe absorption enhancing additive. Possible action mechanisms proposed for citric acid included altered epithelium membrane integrity of the lungs, decreased insulin degradation by suppressing enzyme activity and phagocytic activity of alveolar macrophages [110].

5.4. Cyclodextrins (CDs)

An in vitro permeability study of chemically modified cyclodextrins (CDs), namely hydroxypropyl-β-cyclodextrin (HPβCD), hydroxypropyl-γ-cyclodextrin (HPγCD), randomly methylated β-cyclodextrin (Rameb), and 2-0-methyl-β-cyclodextrin (Crysmeb), was conducted using Calu-3 cells [111]. Results from this study showed a concentration-dependent increase in ^{14}C-mannitol flux across Calu-3 layers in the presence of each of the βCD derivatives, while no change in permeability was caused by HPγCD. Rameb was the only CD that enhanced mannitol transport at the lowest concentration (10 mM), whilst increasing mannitol flux 10-fold at the highest concentration (50 mM). Crysmeb and HPβCD were able to increase mannitol permeability at 25 and 50 mM. A reduction in TEER was observed for all increases in mannitol transport across the Calu-3 cell layers. Confocal microscopy revealed that Crysmeb (25 mM) was able to reversibly disrupt the tight junctional complexes [111].

Similarly, a previous study demonstrated that tetradecyl-β-maltoside (TDM) and dimethyl-β-cyclodextrin (DMβCD) could enhance the pulmonary absorption of low molecular weight heparin (LMWH) both in vitro and in vivo, mainly by acting on the membrane rather than interacting with the drug [115]. Calu-3 cells were used to conduct transport studies with ^{3}H-enoxaparin and ^{14}C-mannitol with or without different concentrations (0.0625%, 0.125%, and 0.25% (*w/v*)) of TDM or DMβCD at pH 7.4. TEER was measured during the transport experiments. For the in vivo pulmonary absorption studies, TDM and DMβCD were dissolved in saline to prepare 1% stock solutions of each. Enoxaparin, dalteparin (MW: 5000 Da), and unfractionated heparin (MW: 15,000–20,000 Da) were respectively mixed with either saline or TDM and DMβCD (0.0625%, 0.125%, and 0.25% (*w/v*)) to yield a final concentration of 15 U of anti-factor Xa activity per 100 μL formulation. These formulations (50 U/kg) were intratracheally or subcutaneously administered to rats for the absorption and bioavailability studies, respectively. Subsequently, blood samples (300 μL) were collected at 0, 15, 30, 60, 120, 240, 360, and 480 min. Enoxaparin absorption was determined by measuring plasma anti-factor Xa levels using a colorimetric assay, followed by standard pharmacokinetic analysis [115].

Results demonstrated a dose-dependent increase in enoxaparin in the presence of TDM or DMCD (0.0625–0.25%) in the apical fluid. With an increase in TDM concentration from 0.0625% to 0.25%, a statistically significant 4-fold increase in the P_{app} of enoxaparin was observed. Similar results were obtained with the transport of mannitol. Increase in the overall permeability of mannitol in the presence of TDM or DMβCD suggest that the action mechanism is loosening of tight junctions and therefore enhanced paracellular transport. This was confirmed with TEER values that were decreased to 51.9% and 70.7% of the initial value in the presence of 0.25% TDM and 0.25% DMβCD, respectively, after 2 h. However, the effect on TEER reduction was reversible, indicating that these bioenhancers are not likely to cause extensive damage or cellular toxicity in respiratory epithelial cells. Increased concentrations of TDM and DMβCD resulted in increased C_{max} and decreased T_{max} for enoxaparin. Altogether, results from the pharmacokinetic analysis suggested that TDM enhanced pulmonary absorption of enoxaparin. Bioavailability data showed that TDM was more efficacious in enhancing pulmonary absorption of LMWH when compared to DMβCD. Interestingly, pharmacokinetic profiles of pulmonary administered enoxaparin showed a quicker onset of anti-factor Xa activity compared to subcutaneous enoxaparin. Dalteparin also increased the anti-factor Xa levels rapidly and substantially in the presence of 0.125% TDM or DMβCD, whereas unfractionated heparin only produced a modest increase in anti-factor Xa activity. Reduced absorption of unfractionated heparin was observed, which could be due to the fact that it is larger and bulkier than LMWHs (enoxaparin and dalteparin). Results from this study are in agreement with previous studies on the nasal delivery of LMWHs [217]. Furthermore, comparative analysis demonstrated that the relative bioavailability of enoxaparin was 4- to 6-fold higher with pulmonary administration compared to nasally administered enoxaparin, and the amounts of bioenhancers required to produce therapeutic anti-factor Xa activity from pulmonary administered LMWHs were 2-5 times less [115].

5.5. Lanthanides

The absorption of insulin pre-administered or co-administered with lanthanides (Ln^{3+}), namely lanthanum, cerium and gadolinium, from rat lung was investigated by means of an in situ pulmonary absorption experiment [112]. Lanthanide ion solutions were prepared by dissolving the oxide in 5 mol/L HCl solution, followed by heating to deplete excess acid. Residue was then diluted with saline water and Ln^{3+} concentrations were determined. For pre-administered intratracheal drug delivery, Ln^{3+} (0.2 mg/kg) in 25 μL saline water (pH 7) was first injected, followed by insulin (1 IU/kg in 40 μL saline water, pH 7) administration 30 min later. In the other experiments, insulin and Ln^{3+} were co-administered. Blood samples (0.5 mL) were collected at predetermined time intervals after insulin administration, and serum insulin levels were measured [112].

Results demonstrated that serum insulin levels increased significantly in the presence of $CeCl_3$ and $GdCl_3$, with relative bioavailabilities of 57.9% and 59.5%, respectively. Furthermore, the anionic form of gadolinium showed greater enhancement of pulmonary insulin absorption than its cationic form (Gd^{3+}). The relative bioavailabilities of co-administered and pre-administered $GdCl_3$ were 80.1% and 59.5%, respectively. In comparison, $LaCl_3$ showed weak enhancement in pulmonary absorption of insulin, with a relative bioavailability of 30.9%, while $LuCl_3$ had no enhancing effect [112]. Co-administration of Gd^{3+} (0.2 mg/kg) with insulin (Fr = 80.1%) showed the greatest insulin absorption enhancement from the lung. Interestingly, higher concentrations of Gd^{3+} (0.6 mg/kg) showed decreased insulin absorption, possibly due to partial hydrolysis of Gd^{3+} upon entrance of the lung. The action mechanism proposed for Ln^{3+} is local mucosal tissue modulation, whereby lanthanides bind to membrane lipids and proteins to induce conformational changes and micropore formation to enhance the permeability of intracellular and exogenous matter flux [218,219]. Another action mechanism is the favorable absorption of insulin from the lung when a conformational change of insulin is induced when Ln^{3+} binds to zinc(II) binding sites. Additionally, increased interaction of insulin with its receptor in the cell membrane might be increased with insulin-bound Ln^{3+} in the serum [112].

5.6. Protease Inhibitors

The effects of protease inhibitors were evaluated as absorption enhancers for the pulmonary absorption of recombinant human colony-stimulating factor (rhG-CSF) in rats [108]. Protease inhibitors included (*p*-amidinophenyl) methanesulfonyl fluoride-HCl (*p*-APMSF), aprotinin and bestatin. The respective protease inhibitors (10 mM *p*-APMSF, 500 IU/mL aprotinin, 1 mM bestatin) were added to rhG-CSF solution (pH 6.5), after which the final rhG-CSF concentration was adjusted to 250 µg/mL. After intravenous, subcutaneous and intratracheal administration of the test solutions (containing protease inhibitors) and the control solution (rhG-CSF only), blood samples were collected periodically for 8h to determine the rhG-CSF plasma concentration by enzyme immunoassay.

The plasma rhG-CSF concentration was greatly enhanced in the presence of protease inhibitors, with *p*-APMSF showing the greatest enhancement with a ~3-fold increase in plasma rhG-CSF concentration from 3.9 to 11.7 ng/mL 30 min after intratracheal administration [108]. In order to determine the mechanism of enhanced absorption, a surfactant, polyoxyethylene 9-lauryl ether (Laureth-9) and the protease inhibitor *p*-APMSF were administered with rhG-CSF. The rhG-CSF concentration increased ~123-fold from 3.9 ± 1.4 ng/mL to 481.5 ± 96.7 ng/mL with the simultaneous intratracheal administration of Laureth-9 and *p*-APMSF. As a result, the proposed mechanism of action entails enhanced membrane permeation and inhibition of enzymatic degradation of rhG-CSF [108].

Similarly, a previous study demonstrated that the tracheal permeability of insulin was significantly increased by bestatin (aminopeptidase B and leucine aminopeptidase inhibitor), and aprotinin (trypsin and chymotrypsin inhibitor) [113]. Non-everted sac (2 cm) segments of excised rabbit trachea were used. Briefly, test solutions, with or without protease inhibitors (0.1 and 1 mM bestatin; 1000 and 10,000 KIU/mL aprotinin), in HEPES-buffered solution (0.2 mL, pH 7.4) was infused into the sac mucosal side, which was then placed in serosal medium consisting of oxygenated (O_2/CO_2, 95%:5%) HEPES (7 mL, pH 7.4). Samples (0.2 mL) were removed from the serosal fluid at pre-determined times for 150 min, and replaced with 0.2 mL fresh fluid. In another experiment, 10 µL samples were removed from the mucosal fluid at pre-determined times to calculate the degradation rate of insulin in the mucosal fluid of the trachea using the RIA method. Additionally, the peptidase activities in the trachea and jejunum were measured and compared to examine the enzymatic barrier for TRH and insulin permeation across rabbit tracheal epithelium [113].

Results demonstrated that the permeability of insulin (10 IU/mL) significantly increased in the presence of 1 mM bestatin and 10,000 KIU/mL aprotinin. However, the half-life of insulin was about 14 h, and only showed slight degradation by luminal secreted enzymes for the duration (150 min) of the experiment [113]. The tracheal and jejunal peptidases showed the following decreasing order of activity: DPP IV > Leu-aminopeptidase > cathepsin-B > trypsin. These four peptidases had significantly lower activities in the tracheal epithelial cells compared to jejunal epithelial cells. However, insulin was slightly degraded during tracheal permeation. It is suggested that insulin (MW: 5814 Da) is mainly transported via paracellular diffusion with slight metabolism by proteolytic enzymes such as trypsin-like and aminopeptidase-like enzymes through isolated rabbit tracheal epithelium. In summary, pulmonary administration of some peptide drugs, such as insulin, by intratracheal insufflation and instillation may contribute to the systemic absorption of these drugs [113].

5.7. Surfactants

The effects of surfactants of natural origin were evaluated as absorption enhancers for the pulmonary absorption of recombinant human colony-stimulating factor (rhG-CSF) in rats [108]. Surfactants included polyoxyethylene 9-lauryl ether (Laureth-9) and sodium glycocholate (SGC). Surfactants (1% *w/v*) were respectively added to rhG-CSF solution (pH 6.5), after which the final rhG-CSF concentration was adjusted to 250 μg/mL. After intravenous and intratracheal administration of the test solutions (containing surfactants) and the control solution (rhG-CSF only), blood samples were collected periodically for 8 h to determine the rhG-CSF plasma concentration by enzyme immunoassay.

The plasma rhG-CSF concentration was greatly enhanced in the presence of the surfactants. Relative bioavailabilities of rhG-CSF achieved with intravenous and intratracheal administration of Laureth-9 and SGC were 37% (intravenous), 88% (intratracheal), 84% (intravenous), and 197% (intratracheal), respectively [108]. In order to determine the mechanism of enhanced absorption, both the surfactant Laureth-9 and a protease inhibitor (*p*-amidinophenyl) methanesulfonyl fluoride-HCl (*p*-APMSF) were administered with rhG-CSF. The rhG-CSF concentration increased ~123-fold from 3.9 ± 1.4 ng/mL to 481.5 ± 96.7 ng/mL with the simultaneous intratracheal administration of Laureth-9 and *p*-APMSF. As a result, the proposed mechanism of action entails enhanced membrane permeation and inhibition of enzymatic degradation of rhG-CSF [108].

6. Conclusions

A comprehensive list of bioenhancers of natural origin is given in Table 1 with their mechanisms of action for four specific routes of drug administration, namely nasal, buccal, pulmonary, and oral. From all the described bioenhancing studies it is evident that inhibition of pre-systemic metabolism as well as efflux transporters and tight junction modulation is the predominant mechanism of drug bioavailability enhancement for the oral route of drug administration. Tight junction modulation and membrane disruption are the pre-dominant mechanisms of drug absorption enhancement for the nasal, buccal and pulmonary routes of administration. Since various factors can influence dissolution and absorption of drugs across different mucosal surfaces, studies on bioenhancers should be conducted for each specific drug for which bioavailability enhancement is needed. Although many studies have shown the potential of absorption enhancing agents, very few have been included in commercially available drugs.

Author Contributions: Conceptualization, J.H.H.; writing-original draft preparation, B.P., M.W., C.G., J.D.S., J.H.S. and J.H.H.; writing-review and editing, B.P. and J.H.H.; supervision, J.H.S., J.D.S. and J.H.H.

Acknowledgments: The authors would like to thank Marioné van der Merwe for drawing the anatomical figures.

References

1. Navia, M.A.; Chaturvedi, P.R. Design principles for orally bioavailable drugs. *Drug Discov. Today* **1996**, *1*, 179–189. [CrossRef]
2. Chillistone, S.; Hardman, J. Factors affecting drug absorption and distribution. *Anaesth. Intensive Care Med.* **2008**, *9*, 167–171. [CrossRef]
3. Klein, I.; Sarkadi, B.; Váradi, A. An inventory of the human abc proteins. *Biochim. Biophys. Acta* **1999**, *1461*, 237–262. [CrossRef]
4. Higgins, C.F.; Gottesman, M.M. Is the multidrug transporter a flippase? *Trends Biochem. Sci.* **1992**, *17*, 18–21. [CrossRef]
5. Sikic, B.I. Modulation of multidrug resistance: A paradigm for translational clinical research. *Oncology* **1999**, *13*, 183–187. [PubMed]
6. Juliano, R.L.; Ling, V. A surface glycoprotein modulating drug permeability in chinese hamster ovary cell mutants. *Biochim. Biophys. Acta* **1976**, *455*, 152–162. [CrossRef]

7. Maliepaard, M.; Scheffer, G.L.; Faneyte, I.F.; van Gastelen, M.A.; Pijnenborg, A.C.; Schinkel, A.H.; van de Vijver, M.J.; Scheper, R.J.; Schellens, J.H. Subcellular localization and distribution of the breast cancer resistance protein transporter in normal human tissues. *Cancer Res.* **2001**, *61*, 3458–3464.
8. Lazzari, P.; Serra, V.; Marcello, S.; Pira, M.; Mastinu, A. Metabolic side effects induced by olanzapine treatment are neutralized by cb1 receptor antagonist compounds co-administration in female rats. *Eur. Neuropsychopharmacol.* **2017**, *27*, 667–678. [CrossRef]
9. Dresser, G.K.; Spence, J.D.; Bailey, D.G. Pharmacokinetic-pharmacodynamic consequences and clinical relevance of cytochrome p450 3a4 inhibition. *Clin. Pharmacokinet.* **2000**, *38*, 41–57. [CrossRef]
10. Schinkel, A.H.; Jonker, J.W. Mammalian drug efflux transporters of the atp binding cassette (abc) family: An overview. *Adv. Drug Deliv. Rev.* **2012**, *64*, 138–153. [CrossRef]
11. Khajuria, A.; Thusu, N.; Zutshi, U. Piperine modulates permeability characteristics of intestine by inducing alterations in membrane dynamics: Influence on brush border membrane fluidity, ultrastructure and enzyme kinetics. *Phytomedicine* **2002**, *9*, 224–231. [CrossRef] [PubMed]
12. Kumar-Sarangi, M.; Chandra-Joshi, B.; Ritchie, B. Natural bioenhancers in drug delivery: An overview. *Puerto Rico Health Sci. J.* **2018**, *37*, 12–18.
13. Bitter, C.; Suter-Zimmermann, K.; Surber, C. Nasal drug delivery in humans. *Curr. Probl. Dermatol.* **2011**, *40*, 20–35. [PubMed]
14. Liu, Z.; Wang, S.; Hu, M. Oral absorption basics: Pathways, physico-chemical and biological factors affecting absorption. In *Developing Solid Oral Dosage Forms*; Elsevier: Amsterdam, The Netherlands, 2009; pp. 263–288.
15. Crowley, P.; Martini, L. Optimising drug delivery: The challenges and opportunities. *Ondrugdelivery* **2015**, *2015*, 4–11.
16. Mastinu, A.; Premoli, M.; Maccarinelli, G.; Grilli, M.; Memo, M.; Bonini, S.A. Melanocortin 4 receptor stimulation improves social deficits in mice through oxytocin pathway. *Neuropharmacology* **2018**, *133*, 366–374. [CrossRef] [PubMed]
17. Sarkar, M.A. Drug metabolism in the nasal mucosa. *Pharm. Res.* **1992**, *9*, 1–9. [CrossRef] [PubMed]
18. Johnson, P.H.; Quay, S.C. Advances in nasal drug delivery through tight junction technology. *Expert Opin. Drug Deliv.* **2005**, *2*, 281–298. [CrossRef]
19. Bonini, S.A.; Premoli, M.; Tambaro, S.; Kumar, A.; Maccarinelli, G.; Memo, M.; Mastinu, A. Cannabis sativa: A comprehensive ethnopharmacological review of a medicinal plant with a long history. *J. Ethnopharmacol.* **2018**, *227*, 300–315. [CrossRef]
20. Ojewole, E.; Mackraj, I.; Akhundov, K.; Hamman, J.; Viljoen, A.; Olivier, E.; Wesley-Smith, J.; Govender, T. Investigating the effect of aloe vera gel on the buccal permeability of didanosine. *Planta Med.* **2012**, *78*, 354–361. [CrossRef]
21. Portero, A.; Remuñán-López, C.; Nielsen, H.M. The potential of chitosan in enhancing peptide and protein absorption across the tr146 cell culture model—An in vitro model of the buccal epithelium. *Pharm. Res.* **2002**, *19*, 169–174. [CrossRef]
22. Şenel, S.; Kremer, M.; Kaş, S.; Wertz, P.; Hıncal, A.; Squier, C. Enhancing effect of chitosan on peptide drug delivery across buccal mucosa. *Biomaterials* **2000**, *21*, 2067–2071. [CrossRef]
23. Langoth, N.; Kahlbacher, H.; Schöffmann, G.; Schmerold, I.; Schuh, M.; Franz, S.; Kurka, P.; Bernkop-Schnürch, A. Thiolated chitosans: Design and in vivo evaluation of a mucoadhesive buccal peptide drug delivery system. *Pharm. Res.* **2006**, *23*, 573–579. [CrossRef] [PubMed]
24. Langoth, N.; Bernkop-Schnürch, A.; Kurka, P. In vitro evaluation of various buccal permeation enhancing systems for pacap (pituitary adenylate cyclase-activating polypeptide). *Pharm. Res.* **2005**, *22*, 2045. [CrossRef] [PubMed]
25. Tsutsumi, K.; Obata, Y.; Takayama, K.; Loftsson, T.; Nagai, T. Effect of cod-liver oil extract on the buccal permeation of ergotamine tartrate. *Drug Dev. Ind. Pharm.* **1998**, *24*, 757–762. [CrossRef] [PubMed]
26. Shojaei, A.H.; Khan, M.; Lim, G.; Khosravan, R. Transbuccal permeation of a nucleoside analog, dideoxycytidine: Effects of menthol as a permeation enhancer. *Int. J. Pharm.* **1999**, *192*, 139–146. [CrossRef]
27. Morishita, M.; Barichello, J.M.; Takayama, K.; Chiba, Y.; Tokiwa, S.; Nagai, T. Pluronic® f-127 gels incorporating highly purified unsaturated fatty acids for buccal delivery of insulin. *Int. J. Pharm.* **2001**, *212*, 289–293. [CrossRef]
28. Xiang, J.; Fang, X.; Li, X. Transbuccal delivery of 2′, 3′-dideoxycytidine: In vitro permeation study and histological investigation. *Int. J. Pharm.* **2002**, *231*, 57–66. [CrossRef]

29. Sandri, G.; Rossi, S.; Bonferoni, M.C.; Ferrari, F.; Zambito, Y.; Di Colo, G.; Caramella, C. Buccal penetration enhancement properties of n-trimethyl chitosan: Influence of quaternization degree on absorption of a high molecular weight molecule. *Int. J. Pharm.* **2005**, *297*, 146–155. [CrossRef] [PubMed]
30. Hinchcliffe, M.; Jabbal-Gill, I.; Smith, A. Effect of chitosan on the intranasal absorption of salmon calcitonin in sheep. *J. Pharm. Pharmacol.* **2005**, *57*, 681–687. [CrossRef]
31. Illum, L.; Watts, P.; Fisher, A.; Hinchcliffe, M.; Norbury, H.; Jabbal-Gill, I.; Nankervis, R.; Davis, S. Intranasal delivery of morphine. *J. Pharmacol. Exp. Ther.* **2002**, *301*, 391–400. [CrossRef] [PubMed]
32. Krauland, A.H.; Guggi, D.; Bernkop-Schnürch, A. Thiolated chitosan microparticles: A vehicle for nasal peptide drug delivery. *Int. J. Pharm.* **2006**, *307*, 270–277. [CrossRef] [PubMed]
33. Hamman, J.; Stander, M.; Kotze, A. Effect of the degree of quaternisation of *N*-trimethyl chitosan chloride on absorption enhancement: In vivo evaluation in rat nasal epithelia. *Int. J. Pharm.* **2002**, *232*, 235–242. [CrossRef]
34. Mizuma, T.; Awazu, S. Dietary polyphenols (−)-epicatechin and chrysin inhibit intestinal glucuronidation metabolism to increase drug absorption. *J. Pharm. Sci.* **2004**, *93*, 2407–2410. [CrossRef] [PubMed]
35. Beneke, C.; Viljoen, A.; Hamman, J.H. In vitro drug absorption enhancement effects of aloe vera and aloe ferox. *Sci Pharm.* **2012**, *80*, 475–486. [CrossRef] [PubMed]
36. Chen, W.; Lu, Z.; Viljoen, A.; Hamman, J. Intestinal drug transport enhancement by aloe vera. *Planta Med.* **2009**, *75*, 587–595. [CrossRef] [PubMed]
37. Vinson, J.A.; Al Kharrat, H.; Andreoli, L. Effect of aloe vera preparations on the human bioavailability of vitamins c and e. *Phytomedicine* **2005**, *12*, 760–765. [CrossRef] [PubMed]
38. Wallis, L.; Malan, M.; Gouws, C.; Steyn, D.; Ellis, S.; Abay, E.; Wiesner, L.; P Otto, D.; Hamman, J. Evaluation of isolated fractions of aloe vera gel materials on indinavir pharmacokinetics: In vitro and in vivo studies. *Curr. Drug Deliv.* **2016**, *13*, 471–480. [CrossRef]
39. Yago, M.R.; Frymoyer, A.; Benet, L.Z.; Smelick, G.S.; Frassetto, L.A.; Ding, X.; Dean, B.; Salphati, L.; Budha, N.; Jin, J.Y. The use of betaine hcl to enhance dasatinib absorption in healthy volunteers with rabeprazole-induced hypochlorhydria. *AAPS J.* **2014**, *16*, 1358–1365. [CrossRef]
40. Choudhary, N.; Khajuria, V.; Gillani, Z.H.; Tandon, V.R.; Arora, E. Effect of carum carvi, a herbal bioenhancer on pharmacokinetics of antitubercular drugs: A study in healthy human volunteers. *Perspect. Clin. Res.* **2014**, *5*, 80.
41. Rosenthal, R.; Günzel, D.; Finger, C.; Krug, S.M.; Richter, J.F.; Schulzke, J.-D.; Fromm, M.; Amasheh, S. The effect of chitosan on transcellular and paracellular mechanisms in the intestinal epithelial barrier. *Biomaterials* **2012**, *33*, 2791–2800. [CrossRef]
42. Schipper, N.G.; Olsson, S.; Hoogstraate, J.A.; Vårum, K.M.; Artursson, P. Chitosans as absorption enhancers for poorly absorbable drugs 2: Mechanism of absorption enhancement. *Pharm. Res.* **1997**, *14*, 923–929. [CrossRef] [PubMed]
43. Bernkop-Schnürch, A.; Guggi, D.; Pinter, Y. Thiolated chitosans: Development and in vitro evaluation of a mucoadhesive, permeation enhancing oral drug delivery system. *J. Control. Release* **2004**, *94*, 177–186. [CrossRef] [PubMed]
44. Krauland, A.H.; Guggi, D.; Bernkop-Schnürch, A. Oral insulin delivery: The potential of thiolated chitosan-insulin tablets on non-diabetic rats. *J. Control. Release* **2004**, *95*, 547–555. [CrossRef] [PubMed]
45. Basu, N.K.; Kole, L.; Kubota, S.; Owens, I.S. Human udp-glucuronosyltransferases show atypical metabolism of mycophenolic acid and inhibition by curcumin. *Drug Metab. Dispos.* **2004**, *32*, 768–773. [CrossRef] [PubMed]
46. Pavithra, B.; Prakash, N.; Jayakumar, K. Modification of pharmacokinetics of norfloxacin following oral administration of curcumin in rabbits. *J. Vet. Sci.* **2009**, *10*, 293–297. [CrossRef] [PubMed]
47. Zhang, W.; Lim, L.-Y. Effects of spice constituents on p-gp-mediated transport and cyp3a4-mediated metabolism in vitro. *Drug Metab. Dispos.* **2008**, *36*, 1283–1290. [CrossRef] [PubMed]
48. Zhang, W.; Tan, T.M.C.; Lim, L.-Y. Impact of curcumin-induced changes in p-glycoprotein and cyp3a expression on the pharmacokinetics of peroral celiprolol and midazolam in rats. *Drug Metab. Dispos.* **2007**, *35*, 110–115. [CrossRef]
49. Lee, J.H.; Shin, Y.-J.; Oh, J.-H.; Lee, Y.-J. Pharmacokinetic interactions of clopidogrel with quercetin, telmisartan, and cyclosporine a in rats and dogs. *Arch. Pharm. Res.* **2012**, *35*, 1831–1837. [CrossRef]

50. Yoo, H.H.; Lee, M.; Chung, H.J.; Lee, S.K.; Kim, D.-H. Effects of diosmin, a flavonoid glycoside in citrus fruits, on p-glycoprotein-mediated drug efflux in human intestinal caco-2 cells. *J. Agric. Food Chem.* **2007**, *55*, 7620–7625. [CrossRef]
51. Li, X.; Hu, J.; Wang, B.; Sheng, L.; Liu, Z.; Yang, S.; Li, Y. Inhibitory effects of herbal constituents on p-glycoprotein in vitro and in vivo: Herb–drug interactions mediated via p-gp. *Toxicol. Appl. Pharmacol.* **2014**, *275*, 163–175. [CrossRef]
52. Ghosal, S. Delivery System for Pharmaceutical, Nutritional and Cosmetic Ingredients. U.S. Patent 6,558,712, 6 May 2003.
53. Wacher, V.J.; Benet, L.Z. Use of Gallic Acid Esters to Increase Bioavailability of Orally Administered Pharmaceutical Compounds. U.S. Patent 5,962,522, 5 October 1999.
54. Lambert, J.D.; Kwon, S.-J.; Ju, J.; Bose, M.; Lee, M.-J.; Hong, J.; Hao, X.; Yang, C.S. Effect of genistein on the bioavailability and intestinal cancer chemopreventive activity of (−)-epigallocatechin-3-gallate. *Carcinogenesis* **2008**, *29*, 2019–2024. [CrossRef] [PubMed]
55. Li, X.; Choi, J.-S. Effect of genistein on the pharmacokinetics of paclitaxel administered orally or intravenously in rats. *Int. J. Pharm.* **2007**, *337*, 188–193. [CrossRef] [PubMed]
56. Ayyanna, C.; Mohan Rao, G.; Sasikala, M.; Somasekhar, P.; Arun Kumar, N.; Pradeep Kumar, M. Absorption enhancement studies of metformin hydrochloride by using tribulus terrestris plant extract. *Int. J. Pharm. Technol.* **2012**, *4*, 4119–4125.
57. Kumar, A.; Bansal, M. Formulation and evaluation of antidiabetic tablets: Effect of absorption enhancser. *World J. Pharm. Res.* **2014**, *3*, 1426–1445.
58. Dresser, G.; Bailey, D. The effects of fruit juices on drug disposition: A new model for drug interactions. *Eur. J. Clin. Investig.* **2003**, *33*, 10–16. [CrossRef]
59. Rekha, M.; Sharma, C.P. Synthesis and evaluation of lauryl succinyl chitosan particles towards oral insulin delivery and absorption. *J. Control. Release* **2009**, *135*, 144–151. [CrossRef]
60. Petyaev, I.M. Improvement of hepatic bioavailability as a new step for the future of statin. *Arch. Med Sci.* **2015**, *11*, 406. [CrossRef]
61. Patil, S.; Dash, R.P.; Anandjiwala, S.; Nivsarkar, M. Simultaneous quantification of berberine and lysergol by hplc-uv: Evidence that lysergol enhances the oral bioavailability of berberine in rats. *Biomed. Chromatogr.* **2012**, *26*, 1170–1175. [CrossRef]
62. Shukla, M.; Malik, M.; Jaiswal, S.; Sharma, A.; Tanpula, D.; Goyani, R.; Lal, J. A mechanistic investigation of the bioavailability enhancing potential of lysergol, a novel bioenhancer, using curcumin. *RSC Adv.* **2016**, *6*, 58933–58942. [CrossRef]
63. Pal, A.; Bawankule, D.U.; Darokar, M.P.; Gupta, S.C.; Arya, J.S.; Shanker, K.; Gupta, M.M.; Yadav, N.P.; Singh Khanuja, S.P. Influence of moringa oleifera on pharmacokinetic disposition of rifampicin using hplc-pda method: A pre-clinical study. *Biomed. Chromatogr.* **2011**, *25*, 641–645. [CrossRef]
64. Choi, J.-S.; Han, H.-K. Enhanced oral exposure of diltiazem by the concomitant use of naringin in rats. *Int. J. Pharm.* **2005**, *305*, 122–128. [CrossRef] [PubMed]
65. Choi, J.-S.; Kang, K.W. Enhanced tamoxifen bioavailability after oral administration of tamoxifen in rats pretreated with naringin. *Arch. Pharm. Res.* **2008**, *31*, 1631–1636. [CrossRef] [PubMed]
66. Choi, J.-S.; Shin, S.-C. Enhanced paclitaxel bioavailability after oral coadministration of paclitaxel prodrug with naringin to rats. *Int. J. Pharm.* **2005**, *292*, 149–156. [CrossRef] [PubMed]
67. Lassoued, M.A.; Sfar, S.; Bouraoui, A.; Khemiss, F. Absorption enhancement studies of clopidogrel hydrogen sulphate in rat everted gut sacs. *J. Pharm. Pharmacol.* **2012**, *64*, 541–552. [CrossRef] [PubMed]
68. Yeum, C.-H.; Choi, J.-S. Effect of naringin pretreatment on bioavailability of verapamil in rabbits. *Arch. Pharm. Res.* **2006**, *29*, 102. [CrossRef] [PubMed]
69. Raiman, J.; Törmälehto, S.; Yritys, K.; Junginger, H.E.; Mönkkönen, J. Effects of various absorption enhancers on transport of clodronate through caco-2 cells. *Int. J. Pharm.* **2003**, *261*, 129–136. [CrossRef]
70. Wacher, V.J.; Wong, S.; Wong, H.T. Peppermint oil enhances cyclosporine oral bioavailability in rats: Comparison with D-α-tocopheryl poly (ethylene glycol 1000) succinate (tpgs) and ketoconazole. *J. Pharm. Sci.* **2002**, *91*, 77–90. [CrossRef] [PubMed]
71. Badmaev, V.; Majeed, M.; Norkus, E.P. Piperine, an alkaloid derived from black pepper increases serum response of β-carotene during 14-days of oral β-carotene supplementation. *Nutr. Res.* **1999**, *19*, 381–388. [CrossRef]

72. Badmaev, V.; Majeed, M.; Prakash, L. Piperine derived from black pepper increases the plasma levels of coenzyme q10 following oral supplementation. *J. Nutr. Biochem.* **2000**, *11*, 109–113. [CrossRef]
73. Bajad, S.; Bedi, K.; Singla, A.; Johri, R. Piperine inhibits gastric emptying and gastrointestinal transit in rats and mice. *Planta Med.* **2001**, *67*, 176–179. [CrossRef]
74. Bano, G.; Raina, R.; Zutshi, U.; Bedi, K.; Johri, R.; Sharma, S. Effect of piperine on bioavailability and pharmacokinetics of propranolol and theophylline in healthy volunteers. *Eur. J. Clin. Pharmacol.* **1991**, *41*, 615–617. [CrossRef]
75. Gupta, S.; Bansal, P.; Bhardwaj, R.; Velpandian, T. Comparative anti-nociceptive, anti-inflammatory and toxicity profile of nimesulide vs nimesulide and piperine combination. *Pharmacol. Res.* **2000**, *41*, 657–662. [CrossRef]
76. Jin, M.J.; Han, H.K. Effect of piperine, a major component of black pepper, on the intestinal absorption of fexofenadine and its implication on food–drug interaction. *J. Food Sci.* **2010**, *75*, H93–H96. [CrossRef]
77. Johnson, J.J.; Nihal, M.; Siddiqui, I.A.; Scarlett, C.O.; Bailey, H.H.; Mukhtar, H.; Ahmad, N. Enhancing the bioavailability of resveratrol by combining it with piperine. *Mol. Nutr. Food Res.* **2011**, *55*, 1169–1176. [CrossRef]
78. Kasibhatta, R.; Naidu, M. Influence of piperine on the pharmacokinetics of nevirapine under fasting conditions. *Drugs R D* **2007**, *8*, 383–391. [CrossRef]
79. Lambert, J.D.; Hong, J.; Kim, D.H.; Mishin, V.M.; Yang, C.S. Piperine enhances the bioavailability of the tea polyphenol (−)-epigallocatechin-3-gallate in mice. *J. Nutr.* **2004**, *134*, 1948–1952. [CrossRef]
80. Mujumdar, A.; Dhuley, J.; Deshmukh, V.; Raman, P.; Thorat, S.; Naik, S. Effect of piperine on pentobarbitone induced hypnosis in rats. *Indian J. Exp. Boil.* **1990**, *28*, 486–487.
81. Pattanaik, S.; Hota, D.; Prabhakar, S.; Kharbanda, P.; Pandhi, P. Pharmacokinetic interaction of single dose of piperine with steady-state carbamazepine in epilepsy patients. *Phytother. Res. Int. J. Devoted Pharmacol. Toxicol. Eval. Nat. Prod. Deriv.* **2009**, *23*, 1281–1286. [CrossRef]
82. Sama, V.; Nadipelli, M.; Yenumula, P.; Bommineni, M.; Mullangi, R. Effect of piperine on antihyperglycemic activity and pharmacokinetic profile of nateglinide. *Arzneimittelforschung* **2012**, *62*, 384–388. [CrossRef]
83. Shoba, G.; Joy, D.; Joseph, T.; Majeed, M.; Rajendran, R.; Srinivas, P. Influence of piperine on the pharmacokinetics of curcumin in animals and human volunteers. *Planta Med.* **1998**, *64*, 353–356. [CrossRef]
84. Singh, M.; Varshneya, C.; Telang, R.; Srivastava, A. Alteration of pharmacokinetics of oxytetracycline following oral administration of piper longum in hens. *J. Vet. Sci.* **2005**, *6*, 197–200.
85. Babu, P.R.; Babu, K.N.; Peter, P.H.; Rajesh, K.; Babu, P.J. Influence of quercetin on the pharmacokinetics of ranolazine in rats and in vitro models. *Drug Dev. Ind. Pharm.* **2013**, *39*, 873–879. [CrossRef]
86. Bansal, T.; Awasthi, A.; Jaggi, M.; Khar, R.K.; Talegaonkar, S. Pre-clinical evidence for altered absorption and biliary excretion of irinotecan (cpt-11) in combination with quercetin: Possible contribution of p-glycoprotein. *Life Sci.* **2008**, *83*, 250–259. [CrossRef]
87. Challa, V.R.; Ravindra Babu, P.; Challa, S.R.; Johnson, B.; Maheswari, C. Pharmacokinetic interaction study between quercetin and valsartan in rats and in vitro models. *Drug Dev. Ind. Pharm.* **2013**, *39*, 865–872. [CrossRef]
88. Choi, J.S.; Han, H.K. The effect of quercetin on the pharmacokinetics of verapamil and its major metabolite, norverapamil, in rabbits. *J. Pharm. Pharmacol.* **2004**, *56*, 1537–1542. [CrossRef]
89. Choi, J.-S.; Li, X. Enhanced diltiazem bioavailability after oral administration of diltiazem with quercetin to rabbits. *Int. J. Pharm.* **2005**, *297*, 1–8. [CrossRef]
90. Choi, J.-S.; Piao, Y.-J.; Kang, K.W. Effects of quercetin on the bioavailability of doxorubicin in rats: Role of cyp3a4 and p-gp inhibition by quercetin. *Arch. Pharm. Res.* **2011**, *34*, 607–613. [CrossRef]
91. Kim, K.-A.; Park, P.-W.; Park, J.-Y. Short-term effect of quercetin on the pharmacokinetics of fexofenadine, a substrate of p-glycoprotein, in healthy volunteers. *Eur. J. Clin. Pharmacol.* **2009**, *65*, 609–614. [CrossRef]
92. Li, X.; Choi, J.-S. Effects of quercetin on the pharmacokinetics of etoposide after oral or intravenous administration of etoposide in rats. *Anticancer. Res.* **2009**, *29*, 1411–1415.
93. Nijveldt, R.J.; Van Nood, E.; Van Hoorn, D.E.; Boelens, P.G.; Van Norren, K.; Van Leeuwen, P.A. Flavonoids: A review of probable mechanisms of action and potential applications. *Am. J. Clin. Nutr.* **2001**, *74*, 418–425. [CrossRef]

94. Scambia, G.; Ranelletti, F.; Panici, P.B.; De Vincenzo, R.; Bonanno, G.; Ferrandina, G.; Piantelli, M.; Bussa, S.; Rumi, C.; Cianfriglia, M. Quercetin potentiates the effect of adriamycin in a multidrug-resistant mcf-7 human breast-cancer cell line: P-glycoprotein as a possible target. *Cancer Chemother. Pharmacol.* **1994**, *34*, 459–464. [CrossRef]
95. Shin, S.-C.; Choi, J.-S.; Li, X. Enhanced bioavailability of tamoxifen after oral administration of tamoxifen with quercetin in rats. *Int. J. Pharm.* **2006**, *313*, 144–149. [CrossRef]
96. Umathe, S.N.; Dixit, P.V.; Bansod, K.U.; Wanjari, M.M. Quercetin pretreatment increases the bioavailability of pioglitazone in rats: Involvement of cyp3a inhibition. *Biochem. Pharmacol.* **2008**, *75*, 1670–1676. [CrossRef]
97. Chan, K.; Liu, Z.Q.; Jiang, Z.H.; Zhou, H.; Wong, Y.F.; Xu, H.-X.; Liu, L. The effects of sinomenine on intestinal absorption of paeoniflorin by the everted rat gut sac model. *J. Ethnopharmacol.* **2006**, *103*, 425–432. [CrossRef]
98. Bedada, S.K.; Yellu, N.R.; Neerati, P. Effect of resveratrol treatment on the pharmacokinetics of diclofenac in healthy human volunteers. *Phytother. Res.* **2016**, *30*, 397–401. [CrossRef]
99. Jia, Y.; Liu, Z.; Wang, C.; Meng, Q.; Huo, X.; Liu, Q.; Sun, H.; Sun, P.; Yang, X.; Ma, X. P-gp, mrp2 and oat1/oat3 mediate the drug-drug interaction between resveratrol and methotrexate. *Toxicol. Appl. Pharmacol.* **2016**, *306*, 27–35. [CrossRef]
100. Liu, Z.Q.; Zhou, H.; Liu, L.; Jiang, Z.H.; Wong, Y.F.; Xie, Y.; Cai, X.; Xu, H.X.; Chan, K. Influence of co-administrated sinomenine on pharmacokinetic fate of paeoniflorin in unrestrained conscious rats. *J. Ethnopharmacol.* **2005**, *99*, 61–67. [CrossRef]
101. Lv, X.-Y.; Li, J.; Zhang, M.; Wang, C.-M.; Fan, Z.; Wang, C.-Y.; Chen, L. Enhancement of sodium caprate on intestine absorption and antidiabetic action of berberine. *AAPS Pharm.* **2010**, *11*, 372–382. [CrossRef]
102. Yu, J.-N.; Zhu, Y.; Wang, L.; Peng, M.; Tong, S.-S.; Cao, X.; Qiu, H.; Xu, X.-M. Enhancement of oral bioavailability of the poorly water-soluble drug silybin by sodium cholate/phospholipid-mixed micelles. *Acta Pharmacol. Sin.* **2010**, *31*, 759. [CrossRef]
103. Chen, Y.; Lu, Y.; Chen, J.; Lai, J.; Sun, J.; Hu, F.; Wu, W. Enhanced bioavailability of the poorly water-soluble drug fenofibrate by using liposomes containing a bile salt. *Int. J. Pharm.* **2009**, *376*, 153–160. [CrossRef]
104. Wang, H.-J.; Pao, L.-H.; Hsiong, C.-H.; Shih, T.-Y.; Lee, M.-S.; Hu, O.Y.-P. Dietary flavonoids modulate cyp2c to improve drug oral bioavailability and their qualitative/quantitative structure–activity relationship. *AAPS J.* **2014**, *16*, 258–268. [CrossRef]
105. Hamman, J.; Schultz, C.; Kotzé, A. N-trimethyl chitosan chloride: Optimum degree of quaternization for drug absorption enhancement across epithelial cells. *Drug Dev. Ind. Pharm.* **2003**, *29*, 161–172. [CrossRef]
106. Kotzé, A.R.; Lueβen, H.L.; de Leeuw, B.J.; Verhoef, J.C.; Junginger, H.E. N-trimethyl chitosan chloride as a potential absorption enhancer across mucosal surfaces: In vitro evaluation in intestinal epithelial cells (caco-2). *Pharm. Res.* **1997**, *14*, 1197–1202. [CrossRef]
107. Cox, D.S.; Raje, S.; Gao, H.; Salama, N.N.; Eddington, N.D. Enhanced permeability of molecular weight markers and poorly bioavailable compounds across caco-2 cell monolayers using the absorption enhancer, zonula occludens toxin. *Pharm. Res.* **2002**, *19*, 1680–1688. [CrossRef]
108. Machida, M.; Hayashi, M.; Awazu, S. The effects of absorption enhancers on the pulmonary absorption of recombinant human granulocyte colony-stimulating factor (rhg-csf) in rats. *Boil. Pharm. Bull.* **2000**, *23*, 84–86. [CrossRef]
109. Florea, B.I.; Thanou, M.; Junginger, H.E.; Borchard, G. Enhancement of bronchial octreotide absorption by chitosan and n-trimethyl chitosan shows linear in vitro/in vivo correlation. *J. Control. Release* **2006**, *110*, 353–361. [CrossRef]
110. Todo, H.; Okamoto, H.; Iida, K.; Danjo, K. Effect of additives on insulin absorption from intratracheally administered dry powders in rats. *Int. J. Pharm.* **2001**, *220*, 101–110. [CrossRef]
111. Salem, L.B.; Bosquillon, C.; Dailey, L.; Delattre, L.; Martin, G.; Evrard, B.; Forbes, B. Sparing methylation of β-cyclodextrin mitigates cytotoxicity and permeability induction in respiratory epithelial cell layers in vitro. *J. Control. Release* **2009**, *136*, 110–116. [CrossRef]
112. Shen, Z.-C.; Cheng, Y.; Zhang, Q.; Wei, S.-L.; Li, R.-C.; Wang, K. Lanthanides enhance pulmonary absorption of insulin. *Boil. Trace Element Res.* **2000**, *75*, 215–225. [CrossRef]
113. Morimoto, K.; Uehara, Y.; Iwanaga, K.; Kakemi, M. Effects of sodium glycocholate and protease inhibitors on permeability of trh and insulin across rabbit trachea. *Pharm. Acta Helv.* **2000**, *74*, 411–415. [CrossRef]
114. Johansson, F.; Hjertberg, E.; Eirefelt, S.; Tronde, A.; Bengtsson, U.H. Mechanisms for absorption enhancement of inhaled insulin by sodium taurocholate. *Eur. J. Pharm. Sci.* **2002**, *17*, 63–71. [CrossRef]

115. Yang, T.; Mustafa, F.; Bai, S.; Ahsan, F. Pulmonary delivery of low molecular weight heparins. *Pharm. Res.* **2004**, *21*, 2009–2016. [CrossRef]
116. Martin, G.P.; El-Hariri, L.M.; Marriott, C. Bile salt-and lysophosphatidylcholine-induced membrane damage in human erythrocytes. *J. Pharm. Pharmacol.* **1992**, *44*, 646–650. [CrossRef]
117. Gibaldi, M.; Feldman, S. Mechanisms of surfactant effects on drug absorption. *J. Pharm. Sci.* **1970**, *59*, 579–589. [CrossRef]
118. Bernkop-Schnürch, A.; Hornof, M.; Zoidl, T. Thiolated polymers—Thiomers: Synthesis and in vitro evaluation of chitosan–2-iminothiolane conjugates. *Int. J. Pharm.* **2003**, *260*, 229–237. [CrossRef]
119. Bechgaard, E.; Gizurarson, S.; Hjortkjær, R.K.; Sørensen, A.R. Intranasal administration of insulin to rabbits using glycofurol as an absorption promoter. *Int. J. Pharm.* **1996**, *128*, 287–289. [CrossRef]
120. Gizurarson, S.; Marriott, C.; Martin, G.P.; Bechgaard, E. The influence of insulin and some excipients used in nasal insulin preparations on mucociliary clearance. *Int. J. Pharm.* **1990**, *65*, 243–247. [CrossRef]
121. Sørensen, A.; Drejer, K.; Engesgaard, A.; Guldhammer, B.; Hansen, P.; Hjortekjaer, R.; Mygind, N. Rabbit model for studies of nasal administration of insulin and glucagon. *Diabet. Res. Clin. Pract. Suppl.* **1988**, *1*, S165.
122. Bagger, M.A.; Nielsen, H.W.; Bechgaard, E. Nasal bioavailability of peptide T in rabbits: Absorption enhancement by sodium glycocholate and glycofurol. *Eur. J. Pharm. Sci.* **2001**, *14*, 69–74. [CrossRef]
123. Shinichiro, H.; Takatsuka, Y.; Hiroyuki, M. Mechanisms for the enhancement of the nasal absorption of insulin by surfactants. *Int. J. Pharm.* **1981**, *9*, 173–184. [CrossRef]
124. Pontiroli, A.; Alberetto, M.; Pajetta, E.; Calderara, A.; Pozza, G. Human insulin plus sodium glycocholate in a nasal spray formulation: Improved bioavailability and effectiveness in normal subjects. *Diabete Metab.* **1987**, *13*, 441–443.
125. Pontiroli, A.; Alberetto, M.; Calderara, A.; Pajetta, E.; Pozza, G. Nasal administration of glucagon and human calcitonin to healthy subjects: A comparison of powders and spray solutions and of different enhancing agents. *Eur. J. Clin. Pharmacol.* **1989**, *37*, 427–430. [CrossRef] [PubMed]
126. Aungst, B.J.; Rogers, N.J.; Shefter, E. Comparison of nasal, rectal, buccal, sublingual and intramuscular insulin efficacy and the effects of a bile salt absorption promoter. *J. Pharmacol. Exp. Ther.* **1988**, *244*, 23–27. [PubMed]
127. Lee, V.H. Mucosal penetration enhancers for facilitation of peptide and protein drug absorption. *Crit. Rev. Ther. Drug Carr. Syst.* **1991**, *8*, 91–192.
128. Illum, L. Nasal drug delivery: New developments and strategies. *Drug Discov. Today* **2002**, *7*, 1184–1189. [CrossRef]
129. Illum, L.; Farraj, N.F.; Davis, S.S. Chitosan as a novel nasal delivery system for peptide drugs. *Pharm. Res.* **1994**, *11*, 1186–1189. [CrossRef] [PubMed]
130. Casettari, L.; Illum, L. Chitosan in nasal delivery systems for therapeutic drugs. *J. Control. Release* **2014**, *190*, 189–200. [CrossRef]
131. Kotze, A.; Luessen, H.; De Boer, A.; Verhoef, J.; Junginger, H. Chitosan for enhanced intestinal permeability: Prospects for derivatives soluble in neutral and basic environments. *Eur. J. Pharm. Sci.* **1999**, *7*, 145–151. [CrossRef]
132. Farraj, N.; Johansen, B.; Davis, S.; Illum, L. Nasal administration of insulin using bioadhesive microspheres as a delivery system. *J. Control. Release* **1990**, *13*, 253–261. [CrossRef]
133. Illum, L. Chitosan and its use as a pharmaceutical excipient. *Pharm. Res.* **1998**, *15*, 1326–1331. [CrossRef]
134. Illum, L.; Fisher, A.; Jabbal-Gill, I.; Davis, S. Bioadhesive starch microspheres and absorption enhancing agents act synergistically to enhance the nasal absorption of polypeptides. *Int. J. Pharm.* **2001**, *222*, 109–119. [CrossRef]
135. Björk, E.; Edman, P. Characterization of degradable starch microspheres as a nasal delivery system for drugs. *Int. J. Pharm.* **1990**, *62*, 187–192. [CrossRef]
136. Sallee, V.L.; Dietschy, J.M. Determinants of intestinal mucosal uptake of short-and medium-chain fatty acids and alcohols. *J. Lipid Res.* **1973**, *14*, 475–484.
137. Westergaard, H.; Dietschy, J.M. The mechanism whereby bile acid micelles increase the rate of fatty acid and cholesterol uptake into the intestinal mucosal cell. *J. Clin. Investig.* **1976**, *58*, 97–108. [CrossRef] [PubMed]
138. Wilson, F.A. Intestinal transport of bile acids. *Am. J. Physiol.-Gastrointest. Liver Physiol.* **1981**, *241*, G83–G92. [CrossRef] [PubMed]

139. Jalali, A.; Moghimipour, E.; Akhgari, A. Enhancing effect of bile salts on gastrointestinal absorption of insulin. *Trop. J. Pharm. Res.* **2014**, *13*, 1797–1802. [CrossRef]
140. Hersey, S.; Jackson, R. Effect of bile salts on nasal permeability in vitro. *J. Pharm. Sci.* **1987**, *76*, 876–879. [CrossRef]
141. Scott-Moncrieff, J.C.; Shao, Z.; Mitra, A.K. Enhancement of intestinal insulin absorption by bile salt–fatty acid mixed micelles in dogs. *J. Pharm. Sci.* **1994**, *83*, 1465–1469. [CrossRef] [PubMed]
142. Ali, B.; Amin, S.; Ahmad, J.; Ali, A.; Ali, M.; Mir, S.R. Bioavailability enhancement studies of amoxicillin with nigella. *Indian J. Med Res.* **2012**, *135*, 555. [PubMed]
143. Sinha, V.; Kaur, M.P. Permeation enhancers for transdermal drug delivery. *Drug Dev. Ind. Pharm.* **2000**, *26*, 1131–1140. [CrossRef]
144. Al-Jenoobi, F.; Al-Suwayeh, S.; Muzaffar, I.; Alam, M.A.; Al-Kharfy, K.M.; Korashy, H.M.; Al-Mohizea, A.M.; Ahad, A.; Raish, M. Effects of nigella sativa and lepidium sativum on cyclosporine pharmacokinetics. *BioMed Res. Int.* **2013**, *2013*. [CrossRef] [PubMed]
145. Bedada, S.K.; Appani, R.; Boga, P.K. Capsaicin pretreatment enhanced the bioavailability of fexofenadine in rats by p-glycoprotein modulation: In vitro, in situ and in vivo evaluation. *Drug Dev. Ind. Pharm.* **2017**, *43*, 932–938. [CrossRef] [PubMed]
146. Tatiraju, D.V.; Bagade, V.B.; Karambelkar, P.J.; Jadhav, V.M.; Kadam, V. Natural bioenhancers: An overview. *J. Pharm. Phytochem.* **2013**, *2*, 55–60.
147. Survase, S.A.; Kagliwal, L.D.; Annapure, U.S.; Singhal, R.S. Cyclosporin A—A review on fermentative production, downstream processing and pharmacological applications. *Biotechnol. Adv.* **2011**, *29*, 418–435. [CrossRef] [PubMed]
148. Thanou, M.; Verhoef, J.; Junginger, H. Oral drug absorption enhancement by chitosan and its derivatives. *Adv. Drug Deliv. Rev.* **2001**, *52*, 117–126. [CrossRef]
149. Prego, C.; Torres, D.; Alonso, M.J. The potential of chitosan for the oral administration of peptides. *Expert Opin. Drug Deliv.* **2005**, *2*, 843–854. [CrossRef] [PubMed]
150. Lueßen, H.L.; de Leeuw, B.J.; Langemeÿer, M.W.; de Boer, A.B.G.; Verhoef, J.C.; Junginger, H.E. Mucoadhesive polymers in peroral peptide drug delivery. Vi. Carbomer and chitosan improve the intestinal absorption of the peptide drug buserelin in vivo. *Pharm. Res.* **1996**, *13*, 1668–1672. [CrossRef]
151. Schipper, N.G.; Vårum, K.M.; Artursson, P. Chitosans as absorption enhancers for poorly absorbable drugs. 1: Influence of molecular weight and degree of acetylation on drug transport across human intestinal epithelial (caco-2) cells. *Pharm. Res.* **1996**, *13*, 1686–1692. [CrossRef]
152. Kotzé, A.F.; Lueßen, H.L.; de Leeuw, B.J.; Verhoef, J.C.; Junginger, H.E. Comparison of the effect of different chitosan salts and n-trimethyl chitosan chloride on the permeability of intestinal epithelial cells (caco-2). *J. Control. Release* **1998**, *51*, 35–46. [CrossRef]
153. Borchard, G.; Lueβen, H.L.; de Boer, A.G.; Verhoef, J.C.; Lehr, C.-M.; Junginger, H.E. The potential of mucoadhesive polymers in enhancing intestinal peptide drug absorption. Iii: Effects of chitosan-glutamate and carbomer on epithelial tight junctions in vitro. *J. Control. Release* **1996**, *39*, 131–138. [CrossRef]
154. Smith, J.; Wood, E.; Dornish, M. Effect of chitosan on epithelial cell tight junctions. *Pharm. Res.* **2004**, *21*, 43–49. [CrossRef] [PubMed]
155. Rosenthal, R.; Heydt, M.S.; Amasheh, M.; Stein, C.; Fromm, M.; Amasheh, S. Analysis of absorption enhancers in epithelial cell models. *Ann. N. Y. Acad. Sci.* **2012**, *1258*, 86–92. [CrossRef] [PubMed]
156. Werle, M.; Takeuchi, H.; Bernkop-Schnürch, A. Modified chitosans for oral drug delivery. *J. Pharm. Sci.* **2009**, *98*, 1643–1656. [CrossRef] [PubMed]
157. Cavaleri, F.; Jia, W. The true nature of curcumin's polypharmacology. *J. Prev. Med.* **2017**, *2*, 5. [CrossRef]
158. Bahramsoltani, R.; Rahimi, R.; Farzaei, M.H. Pharmacokinetic interactions of curcuminoids with conventional drugs: A review. *J. Ethnopharmacol.* **2017**, *209*, 1–12. [CrossRef] [PubMed]
159. Cho, Y.; Lee, W.; Choi, J. Effects of curcumin on the pharmacokinetics of tamoxifen and its active metabolite, 4-hydroxytamoxifen, in rats: Possible role of cyp3a4 and p-glycoprotein inhibition by curcumin. *Die Pharm. Int. J. Pharm. Sci.* **2012**, *67*, 124–130.
160. Abo-El-Sooud, K.; Samar, M.; Fahmy, M. Curcumin ameliorates the absolute and relative bioavailabilities of marbofloxacin after oral administrations in broiler chickens. *Wulfenia* **2017**, *24*, 284–297.
161. Ampasavate, C.; Sotanaphun, U.; Phattanawasin, P.; Piyapolrungroj, N. Effects of curcuma spp. On p-glycoprotein function. *Phytomedicine* **2010**, *17*, 506–512. [CrossRef]

162. Neerati, P.; Bedada, S.K. Effect of diosmin on the intestinal absorption and pharmacokinetics of fexofenadine in rats. *Pharmacol. Rep.* **2015**, *67*, 339–344. [CrossRef]
163. Wang, J.-B.; Zhao, H.-P.; Zhao, Y.-L.; Jin, C.; Liu, D.-J.; Kong, W.-J.; Fang, F.; Zhang, L.; Wang, H.-J.; Xiao, X.-H. Hepatotoxicity or hepatoprotection? Pattern recognition for the paradoxical effect of the chinese herb rheum palmatum l. In treating rat liver injury. *PLoS ONE* **2011**, *6*, e24498. [CrossRef]
164. Lee, M.-H.; Kao, L.; Lin, C.-C. Comparison of the antioxidant and transmembrane permeative activities of the different polygonum cuspidatum extracts in phospholipid-based microemulsions. *J. Agric. Food Chem.* **2011**, *59*, 9135–9141. [CrossRef] [PubMed]
165. Wang, M.; Zhao, R.; Wang, W.; Mao, X.; Yu, J. Lipid regulation effects of polygoni multiflori radix, its processed products and its major substances on steatosis human liver cell line l02. *J. Ethnopharmacol.* **2012**, *139*, 287–293. [CrossRef] [PubMed]
166. Yang, Y.-C.; Lim, M.-Y.; Lee, H.-S. Emodin isolated from cassia obtusifolia (leguminosae) seed shows larvicidal activity against three mosquito species. *J. Agric. Food Chem.* **2003**, *51*, 7629–7631. [CrossRef] [PubMed]
167. Naqvi, S.; Ullah, M.; Hadi, S. *DNA Degradation by Aqueous Extract of Aloe Vera in the Presence Of Copper Ions*; CSIR: New Delhi, India, 2010.
168. Yang, T.; Kong, B.; Kuang, Y.; Cheng, L.; Gu, J.; Zhang, J.; Shu, H.; Yu, S.; Yang, X.; Cheng, J. Emodin plays an interventional role in epileptic rats via multidrug resistance gene 1 (mdr1). *Int. J. Clin. Exp. Pathol.* **2015**, *8*, 3418. [PubMed]
169. Ko, J.-C.; Su, Y.-J.; Lin, S.-T.; Jhan, J.-Y.; Ciou, S.-C.; Cheng, C.-M.; Chiu, Y.-F.; Kuo, Y.-H.; Tsai, M.-S.; Lin, Y.-W. Emodin enhances cisplatin-induced cytotoxicity via down-regulation of ercc1 and inactivation of erk1/2. *Lung Cancer* **2010**, *69*, 155–164. [CrossRef] [PubMed]
170. Tan, W.; Lu, J.; Huang, M.; Li, Y.; Chen, M.; Wu, G.; Gong, J.; Zhong, Z.; Xu, Z.; Dang, Y. Anti-cancer natural products isolated from chinese medicinal herbs. *Chin. Med.* **2011**, *6*, 27. [CrossRef] [PubMed]
171. Guo, J.; Li, W.; Shi, H.; Xie, X.; Li, L.; Tang, H.; Wu, M.; Kong, Y.; Yang, L.; Gao, J. Synergistic effects of curcumin with emodin against the proliferation and invasion of breast cancer cells through upregulation of mir-34a. *Mol. Cell. Biochem.* **2013**, *382*, 103–111. [CrossRef]
172. Min, H.; Niu, M.; Zhang, W.; Yan, J.; Li, J.; Tan, X.; Li, B.; Su, M.; Di, B.; Yan, F. Emodin reverses leukemia multidrug resistance by competitive inhibition and downregulation of p-glycoprotein. *PLoS ONE* **2017**, *12*, e0187971. [CrossRef]
173. Choi, R.J.; Ngoc, T.M.; Bae, K.; Cho, H.-J.; Kim, D.-D.; Chun, J.; Khan, S.; Kim, Y.S. Anti-inflammatory properties of anthraquinones and their relationship with the regulation of p-glycoprotein function and expression. *Eur. J. Pharm. Sci.* **2013**, *48*, 272–281. [CrossRef]
174. Huang, J.; Guo, L.; Tan, R.; Wei, M.; Zhang, J.; Zhao, Y.; Gong, L.; Huang, Z.; Qiu, X. Interactions between emodin and efflux transporters on rat enterocyte by a validated ussing chamber technique. *Front. Pharmacol.* **2018**, *9*, 646. [CrossRef]
175. Mansouri, M.T.; Soltani, M.; Naghizadeh, B.; Farbood, Y.; Mashak, A.; Sarkaki, A. A possible mechanism for the anxiolytic-like effect of gallic acid in the rat elevated plus maze. *Pharmacol. Biochem. Behav.* **2014**, *117*, 40–46. [CrossRef] [PubMed]
176. Stupans, I.; Stretch, G.; Hayball, P. Olive oil phenols inhibit human hepatic microsomal activity. *J. Nutr.* **2000**, *130*, 2367–2370. [CrossRef] [PubMed]
177. Okuda, T.; Yoshida, T.; Hatano, T. Hydrolyzable tannins and related polyphenols. In *Fortschritte der Chemie Organischer Naturstoffe/Progress in the Chemistry of Organic Natural Products*; Springer: New York, NY, USA, 1995; pp. 1–117.
178. Chieli, E.; Romiti, N.; Rodeiro, I.; Garrido, G. In vitro modulation of abcb1/p-glycoprotein expression by polyphenols from mangifera indica. *Chem. Boil. Interact.* **2010**, *186*, 287–294. [CrossRef] [PubMed]
179. Basheer, L.; Kerem, Z. Interactions between cyp3a4 and dietary polyphenols. *Oxidative Med. Cell. Longev.* **2015**, *2015*. [CrossRef]
180. Athukuri, B.L.; Neerati, P. Enhanced oral bioavailability of diltiazem by the influence of gallic acid and ellagic acid in male wistar rats: Involvement of cyp3a and p-gp inhibition. *Phytother. Res.* **2017**, *31*, 1441–1448. [CrossRef]
181. Athukuri, B.L.; Neerati, P. Enhanced oral bioavailability of metoprolol with gallic acid and ellagic acid in male wistar rats: Involvement of cyp2d6 inhibition. *Drug Metab. Pers. Ther.* **2016**, *31*, 229–234. [CrossRef]

182. Kesarwani, K.; Gupta, R. Bioavailability enhancers of herbal origin: An overview. *Asian Pac. J. Trop. Biomed.* **2013**, *3*, 253–266. [CrossRef]
183. Bhadoriya, S.S.; Mangal, A.; Madoriya, N.; Dixit, P. Bioavailability and bioactivity enhancement of herbal drugs by "nanotechnology": A review. *J. Curr. Pharm. Res.* **2011**, *8*, 1–7.
184. Hayeshi, R.; Masimirembwa, C.; Mukanganyama, S.; Ungell, A.-L.B. The potential inhibitory effect of antiparasitic drugs and natural products on p-glycoprotein mediated efflux. *Eur. J. Pharm. Sci.* **2006**, *29*, 70–81. [CrossRef]
185. Limtrakul, P.; Khantamat, O.; Pintha, K. Inhibition of p-glycoprotein function and expression by kaempferol and quercetin. *J. Chemother.* **2005**, *17*, 86–95. [CrossRef]
186. Bobrowska-Hägerstrand, M.; Wróbel, A.; Rychlik, B.; Bartosz, G.; Söderström, T.; Shirataki, Y.; Motohashi, N.; Molnár, J.; Michalak, K.; Hägerstrand, H. Monitoring of mrp-like activity in human erythrocytes: Inhibitory effect of isoflavones. *Blood Cells Mol. Dis.* **2001**, *27*, 894–900. [CrossRef] [PubMed]
187. Dube, A.; Nicolazzo, J.A.; Larson, I. Chitosan nanoparticles enhance the plasma exposure of (−)-epigallocatechin gallate in mice through an enhancement in intestinal stability. *Eur. J. Pharm. Sci.* **2011**, *44*, 422–426. [CrossRef] [PubMed]
188. Perez, M.; Otero, J.A.; Barrera, B.; Prieto, J.G.; Merino, G.; Alvarez, A.I. Inhibition of abcg2/bcrp transporter by soy isoflavones genistein and daidzein: Effect on plasma and milk levels of danofloxacin in sheep. *Vet. J.* **2013**, *196*, 203–208. [CrossRef] [PubMed]
189. Chen, Y.; Huang, C.; Zhou, T.; Chen, G. Genistein induction of human sulfotransferases in hepg2 and caco-2 cells. *Basic Clin. Pharmacol. Toxicol.* **2008**, *103*, 553–559. [CrossRef] [PubMed]
190. Eaton, E.A.; Walle, U.K.; Lewis, A.J.; Hudson, T.; Wilson, A.A.; Walle, T. Flavonoids, potent inhibitors of the human p-form phenolsulfotransferase. Potential role in drug metabolism and chemoprevention. *Drug Metab. Dispos.* **1996**, *24*, 232–237. [PubMed]
191. Reddy, S.A.; Sen, S.; Chakraborty, R.; Parameshappa, B. Effect of gokhru plant extract on intestinal absorption of aspirin using everted sac technique. *Int. J. Pharm. Boil. Arch.* **2011**, *2*, 549–553.
192. Bailey, D.G.; Malcolm, J.; Arnold, O.; Spence, J.D. Grapefruit juice–drug interactions. *Br. J. Clin. Pharmacol.* **1998**, *46*, 101–110. [CrossRef]
193. Mouly, S.; Lloret-Linares, C.; Sellier, P.-O.; Sene, D.; Bergmann, J.-F. Is the clinical relevance of drug-food and drug-herb interactions limited to grapefruit juice and saint-john's wort? *Pharmacol. Res.* **2017**, *118*, 82–92. [CrossRef]
194. Bailey, D.; Spence, J.; Munoz, C.; Arnold, J. Interaction of citrus juices with felodipine and nifedipine. *Lancet* **1991**, *337*, 268–269. [CrossRef]
195. Mertens-Talcott, S.; Zadezensky, I.; Castro, W.; Derendorf, H.; Butterweck, V. Grapefruit-drug interactions: Can interactions with drugs be avoided? *J. Clin. Pharmacol.* **2006**, *46*, 1390–1416. [CrossRef]
196. Ahmed, I.S.; Hassan, M.A.; Kondo, T. Effect of lyophilized grapefruit juice on p-glycoprotein-mediated drug transport in-vitro and in-vivo. *Drug Dev. Ind. Pharm.* **2015**, *41*, 375–381. [CrossRef] [PubMed]
197. Butterweck, V.; Zdrojewski, I.; Galloway, C.; Frye, R.; Derendorf, H. Toxicological and pharmacokinetic evaluation of concomitant intake of grapefruit juice and simvastatin in rats after repeated treatment over 28 days. *Planta Med.* **2009**, *75*, 1196. [CrossRef] [PubMed]
198. Shirasaka, Y.; Shichiri, M.; Mori, T.; Nakanishi, T.; Tamai, I. Major active components in grapefruit, orange, and apple juices responsible for oatp2b1-mediated drug interactions. *J. Pharm. Sci.* **2013**, *102*, 280–288. [CrossRef] [PubMed]
199. Spahn-Langguth, H.; Langguth, P. Grapefruit juice enhances intestinal absorption of the p-glycoprotein substrate talinolol. *Eur. J. Pharm. Sci.* **2001**, *12*, 361–367. [CrossRef]
200. Tian, R.; Koyabu, N.; Takanaga, H.; Matsuo, H.; Ohtani, H.; Sawada, Y. Effects of grapefruit juice and orange juice on the intestinal efflux of p-glycoprotein substrates. *Pharm. Res.* **2002**, *19*, 802–809. [CrossRef] [PubMed]
201. Lown, K.S.; Bailey, D.G.; Fontana, R.J.; Janardan, S.K.; Adair, C.H.; Fortlage, L.A.; Brown, M.B.; Guo, W.; Watkins, P.B. Grapefruit juice increases felodipine oral availability in humans by decreasing intestinal cyp3a protein expression. *J. Clin. Investig.* **1997**, *99*, 2545–2553. [CrossRef]
202. Dresser, G.K.; Kim, R.B.; Bailey, D.G. Effect of grapefruit juice volume on the reduction of fexofenadine bioavailability: Possible role of organic anion transporting polypeptides. *Clin. Pharmacol. Ther.* **2005**, *77*, 170–177. [CrossRef]

203. Tamai, I.; Nakanishi, T. Oatp transporter-mediated drug absorption and interaction. *Curr. Opin. Pharmacol.* **2013**, *13*, 859–863. [CrossRef]
204. Khanuja, S.; Arya, J.; Srivastava, S.; Shasany, A.; Kumar, T.S.; Darokar, M.; Kumar, S. Antibiotic Pharmaceutical Composition with Lysergol as Bio-Enhancer and Method of Treatment. U.S. Patent 11/395,527, 15 March 2007.
205. Alexander, A.; Qureshi, A.; Kumari, L.; Vaishnav, P.; Sharma, M.; Saraf, S.; Saraf, S. Role of herbal bioactives as a potential bioavailability enhancer for active pharmaceutical ingredients. *Fitoterapia* **2014**, *97*, 1–14. [CrossRef]
206. Paine, M.F.; Criss, A.B.; Watkins, P.B. Two major grapefruit juice components differ in intestinal cyp3a4 inhibition kinetic and binding properties. *Drug Metab. Dispos.* **2004**. [CrossRef]
207. Hochman, J.H.; Fix, J.A.; LeCluyse, E.L. In vitro and in vivo analysis of the mechanism of absorption enhancement by palmitoylcarnitine. *J. Pharmacol. Exp. Ther.* **1994**, *269*, 813–822. [PubMed]
208. LeCluyse, E.L.; Appel, L.E.; Sutton, S.C. Relationship between drug absorption enhancing activity and membrane perturbing effects of acylcarnitines. *Pharm. Res.* **1991**, *8*, 84–87. [CrossRef] [PubMed]
209. Duizer, E.; Van Der Wulp, C.; Versantvoort, C.H.; Groten, J.P. Absorption enhancement, structural changes in tight junctions and cytotoxicity caused by palmitoyl carnitine in caco-2 and iec-18 cells. *J. Pharmacol. Exp. Ther.* **1998**, *287*, 395–402. [PubMed]
210. Bhardwaj, R.K.; Glaeser, H.; Becquemont, L.; Klotz, U.; Gupta, S.K.; Fromm, M.F. Piperine, a major constituent of black pepper, inhibits human p-glycoprotein and cyp3a4. *J. Pharmacol. Exp. Ther.* **2002**, *302*, 645–650. [CrossRef] [PubMed]
211. Ahmad, N.; Fazal, H.; Abbasi, B.H.; Farooq, S.; Ali, M.; Khan, M.A. Biological role of piper nigrum l.(black pepper): A review. *Asian Pac. J. Trop. Biomed.* **2012**, *2*, S1945–S1953. [CrossRef]
212. Riedmaier, A.E.; Nies, A.T.; Schaeffeler, E.; Schwab, M. Organic anion transporters and their implications in pharmacotherapy. *Pharmacol. Rev.* **2012**, *64*, 421–449. [CrossRef]
213. Fukuhara, K.; Ikawa, K.; Morikawa, N.; Kumagai, K. Population pharmacokinetics of high-dose methotrexate in japanese adult patients with malignancies: A concurrent analysis of the serum and urine concentration data. *J. Clin. Pharm. Ther.* **2008**, *33*, 677–684. [CrossRef]
214. Li, J.; Liu, Y.; Zhang, J.; Yu, X.; Wang, X.; Zhao, L. Effects of resveratrol on p-glycoprotein and cytochrome p450 3a in vitro and on pharmacokinetics of oral saquinavir in rats. *Drug Des. Dev. Ther.* **2016**, *10*, 3699. [CrossRef]
215. Sharma, P.; Varma, M.V.; Chawla, H.P.; Panchagnula, R. In situ and in vivo efficacy of peroral absorption enhancers in rats and correlation to in vitro mechanistic studies. *IL Farmaco* **2005**, *60*, 874–883. [CrossRef]
216. Fasano, A.; Fiorentini, C.; Donelli, G.; Uzzau, S.; Kaper, J.B.; Margaretten, K.; Ding, X.; Guandalini, S.; Comstock, L.; Goldblum, S.E. Zonula occludens toxin modulates tight junctions through protein kinase c-dependent actin reorganization, in vitro. *J. Clin. Investig.* **1995**, *96*, 710–720. [CrossRef]
217. Yang, T.; Hussain, A.; Paulson, J.; Abbruscato, T.J.; Ahsan, F. Cyclodextrins in nasal delivery of low-molecular-weight heparins: In vivo and in vitro studies. *Pharm. Res.* **2004**, *21*, 1127–1136. [CrossRef] [PubMed]
218. Cheng, Y.; Yao, H.; Lin, H.; Lu, J.; Li, R.; Wang, K. The events relating to lanthanide ions enhanced permeability of human erythrocyte membrane: Binding, conformational change, phase transition, perforation and ion transport. *Chem. Boil. Interact.* **1999**, *121*, 267–289. [CrossRef]
219. Cheng, Y.; Liu, M.; Li, R.; Wang, C.; Bai, C.; Wang, K. Gadolinium induces domain and pore formation of human erythrocyte membrane: An atomic force microscopic study. *Biochim. Biophys. Acta* **1999**, *1421*, 249–260. [CrossRef]

6

Impact of Different Mucoadhesive Polymeric Nanoparticles Loaded in Thermosensitive Hydrogels on Transcorneal Administration of 5-Fluorouracil

Angela Fabiano [1,*], Anna Maria Piras [1], Lorenzo Guazzelli [1], Barbara Storti [2], Ranieri Bizzarri [2,3] and Ylenia Zambito [1,*]

1 Department of Pharmacy, University of Pisa Via Bonanno, 33, 56126 Pisa, Italy; anna.piras@unipi.it (A.M.P.); lorenzo.guazzelli@unipi.it (L.G.)

2 NEST, Scuola Normale Superiore and Istituto Nanoscienze-CNR, Piazza San Silvestro 12, 56127 Pisa, Italy; barbara.storti@nano.cnr.it (B.S.); ranieri.bizzarri@nano.cnr.it (R.B.)

3 Department of Surgical, Medical and Molecular Pathology, and Critical Care Medicine, University of Pisa, Via Roma 67, 56126 Pisa, Italy

* Correspondence: angela.fabiano@unipi.it (A.F.); ylenia.zambito@unipi.it (Y.Z.)

Abstract: In a previous paper a thermosensitive hydrogel formulation based on chitosan or its derivatives (TSOH), containing medicated chitosan nanoparticles (Ch NP) for transcorneal administration of 5-fluorouracil (5-FU) was described. The Ch NP-containing TSOH allowed a time-constant 5-FU concentration in the aqueous for 7 h from instillation. The aim of the present work was to study the impact of the surface characteristics of new NP contained in TSOH on ocular 5-FU bioavailability. The Ch derivatives used to prepare NP were quaternary ammonium-Ch conjugate (QA-Ch), *S*-protected derivative thereof (QA-Ch-*S*-pro), and a sulphobutyl chitosan derivative (SB-Ch). All NP types had 300–400 nm size, 16–18% encapsulation efficiency, and retained the entrapped drug for at least 15 h. Drug release from TSOH containing NP based on QA-Ch or QA-Ch-*S*-pro was virtually equal, whereas with TSOH containing NP based on SB-Ch was significantly slower. Instillation, in rabbit eyes, of NP-containing TSOH based on QA-Ch or SB-Ch led to a plateau in the aqueous concentration vs. time plot in the 1–10 h range with significantly enhanced area under curve (AUC). Negative charges on the NP surface slowed down 5-FU release from TSOH while positive charges increased NP contact with the negatively charged ocular surface. Either results in enhanced ocular bioavailability.

Keywords: thermosensitive hydrogels; mucoadhesive chitosan multifunctional derivatives; mucoadhesive nanoparticles; ocular cancer; microrheology; ocular delivery

---

1. Introduction

Topical ophthalmic preparations such as eyedrops are the most commonly used ocular drug delivery systems. Unfortunately, the intraocular bioavailability of their active substances is generally less than 5%, due to the anatomical and physiological characteristics of the eyes, including tissue barriers, such as cornea, lens, conjunctiva, and sclera, and various physiological functions, such as lacrimation and consequent dilution, and drug expulsion by tear turnover. As a consequence, to obtain the appropriate intraocular drug concentrations, frequent instillations of eyedrops are needed, which can cause toxic side effects and damage to the ocular tissue [1]. Thus, the traditional ophthalmic preparations and relevant therapeutic protocols cannot provide and maintain effective drug concentrations in the corneal tissue, and this results in a poor ocular bioavailability.

The intraocular bioavailability would improve if the drug transcorneal permeability and precorneal residence were increased [2]. One strategy to improve the corneal permeability is the addition of polymeric penetration enhancers to eyedrop formulations [3–5].

Another interesting approach to ocular drug delivery is the use of hydrogel systems. Among hydrogels the most interesting for the ocular administration of drugs are the thermosensitive hydrogels that can be instilled in the form of drops and become gels once in contact with the eyes [6–8]. In particular, chitosan-based thermosensitive hydrogels have proved to be vehicles of choice for biomedical application because they possess mucoadhesive, antibacterial, biodegradable, and biocompatible properties [7,9].

Another approach aimed at increasing the endo-ocular bioavailability of drugs is the use of nanoparticles (NP) or mucoadhesive vesicles capable of prolonging the contact with eye mucosae and promoting the absorption of entrapped drugs [10,11]. Furthermore, the nanoparticles could be internalized by the corneal cells, and form a reservoir from which the drug could be released over time [12].

Recently, innovative formulations based on thermosensitive hydrogels for the sustained ocular delivery of drugs entrapped in nanosize structures have been proposed [13–15]. In all cases such systems were found to have a greater ability than those based on the simple thermosensitive hydrogels to prolong the drug residence in the precorneal area, promote endoocular bioavailability, and prolong the drug halflife in the aqueous. If nanosystem diffusion in hydrogels is excluded, the above results can be explained by the blinking continuously renewing the hydrogel-cornea contact surface, thus bringing new NP into contact with the cornea.

In our previous work we tried to combine the above strategies by preparing thermosensitive hydrogels (TSOH) based on chitosan and its derivatives containing medicated NP based on unmodified chitosan for transcorneal administration of 5-fluorouracil (5-FU) [13]. Chitosan was chosen because cationic polymers have greater interactivity with the negatively charged ocular surface [16], and also, because chitosan has a lower toxicity than other cationic polymers, such as polyarginine or polyethylenimine [17]. Increased bioavailability of 5-FU in the aqueous with respect to control eyedrops resulted from in vivo experiments with rabbit eyes. The NP-containing hydrogels mediated to a zero-order 5-FU absorption, leading to a time-constant anticancer concentration in the aqueous for up to 7 h from instillation. This was ascribed to the ability of this TSOH to control drug release to a zero order and that of NP to be internalized by corneal cells. In that first study the preparation of thermosensitive hydrogels was studied and developed, while the impact of the surface characteristics of the NP they contained on drug ocular bioavailability was not studied. Such an impact has been investigated in the present study.

Nanoparticles differing in mucoadhesivity and surface charge were prepared for this purpose from chitosan (Ch) derivatives, and NP ability to promote the transcorneal penetration of 5-FU was assessed in vivo. The chitosan derivatives consisted in quaternary ammonium-Ch conjugate (QA-Ch), *S*-protected derivative thereof (QA-Ch-*S*-pro), and a sulfobutyl chitosan derivative (SB-Ch). While the properties of quaternary ammonium-Ch conjugate and/or those of the respective *S*-protected derivatives have widely been described in the literature, the properties of Ch modified by sulfate or sulfonate groups is currently under investigation [18]. The NP were dispersed in TSOH in the sol state and compared on the ground of NP size, surface zeta potential, mucoadhesivity, affinity with the drug, and in vitro drug-release properties, in order to select the systems on which to carry out in vivo pharmacokinetic studies.

2. Materials and Methods

2.1. Materials

Low molecular weight Ch (75–85% deacetylated), 5-FU, β-glycerophosphate (β-GP) disodium salt, sodium tripolyphosphate (TPP), 1,4-butane sulphone, and fluorescein isothiocyanate (FITC),

Type II mucin from porcine stomach, were purchased from Sigma-Aldrich (Milan, Italy). The QA-Ch conjugate was synthesized from Ch according to Zambito et al., 2013 [19], the thiolated *S*-protected derivative of QA-Ch was synthesized according to Fabiano et al., 2018 [20]. Reduced molecular weight hyaluronic acid (rHA) (viscosimetric molecular weight 470 kDa) was prepared as described by Zambito et al., 2013 [19]. FITC labelling of QA-Ch, QA-Ch-*S*-pro, and SB-Ch was carried out as previously described [21]. The QA-Ch50 polymer, used to prepare the TSOH, was synthesized according to Zambito et al., 2013 [19]. In the code, 50 means that it was prepared by maintaining the temperature at 50 °C for the entire duration of the reaction. All aqueous solutions/dispersions were prepared with freshly distilled water. QA-Ch was characterized by ^{1}H NMR to determine the degree of substitution with the small side chains containing adjacent quaternary ammonium groups and the length of such chains. Protected thiols present on QA-Ch-*S*-pro chains were determined by polymer reduction and subsequent quantification of the 6-mercaptonicotinamide protecting group. Only polymers that had the same characteristics as previously obtained [20] were used in this work.

2.2. Synthesis and Characterization of Sulphobutyl Chitosan (SB-Ch)

SB-Ch was synthesized from Ch as previously described [22]. Briefly, 1,4-butane sulphone (3 equivalents per *N*-acetylglucosamine unit) was added to a Ch solution in acidic water (1% *w/w* Ch, 2% *w/w* of acid acetic). The mixture was allowed to react at 60 °C for 6 h. The resulting solution was poured into acetone. The precipitated product was resuspended in demineralized water and purified by dialysis 3 days against water. After dialysis, the polymer solution was lyophilized to obtain the purified SB-Ch (Figure 1). ^{1}H NMR spectrum was recorded in D_2O/DCl with a Bruker AC 200 instrument operating at 200.13 MHz (Bruker, Milan, Italy).

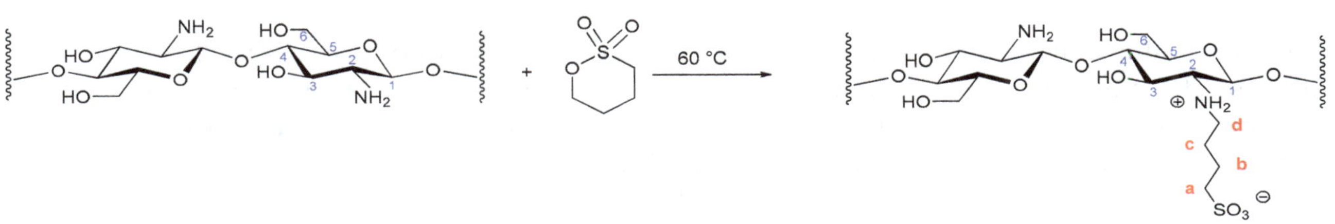

Figure 1. Synthetic route to sulfobutyl chitosan (SB-Ch).

2.3. Preparation of Medicated NP

FITC-labeled or unlabeled NP based on QA-Ch or QA-Ch-*S*-pro were prepared by self-assembly upon addition of rHA. In detail, a solution of rHA 0.2 mg/mL in phosphate buffer (0.13 M, PB pH 7.4) containing 6.25 mg of 5-FU was added dropwise (500 µL) to 5 mL of 2 mg/mL polymer solution in the same buffer, under stirring at room temperature. Similarly, to prepare FITC-labeled or unlabeled NP based on SB-Ch, a solution of TPP 2 mg/mL in demineralized water containing 6.25 mg of FU was added dropwise (700 µL) to 5 mL of 2 mg/mL SB-Ch in demineralized water, under stirring at room temperature. The final 5-FU concentration in NP systems based on QA-Ch, or QA-Ch-*S*-pro, or SB-Ch was 1.25 mg/mL, corresponding to the concentration contained in the commercial 5-FU eyedrops. After their preparation, the NP dispersions were checked for particle size and zeta potential (ζ) at a temperature of 25 °C (Zetasizer Nano ZS, Malvern, UK). The ζ values of medicated NP based on QA-Ch, QA-Ch-*S*-pro, or SB-Ch were determined after NP centrifugation (2000 rpm for 30 min) and their subsequent sediments re-suspended in 1.9 mL of a 0.08 M HCl solution containing 195 µL of NaOH 1 N and 0.8 g/mL of β-GP. Their drug-entrapment efficiency (EE) was evaluated by subjecting the dispersion to centrifugation (20,000 rpm for 30 min at 4 °C) and analyzing the supernatant spectophotometrically at 266 nm. The EE was calculated as follows, using the appropriate calibration curve:

$$EE = (M_t - M_s)/M_t \quad (1)$$

where M_t is the total mass of 5-FU used for the preparation of NP and M_s is the mass found in the supernatant.

2.4. Preparation of Thermosensitive Hydrogels (TSOH) Containing NP Medicated with 5-FU

Thermosensitive ophthalmic hydrogels (TSOH) were prepared according to Fabiano et al. [13]. Briefly, 400 mg of Ch and 100 mg of QA-Ch50 were dissolved in 18 mL of a 0.08 M HCl solution. The resulting solution was kept under magnetic stirring at 4 °C. Then, 5-FU-medicated NP, based on QA-Ch, QA-Ch-*S*-pro, or SB-Ch, freshly prepared, were added in the sol state under magnetic stirring at 4 °C, before the addition of 450 μl β-GP (0.8 g/mL) solution to obtain TSOH.

2.5. Dynamic Dialysis Studies

To study the reversible drug binding by NP in fluid dispersion we used already reported procedure and theory [23,24]. Briefly, a porous cellulose membrane (cut-off 12.5 kDa) was used to separate the donor compartment of the dialysis cell from the receiving phase (100 mL of PB pH 7.4 for 5-FU-loaded QA-Ch or QA-Ch-*S*-pro NP or100 mL of demineralized water for 5-FU-loaded SB-Ch NP). The system was thermostated at 35 °C for 5 h, while maintaining sink conditions. At time $t = 0$, 5 mL of freshly prepared 5-FU loaded NP, or plain drug solution (control), or this solution containing 2 mg/mL of QA-Ch or QA-Ch-*S*-pro dissolved in PB pH 7.4, or 2 mg/mL of SB-Ch in water was introduced in the donor compartment of the cell. In all cases, at the end of experiment, the receiving phase was analyzed spectrophotometrically to determine the drug transport. In the case of NP, the receiving phase was also analyzed for particle size.

2.6. Interrupted-Dialysis Studies

The dynamic dialysis experiment, described in Section 2.5, was stopped after 1, 2, 3, 5, 15, or 24 h, from the start. At each time interval, the donor phase was centrifuged (2000 rpm for 30 min at 4 °C) to determine the drug fraction contained in NP matrix, NP dispersion medium, and acceptor medium, according to reference [25]. The results were plotted as drug fraction in each phase versus time.

2.7. Studies of 5-FU Release from NP-Containing TSOH

5-FU release from TSOH was carried out using a cell and a procedure reported by Fabiano et al. [13]. The gel (0.5 mL) containing medicated NP was introduced in the cylindrical cavity of the cell. A porous cellulose membrane (cut-off 12.5 kDa) was used to separate the gel from the receiving phase (30 mL of PB pH 7.4 for 5-FU-loaded NP based on QA-Ch or QA-Ch-*S*-pro, or 30 mL of demineralized water for 5-FU-loaded NP based on SB-Ch). At time, $t = 0$, the cell was introduced in a beaker containing the receiving phase thermostated at 35 °C and stirred at 300 rpm. The receiving phase was analyzed spectrophotometrically at 30-min intervals to determine the drug transport kinetics.

2.8. Confocal Microscopy and Image Analysis

To evaluate the possibility of re-dispersing NP into the hydrogel system, the FITC-labelled, 5-FU medicated NP, based on QA-Ch, QA-Ch-*S*-pro, or SB-Ch were dispersed in the TSOH at room temperature and observed under a confocal laser-scanning microscope (Zeiss LSM 880 with Airyscan, Carl Zeiss, Jena, Germany). The representative fluorescence confocal micrographs of NP were taken in liquid (21 °C) and gel states (4 °C), using a 63x Apochromat NA = 1.4 oil-immersion objective with the pinhole aperture of the confocal system at 1 Airy unit. The excitation wavelength was set at 488 nm (10–20 μW power emission at objective), whereas emission was in the 500–550 nm range. Pixel dwell time was adjusted to 1.52 μs and 512 × 512 pixel images were collected.

Image analysis was carried out by ImageJ v.1.52o (NIH, Bethesda, MD, USA) software. Particle diameters were calculated by tracing an equatorial line over each bead (average of 5–10 beads), collecting the fluorescence profile and fitting it with a Gaussian function. The full width at half maximum (FWHM) of the best-fitting curve was assumed as particle diameter.

2.9. Micro-Rheological Characterization of NP Mucoadhesive Properties

Micro-rheological measurements were carried out using a Zetasizer Nano ZS, Malvern, with a detection angle of 173 °C and a temperature of 25 °C, applying the theory reported by Dodero et al. [26]. The micro-rheological characterization of 5-FU loaded freshly prepared QA-Ch or SB-Ch NP was performed using mucin from porcine stomach, Type II. Ocular mucins are not commercially available, so porcine gastric mucin was used because it has also been applied as a model substance in other studies, investigating ocular mucoadhesion [27]. In order to obtain reliable micro-rheological data, the conditions about the tracer-sample combination were verified as reported by Dodero et al., 2019 [26]. A dispersion of mucin 3 mg/mL in water, was filtered using a cellulose acetate filter (pore size 0.45 µm). A sample was taken from the filtrate and lyophilized to calculate the concentration of dispersed material (1.85 mg/mL). The filtered mucin dispersion was diluted 10 times with a solution of NaCl 0.9%. Then, 5 µL of tracer sample (polystyrene latex particles, diameter 500 nm, Beckman, 5 µl/mL) and 5 µL of NP dispersions prepared as described in Section 2.4 were added to the diluted mucin dispersion. Micro-rheological tests were performed to evaluate viscoelastic properties and assess NP mucoadhesive properties on the basis of the viscosity changes caused by NP addition to a mucin solution.

2.10. In Vivo Studies

For the in vivo studies we used male New Zealand albino rabbits weighing 3–3.5 kg treated as prescribed in the guidelines from the European Community Council Directive 2010/63, approved by the Animal Care Committee of the University of Pisa (D.L. 2014/26, 12 March 2019). Fifty µL (one drop) of the following two types of ophthalmic formulations were instilled in the lower conjunctival sac: (1) a dispersion of QA-Ch-based NP medicated with 1.25 mg/mL of 5-FU in TSOH and (2) a dispersion of SB-Ch-based NP medicated with 1.25 mg/mL 5-FU in TSOH. For the entire duration of the experiments each rabbit eye was checked for signs of conjunctival/cornea edema and/or hyperemia [28]. Before the aspiration of aqueous humor (~60 µL) from the anterior chamber of the eye, the rabbits were anesthetized with one drop of Novesina®. The 5-FU concentration in aqueous humor was determined by high-performance liquid chromatography (HPLC) using the apparatus and the mobile phase described by Fabiano et al. [13]. An Aeris 3.6 µm, PEPTIDE XB-C18 Å, 250 × 4.6 mm column, equilibrated at 30 °C was used and UV detection was set at 266 nm. Standard curves were obtained analyzing six standard drug solutions (concentration range 0.3–1.25 µg/mL) in acetonitrile mixed with aqueous humor (2:1). The resulting mixtures were centrifuged, and the acetonitrile was removed by evaporation at 50 °C. The resulting aqueous product was lyophilized and re-dispersed in a volume of mobile phase corresponding to the initial volume of standard solution. Standard curves were linear ($r^2 > 0.995$, limit of detection 0.2 µg/mL). The retention time was 8.2 min. The concentration of each unknown sample was determined as described above, using a standard curve produced on the same day.

2.11. Data Treatment

Linear plots were obtained by linear regression analysis of data from in vitro experiments. The relevant slope, intercept, and coefficient of determination (r^2) were calculated. The significance of differences was evaluated by Student's t-test ($p < 0.05$). For the in vivo experiments, the linear trapezoidal rule between 0 and 10 h was used to calculate the area under curve (AUC) and the statistical differences were evaluated using the method reported by Schoenwald et al. [29].

3. Results and Discussion

3.1. *Synthesis of Sulphobutyl Chitosan (SB-Ch)*

^{1}H NMR spectrum (D_2O/DCl) of SB-Ch, seen in Figure 2, shows three sets of signals ascribed to the different methylene groups of the sulfobutyl functionalization at 1.32–1.60 ppm (–CH_{2b} and –CH_{2c}), 2.62–3.72 ppm (–CH_{2d}), and 3.33–3.41 ppm (–CH_{2a} overlapping to protons H-3, H-4, H-5, and H-6 of chitosan). An estimation of the butylsulfonation degree (ca 52%) was possible by comparing the integrals of H-2 of the chitosan backbone, which fell in a quite clean part of the spectrum (2.91–3.20 ppm), and of –CH_{2d} of the sulfobutyl group.

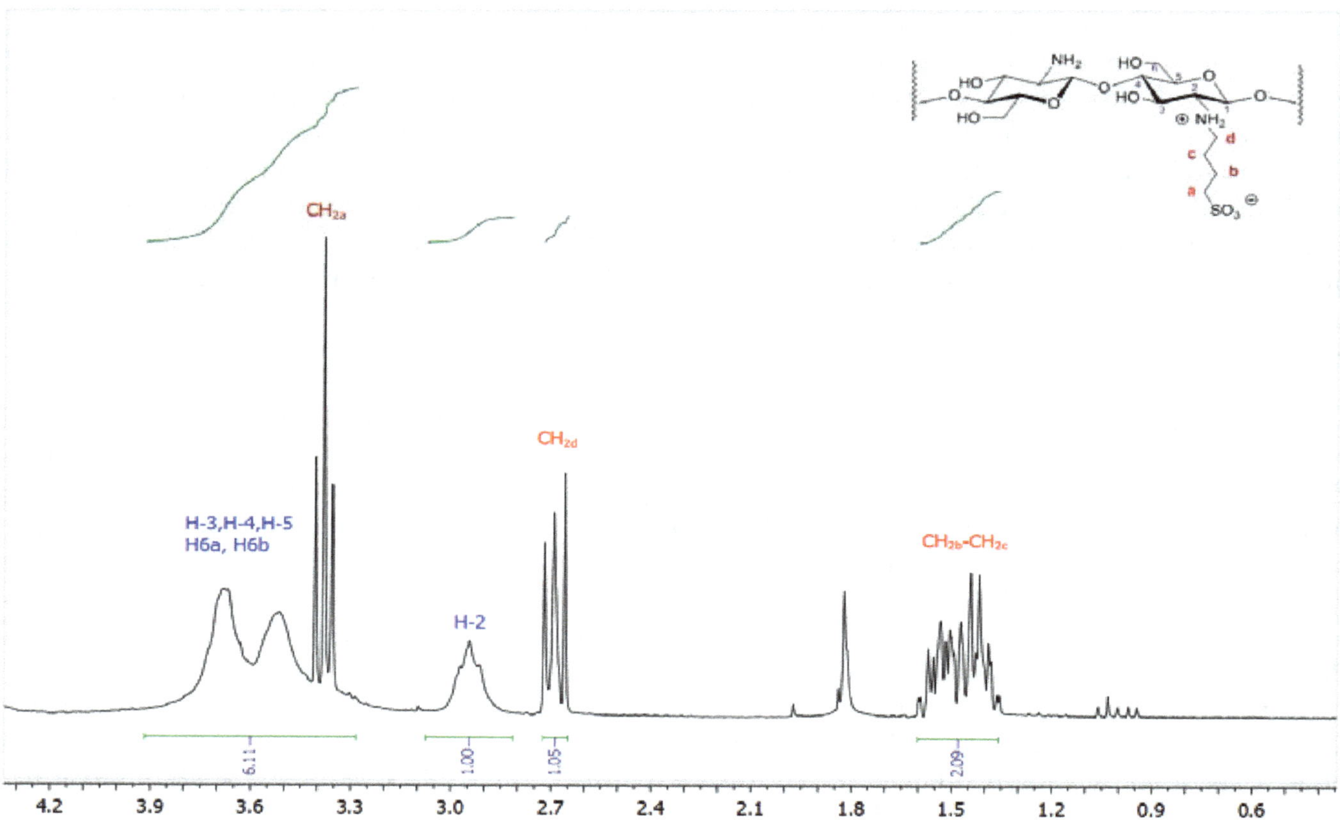

Figure 2. ^{1}H NMR (200.12 MHz, D_2O/DCl) spectral region of SB-Ch.

3.2. *Characteristics of Medicated NP*

The size, polydispersity index, zeta potential (ζ) and encapsulation efficiency (EE) for medicated NP based on QA-Ch, QA-Ch-*S*-pro, or SB-Ch are found in Table 1. The size and polydispersity index values were not significantly different from each other or from those for NP based on Ch prepared in our preceding paper Fabiano et al. [13] (342.5 ± 15.2). The ζ values for medicated NP based on QA-Ch or QA-Ch-*S*-pro were positive in agreement with the presence of ammonium quaternary ions on their surface, whereas for medicated NP based on SB-Ch the ζ value was negative in agreement with the presence of superficial sulfonic groups. The EE was in the range 18–15% with no significant difference between the three cases. The prepared NP only differing for their external charge allowed us to evaluate the impact of this property on the system ability to promote the intraocular absorption of 5-FU.

Table 1. Characteristics of medicated nanoparticles (NP) determined immediately after their preparation.

NP Type	Nanoparticle Size, nm (Polydispersity Index)	ζ, mV	EE%
NP quaternary ammonium-Ch conjugate (QA-Ch)	294.3 ± 60.6 (0.4 ± 0.2)	+9.1 ± 0.4	18.4 ± 4.0
NP QA-Ch-*S*-pro	340.7 ± 100.1 (0.3 ± 0.1)	+9.5 ± 0.1	18.3 ± 0.2
NP SB-Ch	390.6 ± 50.3 (0.2 ± 0.1)	−3.5 ± 0.1	15.6 ± 1.0

3.3. Dynamic Dialysis Studies

Dynamic dialysis data were used to compare reversible drug interactions with the NP in fluid dispersions. According to [23,24], the data obtained were plotted as ln $(C_d/C_{d0}) \times 100$ versus t using the following Equation (2):

$$\ln [(C_d/C_{d0}) \times 100] = 4.605 - K_m F_f t \quad (2)$$

where C_d is the drug concentration in the donor phase, C_{d0} is the drug concentration in donor phase at $t = 0$, F_f is the non-interacting drug fraction in donor phase, and K_m is the dialysis-rate constant. All plots, reported in Figure 3 were significantly linear (r^2 values, 0.90–0.98) which indicated that in all cases (plain 5-FU, control, NP based on QA-Ch, QA-Ch-*S*-pro, or SB-Ch) Equation (2) was obeyed and for plain 5-FU (control) the slope of the relative log-linear plot, used to calculate F_f was equal to K_m. The slopes of the straight lines reported in Table 2 indicated a 5-FU binding with all polymers in solution higher than the binding with NP dispersions. From here, it was deduced that the drug fraction reversibly interacting with the polymers in solution was significantly higher than that adsorbed on NP surface. This was probably due to an interaction between the 5-FU and the polycationic polysaccharide Ch. In the case of NP, the positive groups of Ch could be bound to the crosslinker and, hence, less available for 5-FU binding. This, nevertheless, should not impair the NP effectiveness in vivo, in fact, nanoparticles made of mucoahesive polymers are themselves more mucoahesive than the corresponding parent polymers, hence, likely to strongly adhere to the ocular surface [10,20,30].

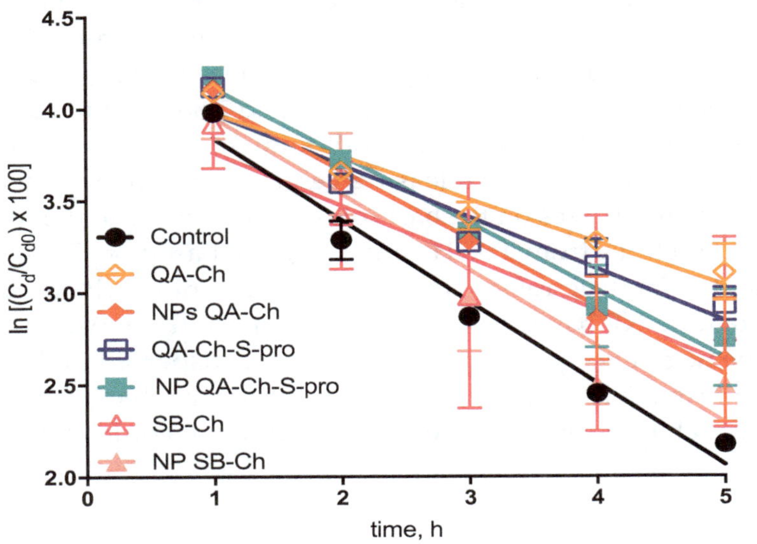

Figure 3. Dynamic dialysis data plotted according to Equation (2). Means ± SD (n = 3–6).

Table 2. Results of dynamic dialysis data plotted in Figure 3 and obtained according to Equation (2).

Formulation	Modulus of Straight-Line Slope ± SD (h^{-1})	r^2	Interaction [a] %
Control	0.44 ± 0.04	0.97	-
QA-Ch	0.23 ± 0.03	0.94	47.7
NP QA-Ch	0.37 ± 0.03	0.98	15.9
QA-Ch-*S*-pro	0.28 ± 0.04	0.93	36.4
NP QA-Ch-*S*-pro	0.37 ± 0.03	0.98	15.9
SB-Ch	0.29 ± 0.06	0.90	34.1
NP SB-Ch	0.41 ± 0.06	0.93	6.8

[a] Bound fraction.

3.4. 5-FU Release from NP

The procedure used to study 5-FU release from NP was based on interrupted dialysis, as described in Section 2.6. A dispersion of each freshly prepared NP type, loaded with 5-FU and not separated from the non-entrapped drug was introduced in the donor compartment of the dialysis cell. Hence, not more than 15–18% of the whole 5-FU amount contained in each dispersion was associated with the NP phase, as shown in Table 1. From knowledge of the drug amount used for each NP preparation, the drug amount determined for the NP dispersion medium in donor compartment (DM phase) at each interruption time, the cumulative amount determined for the drug transferred into the receiving medium (RM phase) during each interruption time, and the relevant % 5-FU contained in the NP matrix, i.e., the NPM data reported in Figure 4, could readily be calculated. This data indicated that the 5-FU fraction immobilized in the NP matrix remained virtually constant at the initial value of 15–18% over the first 15 h of experiment, while it seemed to fade after 24 h probably due to some degradation of the NP. Therefore, it is understood that all NP types are able to retain the 5-FU load for a term sufficient for NP to be internalized by corneal cells. It should be noted that the present NP, prepared from Ch derivatives, were able to retain 5-FU for longer than those prepared by Fabiano et al., from Ch (15 vs. 5 h) [13].

3.5. Drug Release from NP-Containing TSOH

Data on drug release from NP-containing TSOH, obtained as described in Section 2.7 and plotted as percentage of drug released versus t or $\sqrt{t}$ are reported in Figure 5a,b, respectively. The release study lasted 5 h since the 5-FU release study for all NP types had shown that the 5-FU % entrapped in the NP was virtually constant for at least 15 h. The drug amount released vs. $\sqrt{t}$ was in all cases linear with comparatively small ordinate intercepts (between −0.99% and 2.88%) and high r^2 values (between 0.96 and 0.99, $n = 3$). This pattern in all cases fitted a well-known model assuming that the release was entirely governed by drug diffusion in the releasing vehicle. The slope of each straight line allowed comparison between the different cases on the basis of drug diffusivity in the hydrogel. The data listed in Table 3 shows that 5-FU release from TSOH containing NP based on QA-Ch or QA-Ch-*S*-pro was not significantly different from drug release from TSOH containing NP based on Ch, whereas drug release from TSOH containing NP based on SB-Ch was significantly slowed down, with respect to the above, reasonably by the negative charges on the NP surface dispersed in this TSOH. Indeed, TSOH was prepared using a chitosan derivative containing fixed positive charges that could electrostatically interact with the negative charges of SB-Ch, and this interaction could slow down the 5-FU release from TSOH.

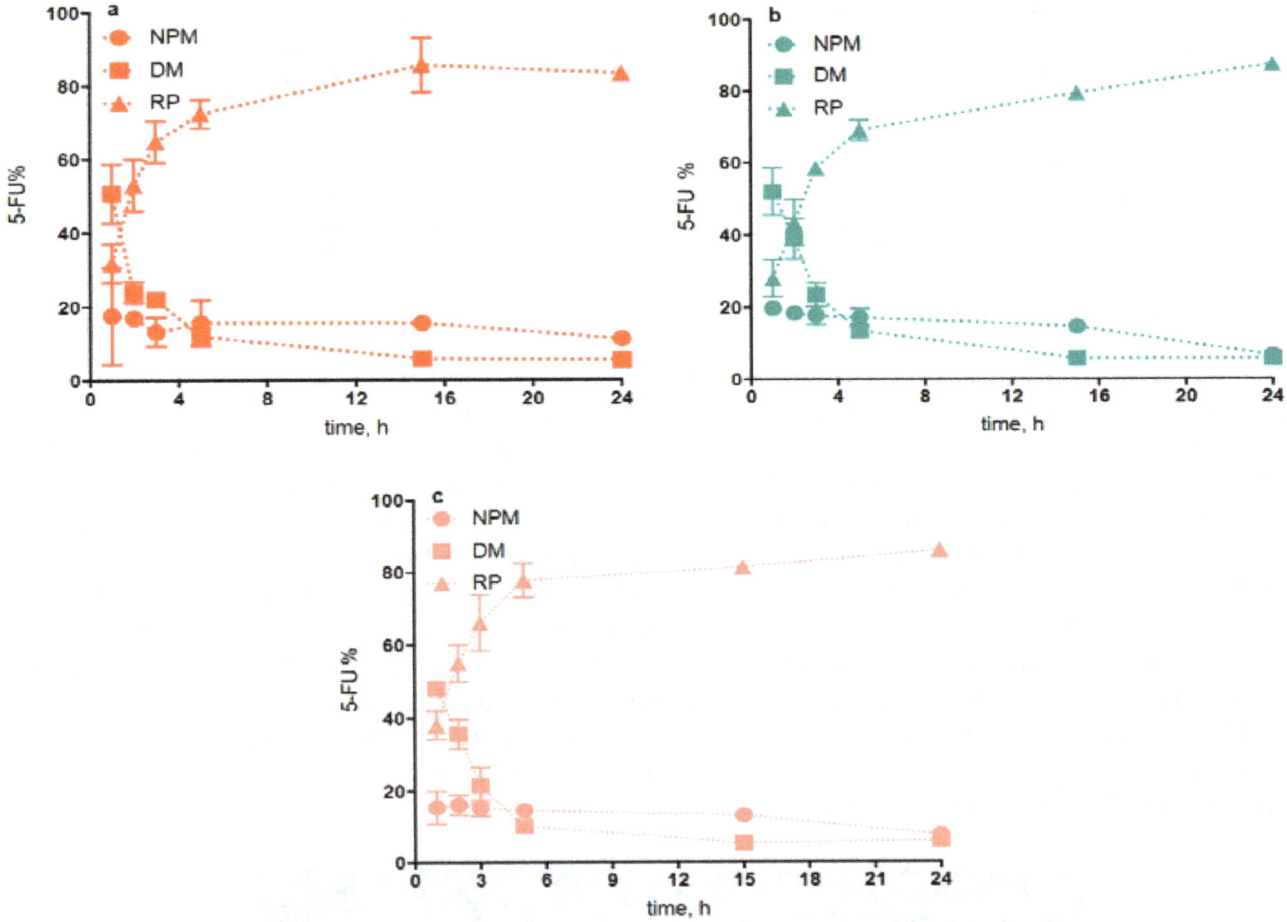

Figure 4. Interrupted dialysis studies: kinetic analysis of dialysis phases for 5-fluorouracil (5-FU)-loaded QA-Ch NP (**a**), QA-Ch-*S*-pro NP (**b**), and SB-Ch NP (**c**). Percent 5-FU in: NP matrix (NPM); NP dispersion medium (DM); and receiving phase (RP). Means ± SD (n = 3).

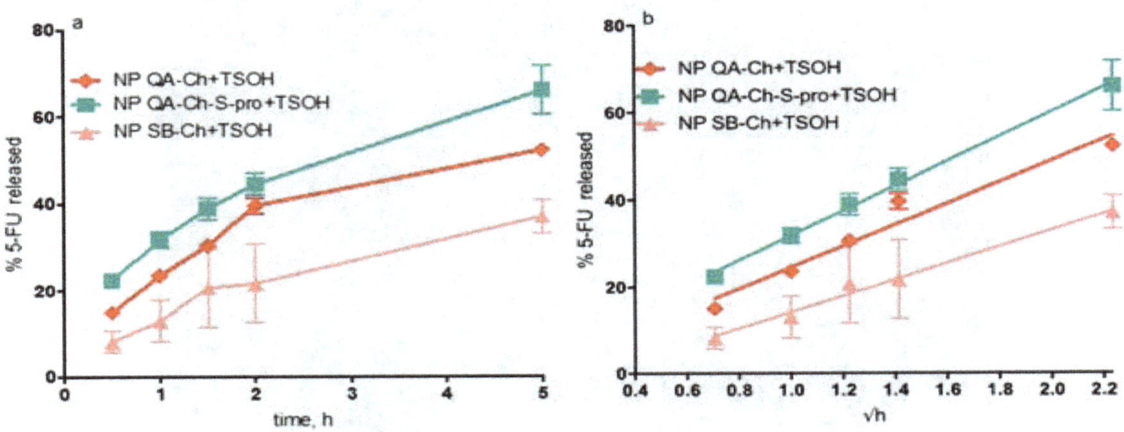

Figure 5. 5-FU released (%) from NP-containing thermosensitive hydrogels (TSOH) vs. time (hours) (**a**) or vs. √t (**b**).

Table 3. Characteristics of 5-FU release from NP-containing TSOH.

Formulation	Slope of √t Plot (%/√h)	Cumulative Release at 5 h (%)
Ch NP+TSOH [a]	3.34 ± 0.32	59.50 ± 0.90
QA-Ch NP+TSOH	3.14 ± 0.39	52.23 ± 1.07
QA-Ch-*S*-pro NP+TSOH	3.64 ± 3.12	65.93 ± 5.70
SB-Ch NP+TSOH	2.43 ± 0.21 *	37.00 ± 3.82 *

[a] Data taken from Fabiano et al., 2017 [13]. * Significantly different from all the others ($p < 0.05$).

3.6. Confocal Microscopy and Image Analysis

Particle fluorescence allowed their visualization in both the sol and gel states by means of fluorescence confocal microscopy [13]. From particle images, their size could be inferred (Table 4, Figure 6) affording interesting information on the role of gelification on their aggregation status. Gelation did not affect the size of SB-Ch NP (Table 4, entries 1,2; Figure 6a,b) which remained close to the optical diffraction limit of the microscopy apparatus (~0.2 μm). Conversely, QA-Ch NP in the gel phase showed the presence of two main particle populations: one, with a size comparable to that of SB-Ch NP, the other twice as large (Table 4, entry 3; Figure 6c). A bimodal pattern was observed also with QA-Ch-*S*-pro NP, although in this case the smaller peak was about 0.6 μm and the larger was, on the average, more than 4 μm with a rather large dispersion as indicated by the relevant standard error (SE) values (Table 4, entry 4; Figure 6d). These findings strongly suggest a moderate aggregation of QA-Ch NP, each aggregate possibly consisting of two particles sticking together, in the sol state, and a much larger aggregate state for QA-Ch-*S*-pro NP in the gel state. These data encouraged us to continue the study only with NP based on QA-Ch and SB-Ch.

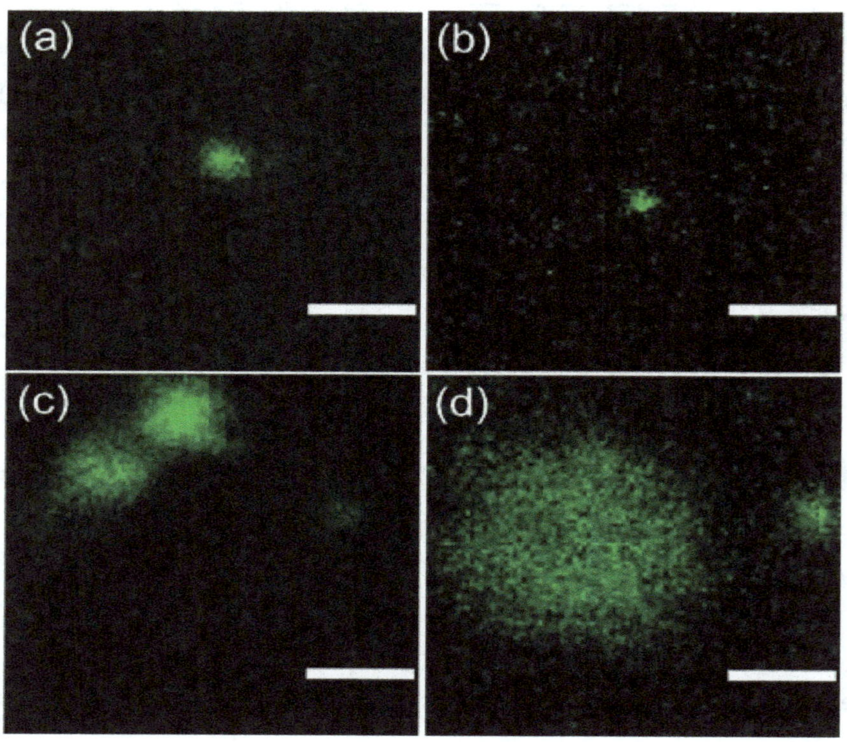

Figure 6. Representative fluorescence confocal micrographs of NP. For all images, the same field of view and pixel size was adopted, to allow a direct visual comparison of NP size. (**a**) SB-Ch NP (sol state), (**b**) SB-Ch NP (gel state), (**c**) QA-Ch NP (gel state), and (**d**) QA-Ch-*S*-pro NP (gel state). Scale bar: 1 μm.

Table 4. Size of the particles as determined by confocal fluorescence microscopy. Each entry refers to one experiment where the size was calculated as the average of five full width at half maximum (FWHM) measurements (see Materials and Methods section).

Entry	Particle (Status)	Mean Size ± SE (μm)
1	SB-Ch NP (sol)	0.27 ± 0.02
2	SB-Ch NP (gel)	0.33 ± 0.02
3	QA-Ch NP (gel)	0.70 ± 0.07; 0.29 ± 0.01
4	QA-Ch-*S*-pro NP (gel)	4.26 ± 1.67; 0.61 ± 0.15

3.7. Micro-Rheological Characterization of NP Mucoadhesive Properties

The elastic (or storage) modulus, G′, the viscous (or loss) modulus, G″, and the complex viscosity, η*, are reported in Figure 7. As can be seen, there was an increase in η* of mucin dispersion in the presence of NP based on either QA-Ch or SB-Ch, compared to plain mucin dispersion. The increase of η* was reflected in the increase of both G′ and G″ moduli. In particular, the increase in G′ is indicative of the development of an inter-connected microstructure between mucin macromolecules and NP based on QA-Ch, resulting in a stronger mucoadhesivity of these NP with respect to the NP based on SB-Ch. However, G′ for NP based on SB-Ch was higher than G′ for mucin, due to the intrinsic mucoadhesivity of Ch, i.e., the pristine material used to prepare SB-Ch. These data demonstrate that the sign of the NP surface charge can actually influence their mucoadhesivity. Moreover, it is known that the mucus glycoproteins bear negatively charged sialic moieties that are capable of forming ionic bonds with oppositely charged chemical species [31].

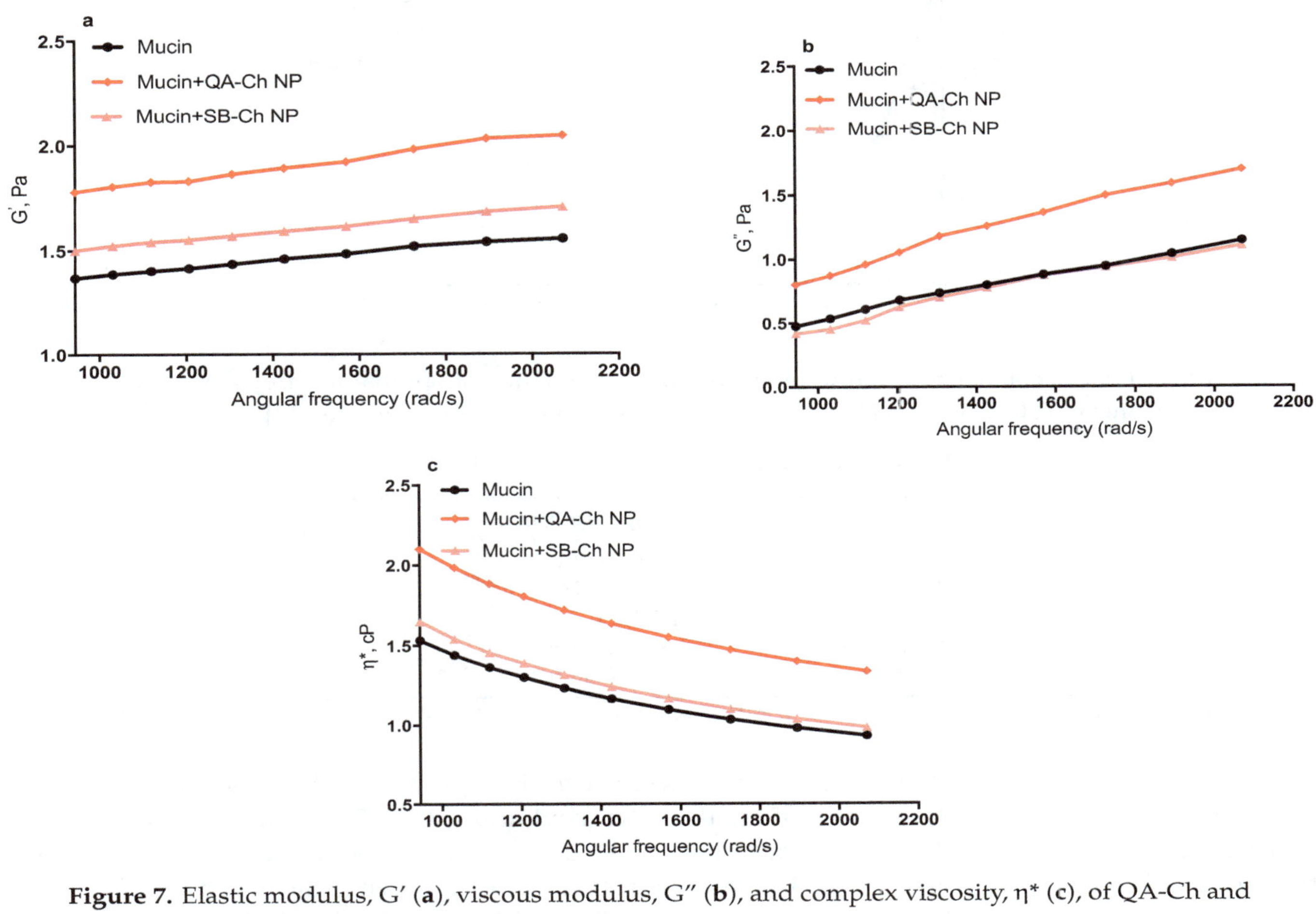

Figure 7. Elastic modulus, G′ (**a**), viscous modulus, G″ (**b**), and complex viscosity, η* (**c**), of QA-Ch and SB-Ch NP with respect to mucin dispersion.

3.8. In Vivo Tests

During each experiment, we observed that all the ophthalmic drops instilled in rabbit eyes caused no conjunctival/corneal edema and/or hyperemia. The pharmacokinetic profiles in the aqueous and the relative AUC values are reported in Figure 8 and Table 5, respectively. The results of the in vivo tests shown in Figure 8 demonstrate the ability of the TSOH containing NP based on QA-Ch or SB-Ch to increase the 5-FU bioavailability with respect to the control, TSOH, and Ch NP-containing TSOH [13]. Indeed, the AUC values relative to QA-Ch NP+TSOH and SB-Ch NP+TSOH listed in Table 5, are significantly higher than those relative to the control, TSOH, and Ch NP+TSOH, with a concentration plateau in the range 1–10 h. These results demonstrate that the QA-Ch NP+TSOH and SB-Ch NP+TSOH systems have much more ability to prolong the drug precorneal residence time than the control, TSOH, or Ch NP-containing TSOH. In view of the ability of NP to retain the drug for longer, the plateau in the 1–10 h range is in-keeping with the hypothesis of an intraocular drug absorption controlled by gel erosion in pre-corneal area accompanied by release of drug-loaded NP that are then internalized in corneal cells.

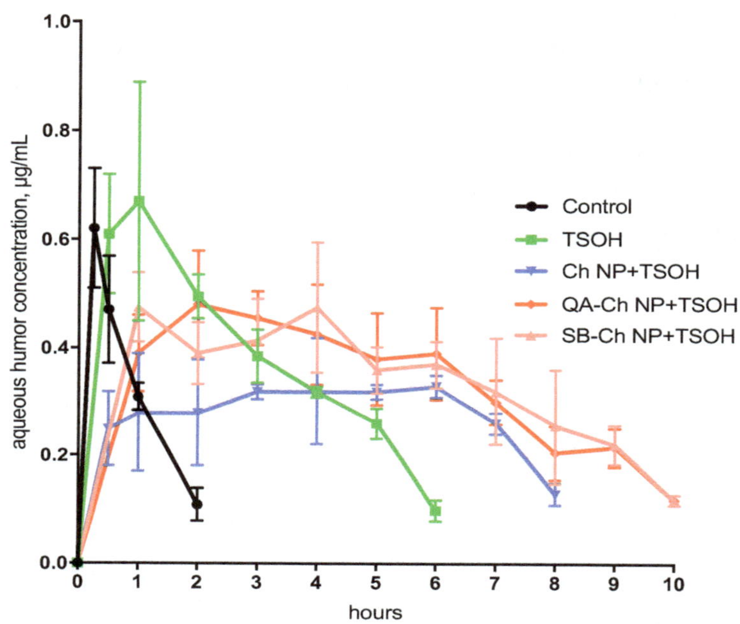

Figure 8. Pharmacokinetics in the aqueous following instillation of ophthalmic drops. Means ± SD ($n = 6$). Control, TSOH, and Ch NP+TSOH profiles are taken from Fabiano et al. [13].

Table 5. AUC data obtained in vivo in rabbit eyes.

Formulation	AUC_{0-10}, µg h/mL	AUC_{rel}
Control [a]	0.62 ± 0.1	-
TSOH [a]	2.32 ± 0.26 *	3.7
Ch NP+TSOH [a]	2.23 ± 0.39 *	3.6
QA-Ch NP+TSOH	3.30 ± 0.52 *,**	5.3
SB-Ch NP+TSOH	3.34 ± 0.53 *,**	5.4

[a] Data taken from Fabiano et al., 2017 [13]; * $p < 0.05$ versus control, ** $p < 0.05$ versus TSOH, and Ch NP+TSOH.

It is interesting to note that no differences were seen, in Figure 8, in the concentration in the aqueous vs. time profiles between any of the three NP-containing TSOH formulations. This can be ascribed to the presence in all formulations of a significant 5-FU dose fraction not entrapped in NP, but free to permeate across the cornea by passive diffusion. Such a drug fraction is unaffected by the different NP ability to be internalized in corneal cells, which can indeed be influenced by the NP surface characteristics.

The data altogether demonstrate the importance of NP mucoadhesion properties and of their ability to interact with the vehicle. In fact, QA-Ch NP-containing TSOH showed an AUC value higher than that for TSOH or Ch NP+ TSOH probably thanks to their fixed positive charges that prolong the drug retention time and increase the drug contact with the anterior surface of the eyes and thereby, enhance ocular absorption via paracellular transport through the tight junctions of corneal epithelia [16]. On the other hand, SB-Ch NP+TSOH showed an AUC value similar to that of QA-Ch NP+TSOH probably due to its ability to slow down the 5-FU release from the vehicle, as demonstrated in Section 3.5.

These present results are in agreement with those shown in a preceding paper where it was found that the more effective NP were able to concurrently adhere to the ocular surface and strongly interact with the drug molecules in solution [10]. After all, although less mucoadhesive than QA-Ch NP, the SB-Ch NP also showed some mucoadhesivity due to the intrinsic mucoadhesivity of the Ch backbone.

4. Conclusions

These results indicate that the present SB-Ch NP-containing thermosensitive hydrogels are able to prolong 5-FU ocular residence thanks to the synergistic effect of negative charges on NP surface and positive charges present in the TSOH. Furthermore, in the case of QA-Ch NP-containing thermosensitive hydrogels the presence of positive charges on NP surface prolongs their contact with corneal and conjunctival surfaces that are negatively charged. As a result, both NP-containing QA-Ch-based and SB-Ch-based TSOH were able to increase the ocular 5-FU bioavailability. NP-containing thermosensitive hydrogels could be administered as conventional eyedrops and still represent an alternative, more effective formulation than the commercial 5-FU eyedrops, with reduced 5-FU applied dose and instillation frequency. However stability studies of the formulations must be carried out in the future to understand if they can really be commercialized.

Author Contributions: Conceptualization, A.F. and Y.Z.; methodology, A.F., A.M.P., R.B. and Y.Z.; validation, A.F., A.M.P., and Y.Z..; formal analysis, A.F., A.M.P., L.G., B.S. and R.B., data curation, A.F., A.M.P., R.B. and Y.Z.; writing—original draft preparation, A.F. and Y.Z.; writing—review and editing, all authors; supervision, Y.Z.

References

1. Gaudana, R.; Ananthula, H.K.; Parenky, A.; Mitra, A.K. Ocular drug delivery. *AAPS J.* **2010**, *12*, 348–360. [CrossRef] [PubMed]
2. Üstündağ-Okur, N.; Gökçe, E.H.; Bozbıyık, D.I.; Eğrilmez, S.; Özer, Ö.; Ertan, G. Preparation and in vitro–in vivo evaluation of ofloxacin loaded ophthalmic nano structured lipid carriers modified with chitosan oligosaccharide lactate for the treatment of bacterial keratitis. *Eur. J. Pharm. Sci.* **2014**, *63*, 204–215. [CrossRef] [PubMed]
3. Di Colo, G.; Zambito, Y.; Zaino, C. Polymeric enhancers of mucosal epithelia permeability: Synthesis, transepithelial penetration-enhancing properties, mechanism of action, safety issues. *J. Pharm. Sci.* **2008**, *97*, 1652–1680. [CrossRef] [PubMed]
4. Zambito, Y.; Di Colo, G. Chitosan and its derivatives as intraocular penetration enhancers. *J. Drug Deliv. Sci. Technol.* **2010**, *20*, 45–52. [CrossRef]
5. Zambito, Y.; Di Colo, G. Thiolated quaternary ammonium–chitosan conjugates for enhanced precorneal retention, transcorneal permeation and intraocular absorption of dexamethasone. *Eur. J. Pharm. Biopharm.* **2010**, *75*, 194–199. [CrossRef] [PubMed]
6. Berger, J.; Reist, M.; Chenite, A.; Felt-Baeyens, O.; Mayer, J.M.; Gurny, R. Pseudo-thermosetting chitosan hydrogels for biomedical application. *Int. J. Pharm.* **2005**, *288*, 197–206. [CrossRef]
7. Chenite, A.; Chaput, C.; Wang, D.; Combes, C.; Buschmann, M.D.; Hoemann, C.D.; Selmani, A. Novel injectable neutral solutions of chitosan form biodegradable gels in situ. *Biomaterials* **2000**, *21*, 2155–2161. [CrossRef]

8. Wang, Q.; Zuo, Z.; Cheung CK, C.; Leung, S.S.Y. Updates on thermosensitive hydrogel for nasal, ocular and cutaneous delivery. *Int. J. Pharm.* **2019**, *559*, 86–101. [CrossRef]
9. Ruel-Gariepy, E.; Leroux, J.C. In situ-forming hydrogels—review of temperature-sensitive systems. *Eur. J. Pharm. Biopharm.* **2004**, *58*, 409–426. [CrossRef]
10. Fabiano, A.; Chetoni, P.; Zambito, Y. Mucoadhesive nano-sized supramolecular assemblies for improved pre-corneal drug residence time. *Drug Dev. Ind. Pharm.* **2015**, *41*, 2069–2076. [CrossRef]
11. Bonferoni, M.C.; Sandri, G.; Dellera, E.; Rossi, S.; Ferrari, F.; Zambito, Y.; Caramella, C. Palmitoyl glycol chitosan micelles for corneal delivery of cyclosporine. *J. Biomed. Nanotechnol.* **2016**, *12*, 231–240. [CrossRef] [PubMed]
12. Diebold, Y.; Jarrín, M.; Saez, V.; Carvalho, E.L.; Orea, M.; Calonge, M.; Alonso, M.J. Ocular drug delivery by liposome–chitosan nanoparticle complexes (LCS-NP). *Biomaterials* **2007**, *28*, 1553–1564. [CrossRef] [PubMed]
13. Fabiano, A.; Bizzarri, R.; Zambito, Y. Thermosensitive hydrogel based on chitosan and its derivatives containing medicated nanoparticles for transcorneal administration of 5-fluorouracil. *Int. J. Nanomed.* **2017**, *12*, 633. [CrossRef] [PubMed]
14. Morsi, N.; Ghorab, D.; Refai, H.; Teba, H. Ketoroloac tromethamine loaded nanodispersion incorporated into thermosensitive in situgel for prolonged ocular delivery. *Int. J. Pharm.* **2016**, *506*, 57–67. [CrossRef] [PubMed]
15. Mo, Z.; Ban, J.; Zhang, Y.; Du, Y.; Wen, Y.; Huang, X.; Xie, Q.; Shen, L.; Zhang, S.; Deng, H.; et al. Nanostructured lipid carriers-based thermosensitive eye drops for enhanced, sustained delivery of dexamethasone. *Nanomedicine* **2018**, *13*, 1239–1253. [CrossRef]
16. Nagarwal, R.C.; Kumar, R.; Pandit, J.K. Chitosan coated sodium alginate–chitosan nanoparticles loaded with 5-FU for ocular delivery: In vitro characterization and in vivo study in rabbit eye. *Eur. J. Pharm. Sci.* **2012**, *47*, 678–685. [CrossRef]
17. Bernkop-Schnürch, A.; Dünnhaupt, S. Chitosan-Based Drug Delivery Systems. *Eur. J. Pharm. Biopharm.* **2012**, *81*, 463–469. [CrossRef]
18. Dimassi, S.; Tabary, N.; Chai, F.; Blanchemain, N.; Martel, B. Sulfonated and sulfated chitosan derivatives for biomedical applications: A review. *Carbohydr. Polym.* **2018**, *202*, 382–396. [CrossRef]
19. Zambito, Y.; Felice, F.; Fabiano, A.; Di Stefano, R.; Di Colo, G. Mucoadhesive nanoparticles made of thiolated quaternary chitosan crosslinked with hyaluronan. *Carbohydr. Polym.* **2013**, *92*, 33–39. [CrossRef] [PubMed]
20. Fabiano, A.; Piras, A.M.; Uccello-Barretta, G.; Balzano, F.; Cesari, A.; Testai, L.; Zambito, Y. Impact of mucoadhesive polymeric nanoparticulate systems on oral bioavailability of a macromolecular model drug. *Eur. J. Pharm. Biopharm.* **2018**, *130*, 281–289. [CrossRef]
21. Felice, F.; Zambito, Y.; Belardinelli, E.; D'Onofrio, C.; Fabiano, A.; Balbarini, A.; Di Stefano, R. Delivery of natural polyphenols by polymeric nanoparticles improves the resistance of endothelial progenitor cells to oxidative stress. *Eur. J. Pharm. Sci.* **2013**, *50*, 393–399. [CrossRef] [PubMed]
22. Tsai, H.S.; Wang, Y.Z.; Lin, J.J.; Lien, W.F. Preparation and properties of sulfopropyl chitosan derivatives with various sulfonation degree. *J. Appl. Polym.* **2010**, *116*, 1686–1693. [CrossRef]
23. Di Colo, G.; Zambito, Y.; Zaino, C.; Sansò, M. Selected polysaccharides at comparison for their mucoadhesiveness and effect on precorneal residence of different drugs in the rabbit model. *Drug Dev. Ind. Pharm.* **2009**, *35*, 941–949. [CrossRef] [PubMed]
24. Uccello-Barretta, G.; Nazzi, S.; Balzano, F.; Di Colo, G.; Zambito, Y.; Zaino, C.; Benvenuti, M. Enhanced affinity of ketotifen toward tamarind seed polysaccharide in comparison with hydroxyethylcellulose and hyaluronic acid: A nuclear magnetic resonance investigation. *Bioorg. Med. Chem.* **2008**, *16*, 7371–7376. [CrossRef]
25. Zambito, Y.; Pedreschi, E.; Di Colo, G. Is dialysis a reliable method for studying drug release from nanoparticulate systems?—A case study. *Int. J. Pharm.* **2012**, *434*, 28–34. [CrossRef]
26. Dodero, A.; Williams, R.; Gagliardi, S.; Vicini, S.; Alloisio, M.; Castellano, M. A micro-rheological and rheological study of biopolymers solutions: Hyaluronic acid. *Carbohydr. Polym.* **2019**, *203*, 349–355. [CrossRef]
27. Ceulemans, J.; Vermeire, A.; Adriaens, E.; Remon, J.P.; Ludwig, A. Evaluation of a mucoadhesive tablet for ocular use. *J. Control. Release* **2001**, *77*, 333–344. [CrossRef]
28. Lallemand, F.; Furrer, P.; Felt-Baeyens, O.; Gex-Fabry, M.; Dumont, J.M.; Besseghir, K.; Gurny, R. A novel water-soluble cyclosporine a prodrug: Ocular tolerance and in vivo kinetics. *Int. J. Pharm.* **2005**, *295*, 7–14. [CrossRef]

29. Schoenwald, R.D.; Harris, R.G.; Turner, D.; Knowles, W.; Chien, D.S. Ophthalmic bioequivalence of steroid/antibiotic combination formulations. *Biopharm. Drug Dispos.* **1987**, *8*, 527–548. [CrossRef]
30. Fabiano, A.; Zambito, Y.; Bernkop-Schnürch, A. About the impact of water movement on the permeation behaviour of nanoparticles in mucus. *Int. J. Pharm.* **2017**, *517*, 279–285. [CrossRef]
31. Bansil, R.; Turner, B.S. The biology of mucus: Composition, synthesis and organization. *Adv. Drug Deliv. Rev.* **2018**, *124*, 3–15. [CrossRef] [PubMed]

7

Electrospun Nanofibers for Tissue Engineering with Drug Loading and Release

Kaiqiang Ye [1], Haizhu Kuang [1], Zhengwei You [2], Yosry Morsi [3] and Xiumei Mo [1,*]

[1] State Key Laboratory for Modification of Chemical Fibers and Polymer Materials, College of Chemistry, Chemical Engineering and Biotechnology, Donghua University, Shanghai 201620, China; yekaiqiang91@gmail.com (K.Y.); kuanghaizhu@gmail.com (H.K.)

[2] State Key Laboratory for Modification of Chemical Fibers and Polymer Materials, College of Materials Science and Engineering, Donghua University, Shanghai 201620, China; zyou@dhu.edu.cn

[3] Faculty of Engineering and Industrial Sciences, Swinburne University of Technology, Boroondara, VIC 3122, Australia; ymorsi@swin.edu.au

* Correspondence: xmm@dhu.edu.cn;

Abstract: Electrospinning technologies have been applied in the field of tissue engineering as materials, with nanoscale-structures and high porosity, can be easily prepared via this method to bio-mimic the natural extracellular matrix (ECM). Tissue engineering aims to fabricate functional biomaterials for the repairment and regeneration of defective tissue. In addition to the structural simulation for accelerating the repair process and achieving a high-quality regeneration, the combination of biomaterials and bioactive molecules is required for an ideal tissue-engineering scaffold. Due to the diversity in materials and method selection for electrospinning, a great flexibility in drug delivery systems can be achieved. Various drugs including antibiotic agents, vitamins, peptides, and proteins can be incorporated into electrospun scaffolds using different electrospinning techniques and drug-loading methods. This is a review of recent research on electrospun nanofibrous scaffolds for tissue-engineering applications, the development of preparation methods, and the delivery of various bioactive molecules. These studies are based on the fabrication of electrospun biomaterials for the repair of blood vessels, nerve tissues, cartilage, bone defects, and the treatment of aneurysms and skin wounds, as well as their applications related to oral mucosa and dental fields. In these studies, due to the optimal selection of drugs and loading methods based on electrospinning, in vitro and in vivo experiments demonstrated that these scaffolds exhibited desirable effects for the repair and treatment of damaged tissue and, thus, have excellent potential for clinical application.

Keywords: electrospinning; tissue engineering; drug delivery

---

1. Introduction

Electrospinning technology has been widely utilized for the preparation of tissue-engineering scaffolds [1]. The set-up of a typical electrospinning apparatus mainly consists of a spinneret (e.g., a medical injector with a blunt tip), a boost pump for controlling the extrusion rate of a polymer solution, a direct-current electric field, and a grounded collector [2]. The electrospinning technique applies electrostatic principles to fabricate electrospun nanofibers [3]. Generally, in the electrospinning process, a polymer solution generates a cone-shaped drop beneath the needle under a strong electric field; then, the polymer drops overcome the surface tension to eject polymer nanofibers into the low electric field [4,5]. Using electrospinning, various polymers including synthetic and natural materials (as well as blends of the two in consideration of the mechanical properties) can be fabricated as diverse tissue-engineering scaffolds possessing nanofibrous structure. Scaffolds prepared by electrospinning have tremendous advantages for tissue engineering, such as a large specific surface area, high porosity, extracellular matrix (ECM)-biomimetic structures, and better biocompatibility [6–10]. Furthermore, the ECM can bind, release, and activate signaling molecules and can also modulate the cell's reaction to soluble factors [11]. In order to functionalize the scaffolds for the promotion of cell adhesion, proliferation, and differentiation, nanofibers of the scaffold can be loaded with many bioactive substances, such as proteins, peptides, and small-molecule drugs [12–18]. Therefore, electrospun scaffolds have remarkable advantages in both ECM-biomimetic structures and the loading of bioactive substances. Electrospun drug delivery scaffolds have emerged as essential applications in the biomedical field [19].

The diversity in material selection and preparation methods gives electrospun scaffolds great flexibility for the application of drug delivery [20]. By utilizing different kinds of electrospinning methods, drugs can be incorporated into electrospun scaffolds in many ways, such as coatings, embedded loading, and encapsulated loading (coaxial and emulsion electrospinning). Traditional electrospinning is the simplest method to prepare electrospun scaffolds. In this method, polymers are directly dissolved into solvent to obtain the electrospinning solution and fabricate the scaffolds. In traditional electrospinning, drugs can be incorporated into the scaffolds either by blending or surface modification. In blending electrospinning, drugs and polymers are simultaneously dissolved in the solvent. Later on, this blended solution is used to fabricate the scaffold [21]. In surface modification, electrospun scaffolds are prepared firstly, then drugs are loaded onto the scaffolds via physical adsorption, covalent binding, and other surface-treatment methods [22]. Accordingly, drugs incorporated into scaffolds via different methods exhibit diverse release characteristics. In blending, the release rate mainly depends on the properties of polymers and drugs in the physiological environment. In physical adsorption, the drug usually shows a faster release rate because of the weaker interaction between drugs and the surface of scaffolds, such as electrostatic adsorption, hydrogen bonding, and hydrophobic interactions [23]. However, drugs covalently bound to the scaffolds hardly release from the scaffolds unless the surface polymers are degraded [24].

Coaxial electrospinning is a special method to generate nanofibers with a core–shell structure. Using a coaxial configuration, two separate polymer solutions (core and shell solutions) flow through two different but coaxial aisles. Core and shell solutions are simultaneously pushed into the configuration. With the slow push of a syringe, the drops are jetted out to form nanofibers under a strong electric field. This technique attracted great attention due to its potential applications in controlled drug delivery [25–27]. In coaxial electrospinning, the shell solutions should have spinnability to form the main part of the nanofibers. However, the core solutions have no need for spinnability; thus, some substances without spinnability, such as drugs, proteins, and some bioactive substances, can be incorporated into the core structure of nanofibers by dissolving in the core solution. In this way, these drugs and bioactive substances can be released from the nanofibers in a sustained manner. Therefore, coaxial electrospinning can prepare electrospun scaffolds with bioactivity and functionality. This method is widely used for the preparation of functional nanofibrous scaffolds. A controlled release of functional molecules from the core layer of core–shell scaffolds loaded with drugs, bio-macromolecules, and growth factors could sustainably exert biological functions. For example, tetracycline hydrochloride encapsulated into electrospun core–shell nanofibers showed a sustained release, and exhibited great antibacterial capability, as shown in *Escherichia coli* growth-inhibiting tests [28]. ZnO and Zn acetate nanoparticles were embedded in polycaprolactone coaxial-fiber and uniaxial-fiber matrices to develop potential antibacterial nanocomposite wound dressings [29]. In order to guide tissue regeneration in an infectious environment, coaxial electrospinning was firstly conducted to fabricate dual drug-loaded fiber mats with a core/shell structure. Naringin-loaded polyvinylpyrrolidone was designed as a core fiber to enrich tissue regeneration, and metronidazole-loaded poly(lactic-*co*-glycolic acid) was designed as a shell fiber to inhibit bacterial growth [30].

In addition, nanofibers prepared via the emulsion electrospinning possess the analogous core–shell structure generated by coaxial electrospinning. Therefore, emulsion electrospinning can also be used to prepare core–shell nanofibers for loading and releasing drugs, proteins, and growth factors.

However, the process and needle used for emulsion electrospinning are different compared to coaxial electrospinning. Emulsion electrospinning has no need for a coaxial configuration, and the spinning solution is made into a uniform emulsifying solution by blending emulsifier into a polymer–drug mixed solution. However, the polymers and drugs are dissolved in different solvents before blending. Then, the solution is used for the electrospinning process via a single syringe needle as in traditional electrospinning. Finally, nanofibers with multicore or core–shell structures can be obtained. In order to verify the controlled delivery of drugs from this novel type of tissue-engineering scaffold, rhodamine B and bovine serum albumin (BSA) were incorporated into nanofibers via emulsion electrospinning [31]. In vitro dual drug-release studies of different types of electrospun mats indicated that the emulsion electrospun mats had the most desirable controllable release behaviors.

Therefore, electrospun scaffolds, due to their ECM-biomimetic structure and diversity of drug delivery applications, are widely applied in the field of tissue engineering [32]. In the upcoming section, we further introduce their specific applications, such as aneurysm treatment, nerve tissue engineering, vascular tissue engineering, wound dressing, and bone tissue engineering.

2. Electrospun Scaffolds for Aneurysm Treatment

Intracranial aneurysms represent one of the most common cerebrovascular diseases, and they cause serious healthcare problems, such as brain damage, hemorrhagic stroke, and even death [33,34]. Many studies demonstrated that a covered stent is a desirable solution to treat aneurysms [35,36]. However, the common problem is that the stent-graft easily causes platelet aggregation when implanted into the blood vessel, leading to thrombosis and intimal hyperplasia. Rapid endothelialization, antithrombotic coatings, and anti-clotting drugs are favorable methods to avoid thrombosis. A covered stent is formed by a covered sheet wrapping a metallic stent, where the anticoagulation properties of the covered sheet play a crucial role in avoiding thrombosis of the covered stent. The emulsion electrospinning technique was used to fabricate heparin-loaded poly(L-lactide-*co*-caprolactone) (PLCL) core–shell nanofibers as an anticoagulant cover sheet. Heparin aqueous solution and emulsifier Span-80 were added dropwise into dichloromethane while stirring until a uniform water-in-oil emulsion formed. PLCL was then added into the emulsion for electrospinning to fabricate PLCL/heparin core–shell nanofibers. The covered stent effectively separated the aneurysm dome in the bloodstream of the rabbit model [37]. In addition, vascular endothelial growth factor (VEGF) was mixed with heparin and loaded into the core of a PLCL nanofiber via emulsion electrospinning to promote rapid endothelialization [38]. An aqueous solution of VEGF, heparin, and Span-80 was mixed in dichloromethane to form a uniform water-in-oil emulsion via consistent stirring. PLCL was then dissolved in the emulsion to obtain a uniform electrospinning solution. Finally, the solution was electrospun to obtain PLCL–Hep–VEGF scaffolds. The release of heparin and VEGF lasted for more than 30 days. That sustained release of heparin and VEGF enhanced cell proliferation and the spread of pig iliac endothelial cells onto the stent. Rosuvastatin calcium can facilitate endothelialization with the ability to enhance the adhesion and proliferation of vascular endothelial cells (VECs). A novel type of covered stent was prepared via coaxial electrospinning to cover the stent with heparin and rosuvastatin calcium-loaded PLCL nanofibers [39]. The fabrication process of the covered stent is shown in Figure 1, showing heparin and rosuvastatin calcium as the core solution and PLCL as the shell solution. The release curves of heparin and rosuvastatin calcium have two stages, including an initial release that occurred during the first 48 h and a slow release that lasted more than 45 days. The covered stent showed remarkable anticoagulation ability, and the HUVECs proliferated well on the covered stent, due to the sustained release of rosuvastatin calcium and heparin from the PLCL coaxial nanofibers.

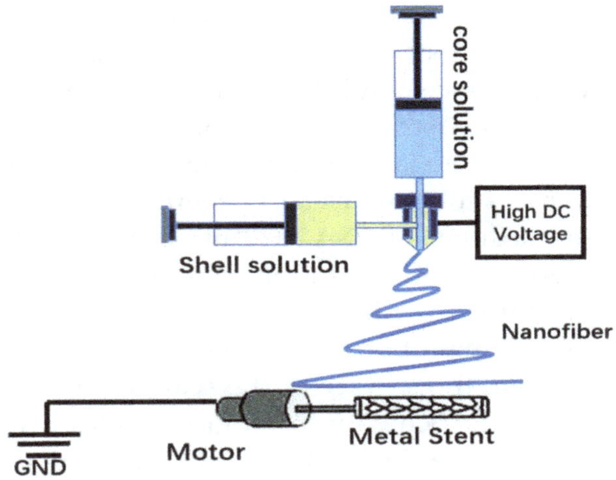

Figure 1. Schematic diagram of the set-up for coaxial electrospinning [39]. Reproduced by permission of The Royal Society of Chemistry (RSC) on behalf of the Centre National de la Recherche Scientifique (CNRS) and the RSC, 2017.

3. Electrospun Scaffolds for Nerve Tissue Engineering

Peripheral nerve defects represent a serious clinical issue which results in high morbidity among trauma patients [40]. To address the limited regenerative ability of the human nervous system and the shortage of therapeutic options, nerve tissue engineered graft transplantation is a potential treatment for peripheral nerve injury [41,42]. Conduit scaffolds, cells, and growth factors are the three elements for nerve tissue engineering [43]. Core–shell poly(D,L-lactide-*co*-glycolide) (PLGA) nanofibrous nerve guidance conduits loaded with nerve growth factor (NGF) were fabricated via coaxial electrospinning and were used to construct nerve guidance conduits for a 13-mm rat sciatic nerve defect. [44]. The shell solution was PLGA, and the core solution was β-NGF with 400 mg of PEG dissolved in distilled water. A rotating wheel drum with a speed of 4000 rpm was used to received nanofibers to form an aligned construct. The release of NGF from nanofibers lasted 30 days. After 12-weeks implantation, the regeneration of nerve cells in the PLGA/NGF conduit was superior to other groups. Another type of nerve guidance conduit (NGC) was fabricated via coaxial electrospinning. NGF in silk solution as a core layer was encapsulated in PLCL via coaxial electrospinning. NGF presented a sustained release and remained biologically active over 60 days because NGF was stabilized by silk fibroin (SF) in the core [45]. The graft was implanted across a 15-mm defect in the sciatic nerve of rats to evaluate nerve regeneration. Results of electrophysiological assessment, histochemistry, and electron microscopy at 12 weeks suggested that the released NGF from nanofibers could effectively promote the regeneration of the peripheral nerve. In order to further promote cell differentiation, the nanofibers with PLCL as the shell and BSA/NGF as the core were fabricated via coaxial electrospinning [46]. Sustained release of BSA/NGF from nanofibers was verified, and it promoted the differentiation of rat pheochromocytoma cells (PC12). Monosialoganglioside (GM1) can promote neuronal development, cell growth, and differentiation, and it plays an essential role in neuronal excitability of myelinated and nonmyelinated fibers. It was reported that the combination of GM1 with NGF can enhance the effects of protecting nerve cells. NGF and GM1 were loaded into the PLCL/silk fibroin (PLCL/SF) nanofibers via a coaxial electrospinning technique [47]. NGF reached 55.8 ± 1.6% release at 71 days. Schwann cell (SC) proliferation and pheochromocytoma (PC12) differentiation were enhanced by the synergistic effect of GM1 and NGF. The graft loading with GM1 and NGF performed good nerve function recovery in a rabbit sciatic nerve defect model. Vitamins play an important role in tissue growth and differentiation. The water-soluble vitamin B5 was blended with PLCL/silk solutions to form an electrospinning solution. Then, the electrospinning solution was aligned with nanofiber meshes via electrospinning technique [48]. Vitamin B5 was added to a PLCL/silk solution and constantly stirred overnight to form the electrospinning solution. Nanofibers with aligned structure were collected by a rotating drum collector with a speed of 3000 rpm. Vitamin B5 was released up to 80% in 24 h. This nanofibrous material might have potential applications in nerve repair or regeneration. A laminin-coated and yarn-encapsulated PLGA nerve guidance conduit (LC-YE-PLGA NGC) was fabricated to perform the cooperative effects of a topological structure promoting Schwann cell (SC) proliferation and migration [49]. The PLGA fiber yarns were fabricated through a double-nozzle electrospinning system; then, the PLGA fibrous outer layer was collected using a general electrospinning method. Subsequently, laminin was coated on the yarn-encapsulated PLGA NGC through covalent bonding (Figure 2). The cell growth test showed that SC growth and SC migration were much better in the LC-YE-PLGA NGCs than in those without yarn encapsulation or laminin coating. Polycaprolactone (PCL) and chitosan were blended and fabricated to form nanofibrous scaffolds via electrospinning. Taking advantage of the amine groups on the chitosan, the surface of the scaffolds was functionalized with laminin via carbodiimide-based cross-linking. Schwann cells grew well on PCL–chitosan scaffolds with excellent mechanical and surface properties [50]. NGF and GDNF were encapsulated in poly(D,L-lactic acid) (PDLLA) and poly(lactic-*co*-glycolic acid) (PLGA) nanofibers, respectively, via a dual-source dual-power (DS-DP) emulsion electrospinning technique. Scaffolds were developed providing dual GF delivery, and sustained release of both types of GFs was also achieved [51].

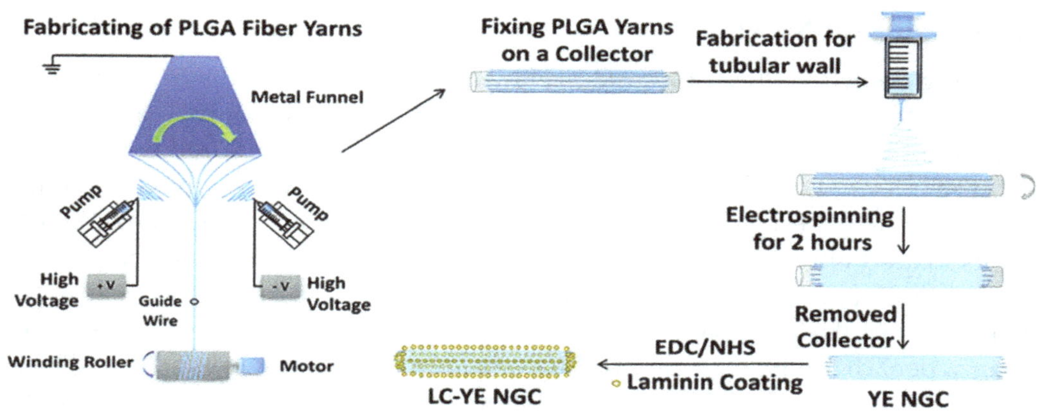

Figure 2. A schematic diagram of the fabrication of the laminin-coated and yarn-encapsulated PLGA (LC-YE-PLGA) nerve guidance conduit (YE NGC: yarn-encapsulated nerve guidance conduit; LC-YE NGC: laminin-coated and yarn-encapsulated nerve guidance conduit) [49]. Reproduced by permission of The Royal Society of Chemistry, 2017.

4. Electrospun Scaffolds for Vascular Tissue Engineering

Coronary heart and peripheral vascular diseases are now the leading cause of death worldwide [52]. Autologous and allogeneic vascular transplantation has limitations caused by many factors such as donor-site morbidity and the shortage of donors in clinic treatment. Developing artificial blood vessels shows increasing significance [53]. Electrospinning is an ideal technique to prepare grafts for small-diameter blood vessels. Heparin-loaded PLCL nanofibers were prepared via a coaxial electrospinning technique, fabricating tubular grafts with an inner diameter of 4 mm [54]. The release of heparin experienced two stages: an initial burst release of 50% followed by continuous release up to 72% from day 2 to 14. Evaluation with a canine artery model demonstrated that heparin loading could greatly enhance the patency rate of small-diameter grafts. To promote endothelial progenitor cell proliferation, vascular endothelial growth factors (VEGFs) are often loaded into scaffolds. Heparin and VEGF were encapsulated into a PLCL nanofiber via emulsion electrospinning to construct vascular grafts for anticoagulation and rapid endothelization [55]. Heparin/VEGF aqueous solution and Span-80 were added dropwise into methylene dichloride and stirred magnetically to form a uniform water-in-oil emulsion. Then, PLCL was dissolved in the emulsion and stirred overnight to obtain the electrospinning solution. Finally, electrospun vascular grafts were prepared using the electrospinning solution. Heparin and VEGF exhibited sustained release for 29 days. The controlled release of heparin and VEGF from the grafts showed good capability for anticoagulation and promoted EPC growth. Platelet-rich growth factor (PRGF) was added into PLCL/SF solutions at a concentration of 20 mg/mL to obtain the electrospinning solution; then, a tubular graft 4 nm in diameter was prepared via an electrospinning process. The graft promoted fast SMC growth and cell penetration into grafts [56]. Salvianolic acid B (SAB), a traditional Chinese plant medicine, can promote the proliferation and migration of endothelial cells. Heparin was dissolved in reverse osmosis (RO) water as a core solution. PLCL and collagen were dissolved in a solution of 1,1,1,3,3,3-hexafluoro-2-propanol (HFIP) with SAB-MSN as a shell solution. Heparin and SAB-MSN were separately encapsulated into the core and the shell of nanofibers via coaxial electrospinning to construct an inner layer of a small-diameter blood vessel graft. The electrospinning process is shown in Figure 3 [57]. SAB was gently released, and no burst release was observed; this is because SAB was adsorbed onto the MSN and blended into the coaxial fiber shell. The total release of 56% was attained within 30 days. The release of heparin was observed, with an initial burst followed by a steady increase up to 30 days. At the end of the test, the cumulative amount of heparin released was 68%. Assessment of the graft in a rat subcutaneous embedding model demonstrated that it possessed good biocompatibility and did not cause significant immune responses, suggesting that the graft is promising for preventing acute thrombosis and for promoting rapid endothelialization. Some findings provide evidence that surface-immobilized growth factors display enhanced stability and induce prolonged function. PCL nano- or microfibers were produced via electrospinning, and they were coated in a radio frequency (RF) plasma process to induce an oxygen functional hydrocarbon layer. Implemented carboxylic acid groups were converted into amine-reactive esters and covalently coupled to VEGF by forming stable amide bonds. Endothelial cell number was significantly enhanced on VEGF-functionalized scaffolds compared to native PCL scaffolds [58].

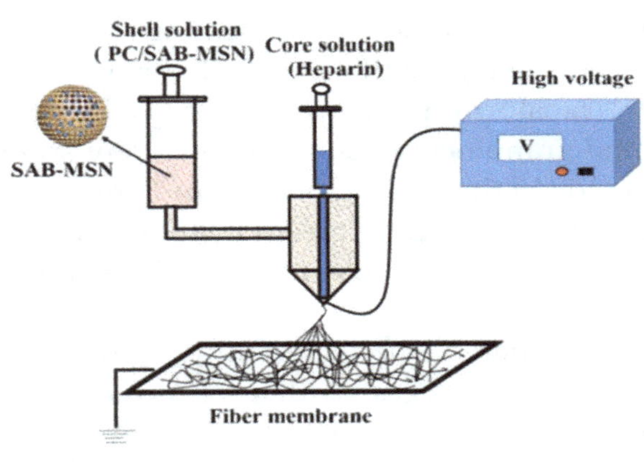

Figure 3. Process of fabricating the core (heparin)−shell (PC/SAB-MSN) fiber. Reprinted with permission from [57].

5. Electrospun Scaffolds for Wound Dressing Application

Skin wounds are a common issue for surgeons. Clinically, the injured skin should be disposed of and carefully protected with wound dressing immediately. Figure 4 exhibits the classic stages of wound repair. There are three classic stages of wound repair: inflammation (a), new tissue formation (b), and remodeling (c) [59]. The effective promotion of the healing of wounds and the prevention of any infection are the functions of wound dressing. Traditional wound dressings are no longer applicable for the required high-quality healing of heavy and chronic skin wounds [60]. In recent years, wound dressings fabricated via electrospinning methods have received a lot of attention in tissue engineering. Electrospinning is a simple and effective technology for preparing materials with a nanofibrous structure which is similar to the ECM. Wound dressing with this structure was proven to promote the repair of injured skin [61–63]. This is because the electrospun mats possess nanofibrous porous webs, which are not only suitable for the volatilization of tissue fluid, but also for the permeation of oxygen from the external environment. In addition, many growth factors and antibacterial substances can be loaded onto the electrospun wound dressings in various ways during the fabrication process.

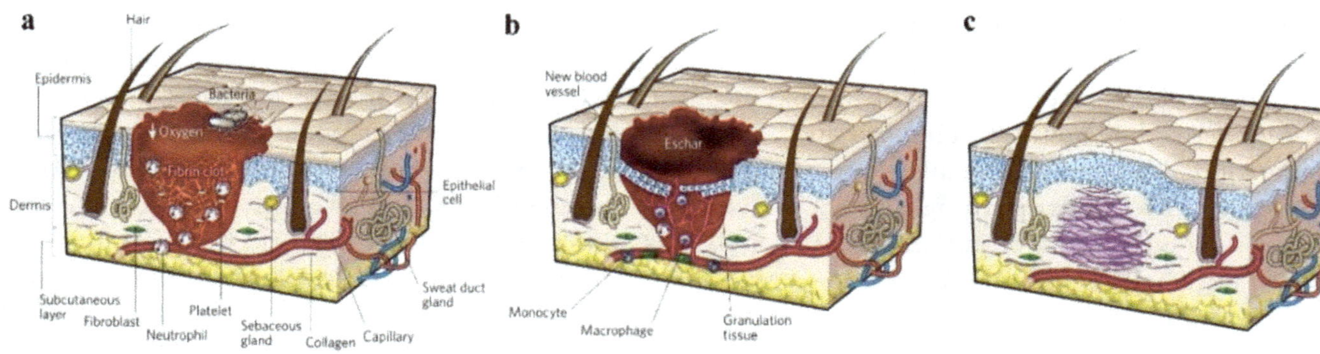

Figure 4. Classic stages of wound repair. There are three classic stages of wound repair: inflammation (**a**), new tissue formation (**b**), and remodeling (**c**) [59]. Reproduced with permission from Springer Nature, 2008.

Generally, electrospun wound dressings are fabricated through a typical electrospinning process to obtain membrane materials. Electrospinning solutions were prepared by dissolving single polymers or by blending natural and synthetic polymers; in some cases, the antibacterial substances could be directly mixed into the solutions [64,65]. Moreover, the healing of skin wounds is a complex biological process. In this process, many cellular pathways are activated to regulate cell behaviors to promote the repair of the wound and reduce the probability of infection [66,67]. Furthermore, different growth factors and important active substances in the wound healing process attracted attention in wound dressing applications, such as epidermal growth factor (EGF), platelet-derived growth factor (PDGF), fibroblast growth factor (FGF), transforming growth factor (TGF), insulin-like growth factor (IGF), and human growth hormone and granulocyte-macrophage colony-stimulating factor (GM-CSF) [60]. Other important active compounds in the healing of a wound are vitamins A, C, and E, zinc, iodine, silver nanoparticles, and copper minerals. Therefore, in many studies, there was a growing tendency to incorporate growth factors or antibacterial molecules into the electrospun materials for enhancing the healing quality of wounds [68–72].

Specifically, Sheng et al. [73] prepared a novel vitamin E (VE)-loaded silk fibroin (SF) nanofiber mat for skin care application. Studies suggested that VE possesses antioxidant and skin barrier stabilizing properties, which make VE a suitable agent for skin protection. In this study, water-soluble VE, RRR-α-tocopherol polyethylene glycol 1000 succinate (VE TPGS), was incorporated into SF nanofibers to investigate its potential application in skin care and tissue regeneration. An in vitro study showed that VE TPGS exhibited sustained-release behavior from the nanofiber mats in a physiological environment. In addition, cell experiments demonstrated that nanofibers containing VE TPGS promoted the proliferation of mouse skin fibroblasts (L929 cells) and protected the cell from oxidation.

El-Aassar et al. [74] developed electrospun polyvinyl alcohol (PVA)/pluronic F127 (Plur)/polyethyleneimine (PEI) composite mats containing titanium dioxide nanoparticles (TiO_2 NPs) for wound dressing application. Titanium ions having wound-healing and antimicrobial properties could be released from TiO_2 nanoparticles in a slow way, so as to accelerate the wound healing. In this study, TiO_2 nanoparticles were used as an antimicrobial agent by directly blending them into the electrospinning solution, and antibacterial tests demonstrated that the fabricated PVA-Plur-PEI/TiO_2 nanofibers exhibited better bactericidal activity than PVA-Plur-PEI nanofibers.

Lv et al. [75] reported an electrospun poly(caprolactone) (PCL)/gelatin scaffold containing silicate-based bioceramic particles (Nagelschmidtite, NAGEL, $Ca_7P_2Si_2O_{16}$) for wound healing. In this study, via a co-electrospinning process, the NAGEL bioceramic particles could be uniformly incorporated into PCL/gelatin fibers, and, with the degradation of the scaffold, the Si ions could be released from the fibers in a sustained way. Figure 5 shows the SEM and TEM images of electrospun fibers containing different amounts of NAGEL bioceramic particles which were well embedded inside polymer fibers [75]. Human umbilical vein endothelial cells (HUVECs) and human keratinocytes (HaCaTs) were cultured into the scaffolds, and cell tests indicated that the scaffolds could significantly promote cell adhesion, proliferation, and migration. Wound healing assessment also displayed that wound sites repaired by these scaffolds exhibited desirable healing results in the aspects of angiogenesis, collagen deposition, re-epithelialization, and inhibiting an inflammation reaction. Furthermore, the mechanism of the high-quality healing of the bioceramic/polymer composite biomaterial was identified as being related to the activation of the epithelial-to-mesenchymal transition (EMT) and endothelial-to-mesenchymal transition (EndMT) pathway.

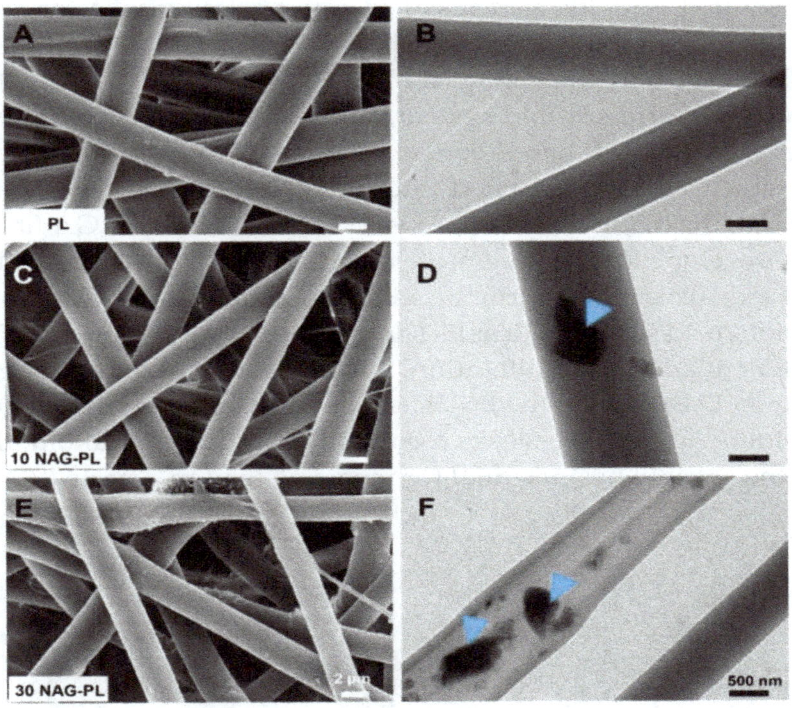

Figure 5. SEM (**A**,**C**,**E**) and TEM (**B**,**D**,**F**) images of the composite electrospun scaffolds with different contents of NAG bioceramic particles: (**A**,**B**) pure polymer (PL); (**C**,**D**) polymer with 10% NAG bioceramic particles (10 NAG-PL); (**E**,**F**) polymer with 30% NAG bioceramic particles (30 NAG-PL). Blue arrows identify the NAG bioceramic particles which were well embedded inside polymer fibers [75]. Reproduced with permission from Elsevier, 2017.

As a result of incorporating various bioactive molecules into the nanofibers, these novel electrospun biomaterials provided strategies to design functional dressings for the rapid and high-quality healing of skin wounds.

6. Electrospun Scaffolds for Tendon Tissue Engineering

Surgical repair utilizing autografts, allografts, xenografts, tendon prostheses, and suture techniques are the main therapies in the current approach to the treatment of tendon injuries [76]. However, tendon grafts clinically used in surgical treatments fail to meet the demands of adaptability, flexibility, and perpetual remodeling. To address these problems, tissue-engineering scaffolds based on electrospun fibers provide potential alternatives for the treatment and regeneration of damaged tendon tissue. The combination of synthetic polymers and natural materials was an easy method to obtain electrospun scaffolds with both biocompatibility and excellent mechanical strength. Electrospun fibers materials have been investigated in tissue engineering for the potential application of tendon treatment [77–79];

these studies revealed that electrospun composite scaffolds for tendon tissue engineering performed much better than conventional tendon materials in the aspects of biocompatibility, cell adhesion, proliferation, and mechanical properties.

A desirable scaffold that possesses both suitable mechanical properties and biological signals is required for tendon tissue engineering [80]. In recent years, novel spinning approaches were used to fabricate scaffolds mimicking the hierarchical structures of natural tendon tissue [81,82], and to accelerate the healing of tendon defects and further induce tendon regeneration. In addition to varying the preparation method, tendon scaffolds containing various bioactive molecules were also fabricated [83,84].

Sahoo et al. [85]. developed a hybrid scaffold containing both microfibers and nanofibers. Specifically speaking, the knitted silk scaffolds were firstly prefabricated and coated with an aqueous silk solution; then, the knitted scaffolds were installed onto a rotating collector during electrospinning, and the solution for electrospinning was prepared by dissolving PLGA and basic fibroblast growth factor (bFGF) into HFIP. As a result, the knitted scaffolds were wrapped around the electrospun PLGA ultrafine fibers. In this biohybrid scaffold system, silk microfibers were responsible for enhancing mechanical properties, while PLGA nanofibers, coated on the silk scaffolds, could release bFGF in a sustained manner, which was incorporated into PLGA nanofibers via blending electrospinning. As shown in Figure 6A,B, the bFGF was randomly distributed in the PLGA fibers; Figure 6C shows the biohybrid scaffold developed by coating protein-containing (FGF+ group) electrospun fibers (eF) onto microfibrous knitted silk scaffolds (μF). In cell evaluation, mesenchymal progenitor cell (MPC) was seeded into the biohybrid scaffold. Results showed that the biohybrid scaffold system not only promoted MPC attachment and cell proliferation, but also stimulated the tenogeneic differentiation of seeded MPCs. Figure 6D,E exhibits the BMSC-seeded ligament/tendon analogs after seven days of culture. Moreover, following a three-week co-culture of MPCs and scaffold, the generated tendon analog indicated that the scaffold has potential for repairing tendon defects.

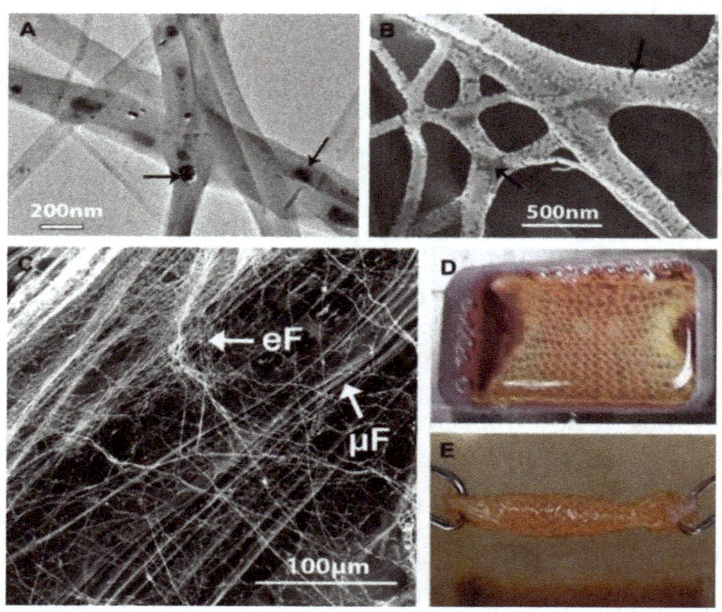

Figure 6. (**A**) TEM and (**B**) back-scattered SEM images of electrospun bFGF-containing PLGA fibers showing the random distribution of proteins (indicated by black arrows) in the fibers; (**C**) SEM image of biohybrid scaffold developed by coating FGF(+) electrospun fibers (eF) on microfibrous knitted silk scaffolds (mF); (**D**,**E**) BMSC-seeded biohybrid scaffold cultured in a custom-made chamber before being rolled up into cylindrical ligament/tendon analogs after seven days of culture [85]. Reproduced with permission from Elsevier, 2010.

Manning et al. [86] reported a scaffold with the capacity for controlled delivery of growth factors and cells for tendon tissue engineering. Platelet-derived growth factor BB (PDGF-BB), together with adipose-derived mesenchymal stem cells (ASCs), was firstly incorporated into a heparin/fibrin-based delivery system (HBDS). Then, the hydrogel was layered with electrospun nanofibers to obtain the resulting composite scaffold. In vitro and in vivo studies verified that this fabricating strategy allowed the novel layered scaffold to simultaneously and effectively deliver growth factors and fulfill cell migration in a controlled manner in the tendon repair environment so as to promote the tendon healing. Figure 7 shows the fluorescence dyed cells on the scaffold and the schematic of the scaffold structure and ingredients.

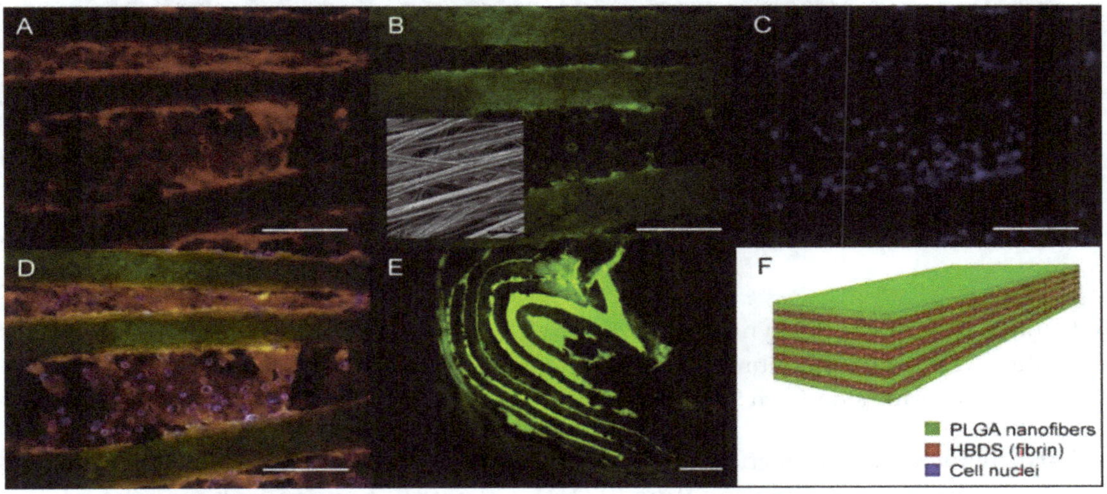

Figure 7. A representative HBDS/nanofiber scaffold with 11 alternating layers of aligned electrospun PLGA nanofiber mats separated by HBDS containing 1×10^6 ASCs is shown. (**A–D**) Micrograph showing the HBDS/nanofiber scaffold in vitro; the PLGA is labeled with FITC (green), the HBDS is labeled with Alexa Fluor 546 (red), and the ASC nuclei are labeled with Hoescht 33258 (blue) (scale bar = 200 μm). (**B**, inset) SEM image of the scaffold showing PLGA nanofiber alignment. (**E**) Micrograph showing the HBDS/nanofiber scaffold in vivo nine days after implantation in tendon repair. Eleven alternating layers of PLGA and HBDS can be seen (i.e., six layers of PLGA and five layers of fibrin); the PLGA is labeled with FITC (green) (scale bar = 100 μm). (**F**) A schematic of the layered scaffold is shown [86]. Reproduced with permission from Elsevier, 2013.

7. Electrospun Scaffolds for Bone Tissue Engineering

Bone tissue-engineering scaffolds are applied to repair bone defects mainly caused by tumors, trauma, osteoporosis, and infection. Due to a limited donor site in autografting treatment, bone tissue engineering aims to produce functional bone scaffolds as alternatives for clinical treatments [87]. An ideal bone scaffold should mimic the architecture of the native ECM to provide a three-dimensional (3D) environment for cell adhesion, proliferation, and differentiation [88]. However, nanofiber materials prepared via traditional electrospinning only possess nanofibrous structure on a two-dimensional level, lacking a 3D porous structure essential for nutrient transport and tissue regeneration; it is estimated that the interconnected spaces >100 μm are required for vascularized bone tissue growth [89]. Recently, emerging strategies were applied to prepare 3D nanofibrous scaffolds based on electrospun nanofibers, which have attracted attention in tissue engineering, especially bone tissue engineering [90–92]. Figure 8 shows the typical strategy of the preparation of electrospun 3D nanofibrous scaffolds; this method mainly consists of nanofiber preparation, homogenization, freeze-drying, and cross-linking processes. These scaffolds possess nanofibrous morphologies and interconnected pores. In addition, a prevailing strategy in bone engineering is the combination of growth factors and scaffolds to facilitate the osteogenic differentiation of stem cells in vitro, and bone regeneration in vivo.

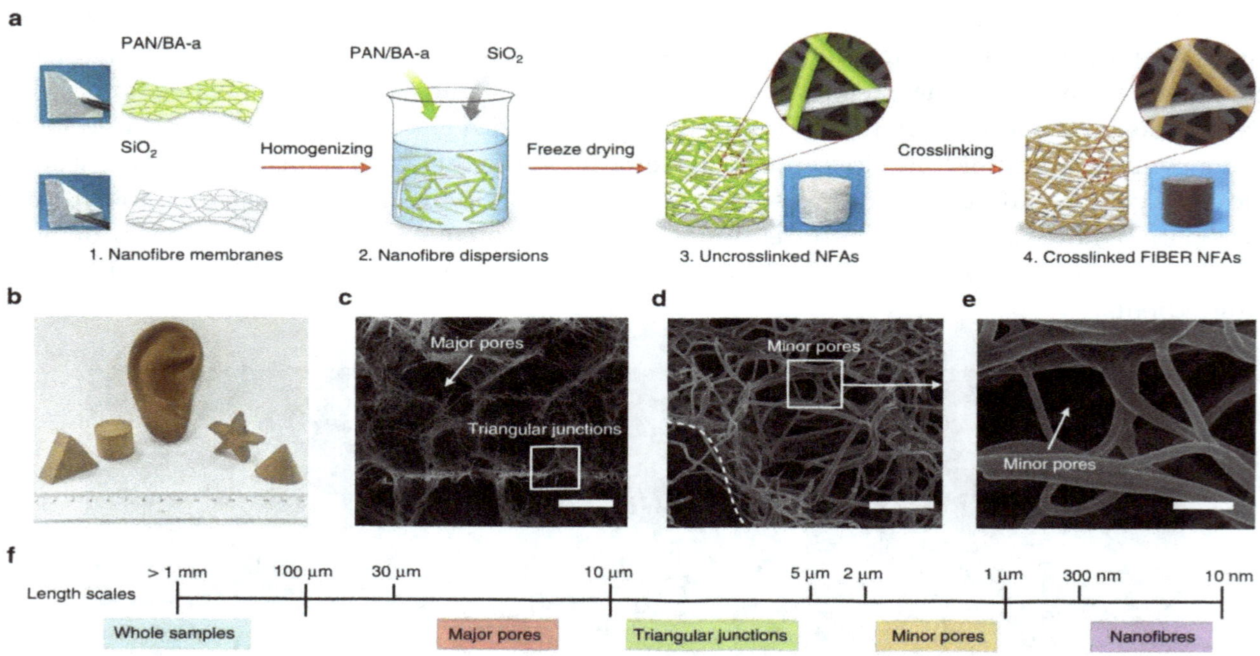

Figure 8. (**a**) Schematic of the synthetic steps. (**b**) The pictures of fabricated scaffolds. (**c**–**e**) SEM images of the electrospun nanofibrous scaffolds. (**f**) Length scales: 20 μm (**c**), 5 μm (**d**), 1 μm (**e**) [92]. Reproduced with permission from Springer Nature, 2014.

Several studies verified the crucial role of growth factors in regulating cell behaviors, such as recruitment, proliferation, and differentiation [93,94]. Currently, bone morphogenetic proteins (BMPs) are the most effective osteoinductive growth factors investigated in bone tissue engineering [24]. In particular, BMP-2 was approved for clinical application by the FDA. Su et al. [95] developed a BMP-2-and dexamethasone (DEX)-loaded core–shell electrospun mat for use in bone tissue engineering. BMP-2 and DEX were successfully incorporated into nanofibers via blending or coaxial electrospinning, and evaluation of release in vitro indicated that coaxial electrospinning nanofibers exhibited better controlled release of the two substances than blending electrospinning nanofibers. Moreover, the BMP-2 and DEX released from nanofibers induced human mesenchymal stromal cells (hMSC) to differentiate into osteogenic cells.

However, BMP-2 has the disadvantages of rapid enzymatic hydrolysis, ectopic bone formation, immune reactions, and high cost [96,97]. Recently, BMP-2-derived peptides gained much attention as alternative bioactive molecules. The sequences of the peptides were synthesized based on the "wrist" epitope and "knuckle" epitope, which are supposed to bind to BMP receptors [98]. Studies based on BMP-2-derived peptides indicated that these peptides had positive impacts on osteogenic differentiation of stem-cell and bone formation in defects [99,100]. For example, Ye et al. [23] developed a scaffold with a 3D nanofibrous porous structure for bone tissue engineering. In this study, by combining homogenization, freeze-drying, and thermal treatment, nano-hydroxyapatite/PLLA/gelatin (nHA/PLA/GEL) 3D nanofibrous scaffolds were fabricated using pre-prepared electrospun nanofibers. Then, utilizing a polydopamine (pDA)-assisted coating strategy, BMP-2-derived peptides (PEP, sequence: $S_{[PO4]}$KIPKASSVPTELSAISTLYLDDD) were immobilized onto the 3D scaffolds to obtain the resulting nHA/PLA/GEL-PEP 3D nanofibrous scaffolds capable of sustained release of BMP-2 peptides. Figure 9 illustrates the highlights of the study from fabrication to animal experiment. In vitro studies demonstrated that nHA/PLA/GEL-PEP scaffolds promoted the activity of alkaline phosphatase of bone mesenchymal stem cells (BMSCs) and gene expression related to osteogenic differentiation. Moreover, in vivo evaluation was performed using a rat cranial bone defect model, and the results of radiology and histology analysis indicated that this scaffold facilitated bone formation in the defects. Therefore, the scaffold has excellent potential in bone defect repair [23].

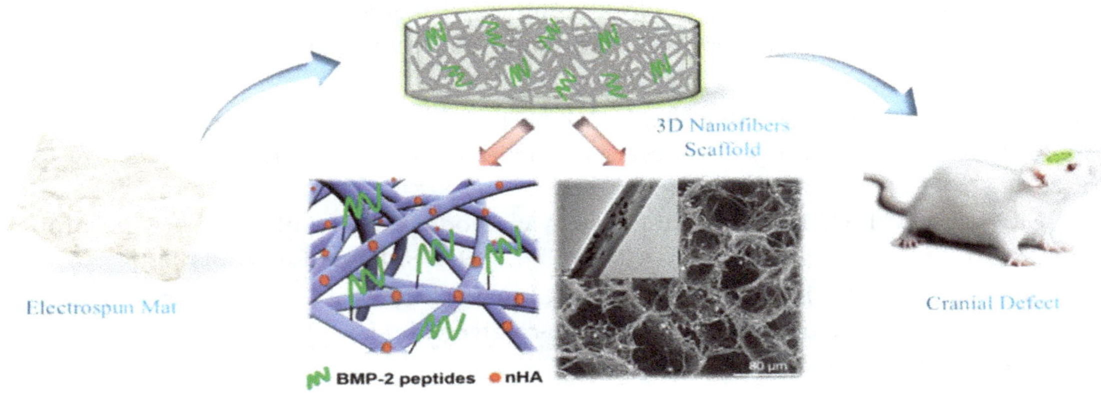

Figure 9. Three-dimensional (3D) electrospun nanofibrous scaffold for rat cranial bone regeneration [23]. Reproduced with permission from Elsevier, 2019.

8. Conclusions

In this review, various scaffolds based on electrospinning for tissue engineering have been discussed, and various strategies for designing novel scaffolds explained. Preparation and delivery methods highlighted indicate that electrospinning technology is a useful tool to fabricate scaffolds with nanofibrous structure. Moreover, bioactive molecules can also be incorporated into the scaffolds via method selection or surface modification for controlling the drug delivery. The ECM-mimicking structure, along with the delivery system based on electrospinning, makes electrospun scaffolds ideal biomaterials for tissue-engineering applications. Key aims going forward should be to address the relationship between mass production and material stability, and the deeper impacts on cells generated by these drug-loaded scaffolds should be illustrated.

References

1. Qasim, S.B.; Zafar, M.S.; Najeeb, S.; Khurshid, Z.; Shah, A.H.; Husain, S.; Rehman, I.U. Electrospinning of chitosan-based solutions for tissue engineering and regenerative medicine. *Int. J. Mol. Sci.* **2018**, *19*, 407.
2. Liu, W.; Thomopoulos, S.; Xia, Y. Electrospun nanofibers for regenerative medicine. *Adv. Healthc. Mater.* **2012**, *1*, 10–25. [PubMed]
3. Zamani, R.; Aval, S.F.; Pilehvar-Soltanahmadi, Y.; Nejati-Koshki, K.; Zarghami, N. Recent advances in cell electrospining of natural and synthetic nanofibers for regenerative medicine. *Drug Res.* **2018**, *68*, 425–435.
4. Greiner, A.; Wendorff, J.H. Electrospinning: A fascinating method for the preparation of ultrathin fibers. *Angew. Chem. Int. Ed.* **2007**, *46*, 5670–5703.
5. Zafar, M.; Najeeb, S.; Khurshid, Z.; Vazirzadeh, M.; Zohaib, S.; Najeeb, B.; Sefat, F. Potential of electrospun nanofibers for biomedical and dental applications. *Materials* **2016**, *9*, 73. [CrossRef] [PubMed]
6. Flemming, R.G.; Murphy, C.J.; Abrams, G.A.; Goodman, S.L.; Nealey, P.F. Effects of synthetic micro- and nano-structured surfaces on cell behavior. *Biomaterials* **1999**, *20*, 573–588. [PubMed]
7. Von Recum, A.F.; Shannon, C.E.; Cannon, C.E.; Long, K.J.; van Kooten, T.G.; Meyle, J. Surface roughness, porosity, and texture as modifiers of cellular adhesion. *Tissue Eng.* **1996**, *2*, 241–253.
8. Green, A.M.; Jansen, J.A.; van der Waerden, J.P.C.M.; Von Recum, A.F. Fibroblast response to microtextured silicone surfaces: Texture orientation into or out of the surface. *J. Biomed. Mater. Res. Part A* **1994**, *28*, 647–653.
9. Mitragotri, S.; Anderson, D.G.; Chen, X.; Chow, E.K.; Ho, D.; Kabanov, A.V.; Karp, J.M.; Kataoka, K.; Mirkin, C.A.; Petrosko, S.H.; et al. Accelerating the translation of nanomaterials in biomedicine. *ACS Nano* **2015**, *9*, 6644–6654.
10. Jiang, L.; Jiang, Y.; Stiadle, J.; Wang, X.; Wang, L.; Li, Q.; Shen, C.; Thibeault, S.L.; Turng, L.-S. Electrospun nanofibrous thermoplastic polyurethane/poly(glycerol sebacate) hybrid scaffolds for vocal fold tissue engineering applications. *Mater. Sci. Eng. C* **2019**, *94*, 740–749. [CrossRef] [PubMed]

11. Campiglio, C.; Marcolin, C.; Draghi, L. Electrospun ECM macromolecules as biomimetic scaffold for regenerative medicine: Challenges for preserving conformation and bioactivity. *AIMS J.* **2017**, *4*, 638–669. [CrossRef]
12. Bölgen, N.; Vargel, I.; Korkusuz, P.; Menceloğlu, Y.Z.; Pişkin, E. In vivo performance of antibiotic embedded electrospun PCL membranes for prevention of abdominal adhesions. *J. Biomed. Mater. Res. Part B Appl. Biomater.* **2010**, *81B*, 530–543.
13. Huang, Z.M.; Yang, C.L.H. Encapsulating drugs in biodegradable ultrafine fibers through co-axial electrospinning. *J. Biomed. Mater. Res. Part A* **2010**, *77A*, 169–179. [CrossRef] [PubMed]
14. Kim, K.; Luu, Y.K.; Chang, C.; Fang, D.; Hsiao, B.S.; Chu, B.; Hadjiargyrou, M. Incorporation and controlled release of a hydrophilic antibiotic using poly(lactide-*co*-glycolide)-based electrospun nanofibrous scaffolds. *J. Control. Release* **2004**, *98*, 47–56. [PubMed]
15. Nie, H.; Wang, C.H. Fabrication and characterization of PLGA/HAp composite scaffolds for delivery of BMP-2 plasmid DNA. *J. Control. Release* **2007**, *120*, 111–121. [CrossRef] [PubMed]
16. Chew, S.Y.; Jie, W.; Yim, E.K.F.; Leong, K.W. Sustained release of proteins from electrospun biodegradable fibers. *Biomacromolecules* **2005**, *6*, 2017–2024. [CrossRef]
17. Sadeghi, A.; Moztarzadeh, F.; Aghazadeh Mohandesi, J. Investigating the effect of chitosan on hydrophilicity and bioactivity of conductive electrospun composite scaffold for neural tissue engineering. *Int. J. Biol. Macromol.* **2019**, *121*, 625–632. [CrossRef]
18. Venugopal, E.; Rajeswaran, N.; Sahanand, K.S.; Bhattacharyya, A.; Rajendran, S. In vitro evaluation of phytochemical loaded electrospun gelatin nanofibers for application in bone and cartilage tissue engineering. *Biomed. Mater.* **2018**, *14*, 015004. [CrossRef]
19. Ding, Y.; Li, W.; Zhang, F.; Liu, Z.; Zanjanizadeh Ezazi, N.; Liu, D.; Santos, H.A. Electrospun fibrous architectures for drug delivery, tissue engineering and cancer therapy. *Adv. Funct. Mater.* **2019**, *29*, 1802852.
20. Sill, T.J.; Von Recum, H.A. Electrospinning: Applications in drug delivery and tissue engineering. *Biomaterials* **2008**, *29*, 1989–2006. [CrossRef]
21. Kenawy, E.R.; Bowlin, G.L.; Mansfield, K.; Layman, J.; Simpson, D.G.; Sanders, E.H.; Wnek, G.E. Release of tetracycline hydrochloride from electrospun poly(ethylene-*co*-vinylacetate), poly(lactic acid), and a blend. *J. Control. Release* **2002**, *81*, 57–64. [CrossRef]
22. Park, K.; Ju, Y.M.; Son, J.S.; Ahn, K.D.; Dong, K.H. Surface modification of biodegradable electrospun nanofiber scaffolds and their interaction with fibroblasts. *J. Biomater. Sci. Polym. Ed.* **2007**, *18*, 369–382. [CrossRef]
23. Ye, K.; Liu, D.; Kuang, H.; Cai, J.; Chen, W.; Sun, B.; Xia, L.; Fang, B.; Morsi, Y.; Mo, X. Three-dimensional electrospun nanofibrous scaffolds displaying bone morphogenetic protein-2-derived peptides for the promotion of osteogenic differentiation of stem cells and bone regeneration. *J. Colloid Interface Sci.* **2019**, *534*, 625–636. [CrossRef]
24. Chen, R.; Wang, J.; Liu, C. Biomaterials act as enhancers of growth factors in bone regeneration. *Adv. Funct. Mater.* **2016**, *26*, 8810–8823. [CrossRef]
25. Zhao, P.; Jiang, H.H.; Zhu, K.; Chen, W. Biodegradable fibrous scaffolds composed of gelatin coated poly(epsilon-caprolactone) prepared by coaxial electrospinning. *J. Biomed. Mater. Res. A* **2010**, *83A*, 372–382. [CrossRef] [PubMed]
26. Zhang, Y.Z.; Wang, X.; Feng, Y.; Li, J.; Lim, C.T.; Ramakrishna, S. Coaxial electrospinning of (fluorescein isothiocyanate-conjugated bovine serum albumin)-encapsulated poly(epsilon-caprolactone) nanofibers for sustained release. *Biomacromolecules* **2006**, *7*, 1049–1057. [CrossRef]
27. Yan, L.I. A facile technique to prepare biodegradable coaxial electrospun nanofibers for controlled release of bioactive agents. *J. Control. Release* **2005**, *108*, 237–243.
28. Su, Y.; Li, X.; Wang, H.; He, C.; Mo, X. Fabrication and characterization of biodegradable nanofibrous mats by mix and coaxial electrospinning. *J. Mater. Sci. Mater. Med.* **2009**, *20*, 2285–2294. [CrossRef]
29. Prado-Prone, G.; Silva-Bermudez, P.; Almaguer-Flores, A.; García-Macedo, J.A.; García, V.I.; Rodil, S.E.; Ibarra, C.; Velasquillo, C. Enhanced antibacterial nanocomposite mats by coaxial electrospinning of polycaprolactone fibers loaded with Zn-based nanoparticles. *Nanomed. Nanotechnol. Biol. Med.* **2018**, *14*, 1695–1706. [CrossRef]

30. He, P.; Zhong, Q.; Ge, Y.; Guo, Z.; Tian, J.; Zhou, Y.; Ding, S.; Li, H.; Zhou, C. Dual drug loaded coaxial electrospun PLGA/PVP fiber for guided tissue regeneration under control of infection. *Mater. Sci. Eng. C* **2018**, *90*, 549–556. [CrossRef]
31. Yan, S.; Li, X.; Liu, S.; Mo, X.; Ramakrishna, S. Controlled release of dual drugs from emulsion electrospun nanofibrous mats. *Colloids Surf. B Biointerfaces* **2009**, *73*, 376–381. [CrossRef] [PubMed]
32. Chen, S.; Li, R.; Li, X.; Xie, J. Electrospinning: An enabling nanotechnology platform for drug delivery and regenerative medicine. *Adv. Drug Deliv. Rev.* **2018**, *132*, 188–213. [CrossRef] [PubMed]
33. Chandra, A.; Suliman, A.; Angle, N. Spontaneous dissection of the carotid and vertebral arteries: The 10-year UCSD experience. *Ann. Vasc. Surg.* **2007**, *21*, 178–185. [CrossRef]
34. Schoder, M.; Cartes-Zumelzu, F.; Grabenwöger, M.; Cejna, M.; Funovics, M.; Krenn, C.G.; Hutschala, D.; Wolf, F.; Thurnher, S.; et al. Elective endovascular stent-graft repair of atherosclerotic thoracic aortic aneurysms: Clinical results and midterm follow-up. *AJR Am. J. Roentgencl.* **2003**, *180*, 709–715. [CrossRef] [PubMed]
35. Grabenwöger, M.; Hutschala, D.; Cartes-Zumelzu, F.; Ehrlich, M.; Grimm, M.; Thurnher, S.; Lammer, J.; Wolner, E.; Havel, M. Behandlung von thorakalen Aortenaneurysmen mit selbstexpandierenden endoluminalen Gefäßprothesen. *Acta Chir. Austriaca* **1999**, *31*, 319–322. [CrossRef]
36. Golshani, K.; Ferrel, A.; Lessne, M.; Shah, P.; Chowdhary, A.; Choulakian, A.; Alexander, M.J.; Smith, T.P.; Enterline, D.S.; Zomorodi, A.R. Stent-assisted coil emboilization of ruptured intracranial aneurysms: A retrospective multicenter review. *Surg. Neurol. Int.* **2012**, *3*, 84.
37. Wu, C.; An, Q.; Li, D.; Jing, W.; He, L.; Chen, H.; Yu, L.; Wei, Z.; Mo, X. A novel heparin loaded poly(L-lactide-*co*-caprolactone) covered stent for aneurysm therapy. *Mater. Lett.* **2014**, *116*, 39–42. [CrossRef]
38. Wang, J.; An, Q.; Li, D.; Wu, T.; Chen, W.; Sun, B.; El-Hamshary, H.; Al-Deyab, S.S.; Zhu, W.; Mo, X. Heparin and vascular endothelial growth factor loaded poly(L-lactide-*co*-caprolactone) nanofiber covered stent-graft for aneurysm treatment. *J. Biomed. Nanotechnol.* **2015**, *11*, 1947–1960. [CrossRef]
39. Feng, W.; Liu, P.; Yin, H.; Gu, Z.; Wu, Y.; Zhu, W.; Liu, Y.; Zheng, H.; Mo, X. Heparin and rosuvastatin calcium loaded ploy(L-lactide-*co*-caprolactone) nanofiber covered stent-graft for aneurysm treatment. *New J. Chem.* **2017**, *41*, 9014–9023. [CrossRef]
40. Raimondo, S.; Fornaro, M.; Tos, P.; Battiston, B.; Giacobini-Robecchi, M.G.; Geuna, S. Perspectives in regeneration and tissue engineering of peripheral nerves. *Ann. Anat.* **2011**, *193*, 334–340.
41. Evans, G.R.D.; Brandt, K.; Widmer, M.S.; Lu, L.; Meszlenyi, R.K.; Gupta, P.K.; Mikos, A.G.; Hodges, J.; Williams, J.; Gürlek, A. In vivo evaluation of poly(L-lactic acid) porous conduits for peripheral nerve regeneration. *Biomaterials* **1999**, *20*, 1109–1115.
42. Hsu, C.-C.; Serio, A.; Amdursky, N.; Besnard, C.; Stevens, M.M. Fabrication of hemin-doped serum albumin-based fibrous scaffolds for neural tissue engineering applications. *ACS Appl. Mater. Interfaces* **2018**, *10*, 5305–5317. [CrossRef] [PubMed]
43. Shao, Z. Application of self-assembling peptide nanofiber scaffold in nerve tissue engineering. *Chin. J. Repar. Reconstr. Surg.* **2009**, *23*, 861–863.
44. Chun-Yang, W.; Jun-Jian, L.; Cun-Yi, F.; Xiu-Mei, M.; Hong-Jiang, R.; Feng-Feng, L. The effect of aligned core-shell nanofibres delivering NGF on the promotion of sciatic nerve regeneration. *J. Biomater. Sci. Polym. Ed.* **2012**, *23*, 167–184.
45. Zhang, K.; Wang, C.; Fan, C.; Mo, X. Aligned SF/P(LLA-CL)-blended nanofibers encapsulating nerve growth factor for peripheral nerve regeneration. *J. Biomed. Mater. Res. Part A* **2014**, *102*, 2680–2691.
46. Su, Y.; Li, X.; Tian, L.; Chen, H.; Xiumei, M. Poly(L-lactide-*co*-ε-caprolactone) electrospun nanofibers for encapsulating and sustained releasing proteins. *Polymer* **2009**, *50*, 4212–4219.
47. Sun, B.; Wu, T.; He, L.; Zhang, J.; Yuan, Y.; Huang, X.; El-Hamshary, H.; Al-Deyab, S.S.; Xu, T.; Mo, X. Development of dual neurotrophins-encapsulated electrosupun nanofibrous scaffolds for peripheral nerve regeneration. *J. Biomed. Nanotechnol.* **2016**, *12*, 1987–2000. [PubMed]
48. Bhutto, M.A.; Wu, T.; Sun, B.; Ei-Hamshary, H.; Al-Deyab, S.S.; Mo, X. Fabrication and characterization of vitamin B5 loaded poly (L-lactide-*co*-caprolactone)/silk fiber aligned electrospun nanofibers for Schwann cell proliferation. *Colloids Surf. B Biointerfaces* **2016**, *144*, 108–117.
49. Tong, W.; Li, D.; Wang, Y.; Sun, B.; Li, D.; Morsi, Y.; Hamshary, H.A.E.; Al-Deyab, S.S.; Mo, X.M. Laminin-coated nerve guidance conduits based on poly(L-lactide-*co*-glycolide) fibers and yarns for promoting Schwann cells proliferation and migration. *J. Mater. Chem. B* **2017**, *5*, 3186–3194.

50. Junka, R.; Valmikinathan, C.M.; Kalyon, D.M.; Yu, X. Laminin functionalized biomimetic nanofibers for nerve tissue engineering. *J. Biomater. Tissue Eng.* **2013**, *3*, 494–502.
51. Liu, C.; Wang, C.; Zhao, Q.; Li, X.; Xu, F.; Yao, X.; Wang, M. Incorporation and release of dual growth factors for nerve tissue engineering using nanofibrous bicomponent scaffolds. *Biomed. Mater.* **2013**, *13*, 044107. [CrossRef] [PubMed]
52. Canver, C.C. Conduit options in coronary artery bypass surgery. *Chest* **1995**, *108*, 1150–1155. [CrossRef] [PubMed]
53. Chlupác, J.; Filová, E.; Bacáková, L. Vascular prostheses: 50 years of advancement from synthetic towards tissue engineering and cell therapy. *Rozhledy* **2010**, *89*, 85–94.
54. Huang, C.; Wang, S.; Qiu, L.; Ke, Q.; Zhai, W.; Mo, X. Heparin loading and pre-endothelialization in enhancing the patency rate of electrospun small-diameter vascular grafts in a canine model. *ACS Appl. Mater. Interfaces* **2013**, *5*, 2220–2226. [CrossRef] [PubMed]
55. Chen, X.; Wang, J.; An, Q.; Li, D.; Liu, P.; Zhu, W.; Mo, X. Electrospun poly(L-lactic acid-*co*-ε-caprolactone) fibers loaded with heparin and vascular endothelial growth factor to improve blood compatibility and endothelial progenitor cell proliferation. *Colloids Surf. B Biointerfaces* **2015**, *128*, 106–114. [CrossRef] [PubMed]
56. Yin, A.; Bowlin, G.L.; Luo, R.; Zhang, X.; Wang, Y.; Mo, X. Electrospun silk fibroin/poly(L-lactide-ε-caplacton) graft with platelet-rich growth factor for inducing smooth muscle cell growth and infiltration. *Regen. Biomater.* **2016**, *3*, 239–245.
57. Kuang, H.; Wang, Y.; Hu, J.; Wang, C.; Lu, S.; Mo, X. A method for preparation of an internal layer of artificial vascular graft co-modified with Salvianolic acid B and heparin. *ACS Appl. Mater. Interfaces* **2018**, *10*, 19365–19372.
58. Guex, A.G.; Hegemann, D.; Giraud, M.N.; Tevaearai, H.T.; Popa, A.M.; Rossi, R.M.; Fortunato, G. Covalent immobilisation of VEGF on plasma-coated electrospun scaffolds for tissue engineering applications. *Colloids Surf. B Biointerfaces* **2014**, *123*, 724–733.
59. Gurtner, G.C.; Sabine, W.; Yann, B.; Longaker, M.T. Wound repair and regeneration. *Nature* **2008**, *453*, 314–321.
60. Zahedi, P.; Rezaeian, I.; Ranaei-Siadat, S.O.; Jafari, S.H.; Supaphol, P. A review on wound dressings with an emphasis on electrospun nanofibrous polymeric bandages. *Polym. Adv. Technol.* **2010**, *21*, 77–95. [CrossRef]
61. Zeng-Xiao, C.; Xiu-Mei, M.; Kui-Hua, Z.; Lin-Peng, F.; An-Lin, Y.; Chuang-Long, H.; Hong-Sheng, W. Fabrication of chitosan/silk fibroin composite nanofibers for wound-dressing applications. *Int. J. Mol. Sci.* **2010**, *11*, 3529–3539.
62. Alhusein, N.; Blagbrough, I.S.; De Bank, P.A. Electrospun matrices for localised controlled drug delivery: Release of tetracycline hydrochloride from layers of polycaprolactone and poly(ethylene-*co*-vinyl acetate). *Drug Deliv. Transl. Res.* **2012**, *2*, 477–488. [CrossRef]
63. Alhusein, N.; Blagbrough, I.S.; Beeton, M.L.; Bolhuis, A.; De Bank, P.A. Electrospun zein/PCL fibrous matrices release tetracycline in a controlled manner, killing *Staphylococcus aureus* both in biofilms and ex vivo on pig skin, and are compatible with human skin cells. *Pharm. Res.* **2016**, *33*, 237–246. [CrossRef] [PubMed]
64. Alhusein, N.; Blagbrough, I.S.; De Bank, P.A. Zein/polycaprolactone electrospun matrices for localised controlled delivery of tetracycline. *Drug Deliv. Transl. Res.* **2013**, *3*, 542–550. [CrossRef] [PubMed]
65. Ghosal, K.; Agatemor, C.; Thomas, S.; Kny, E. Electrospinning tissue engineering and wound dressing scaffolds from polymer–titanium dioxide nanocomposites. *Chem. Eng. J.* **2019**, *358*, 1262–1278. [CrossRef]
66. Li, J.; Zhai, D.; Lv, F.; Yu, Q.; Ma, H.; Yin, J.; Yi, Z.; Liu, M.; Chang, J.; Wu, C. Preparation of copper-containing bioactive glass/eggshell membrane nanocomposites for improving angiogenesis, antibacterial activity and wound healing. *Acta Biomater.* **2016**, *36*, 254–266. [CrossRef] [PubMed]
67. Eming, S.A.; Martin, P.; Tomic-Canic, M. Wound repair and regeneration: Mechanisms, signaling, and translation. *Sci. Transl. Med.* **2014**, *6*, 265sr6. [CrossRef]
68. Gaoxing Luo, M.D.; Jin, T.M.; He, W.; Jun Wu, M.D.; Bing, M.M.; Xihua Wang, M.D.; Chen, X.; Yi, S.; Zhang, X.; Li, X. Antibacterial effect of dressings containing multivalent silver ion carried by zirconium phosphate on experimental rat burn wounds. *Wound Repair Regen.* **2010**, *16*, 800–804.
69. Brett, B.; Sampson, E.M.; Schultz, G.S.; Parnell, L.K.S. Wound dressing components degrade proteins detrimental to wound healing. *Int. Wound J.* **2010**, *5*, 543–551.
70. Ignatova, M.; Manolova, N.; Rashkov, I. Electrospinning of poly(vinyl pyrrolidone)–iodine complex and poly(ethylene oxide)/poly(vinyl pyrrolidone)–iodine complex—A prospective route to antimicrobial wound dressing materials. *Eur. Polym. J.* **2007**, *43*, 1609–1623. [CrossRef]

71. Alhusein, N.; De Bank, P.A.; Blagbrough, I.S.; Bolhuis, A. Killing bacteria within biofilms by sustained release of tetracycline from triple-layered electrospun micro/nanofibre matrices of polycaprolactone and poly(ethylene-co-vinyl acetate). *Drug Deliv. Transl. Res.* **2013**, *3*, 531–541. [CrossRef]
72. Román-Doval, R.; Tellez-Cruz, M.M.; Rojas-Chávez, H.; Cruz-Martínez, H.; Carrasco-Torres, G.; Vásquez-Garzón, V.R. Enhancing electrospun scaffolds of PVP with polypyrrole/iodine for tissue engineering of skin regeneration by coating via a plasma process. *J. Mater. Sci.* **2019**, *54*, 3342–3353. [CrossRef]
73. Sheng, X.; Fan, L.; He, C.; Zhang, K.; Mo, X.; Wang, H. Vitamin E-loaded silk fibroin nanofibrous mats fabricated by green process for skin care application. *Int. J. Biol. Macromol.* **2013**, *56*, 49–56. [CrossRef]
74. El-Aassar, M.R.; El Fawal, G.F.; El-Deeb, N.M.; Hassan, H.S.; Mo, X. Electrospun polyvinyl alcohol/ pluronic F127 blended nanofibers containing titanium dioxide for antibacterial wound dressing. *Appl. Biochem. Biotechnol.* **2015**, *178*, 1–15.
75. Lv, F.; Wang, J.; Xu, P.; Han, Y.; Ma, H.; Xu, H.; Chen, S.; Chang, J.; Ke, Q.; Liu, M. A conducive bioceramic/polymer composite biomaterial for diabetic wound healing. *Acta Biomater.* **2017**, *60*, 128–143. [CrossRef] [PubMed]
76. Bagnaninchi, P.O.; Yang, Y.; El Haj, A.J.; Maffulli, N. Tissue engineering for tendon repair. *Br. J. Sports Med.* **2007**, *41*, e10. [CrossRef]
77. Yang, C.; Deng, G.; Chen, W.; Ye, X.; Mo, X. A novel electrospun-aligned nanoyarn-reinforced nanofibrous scaffold for tendon tissue engineering. *Colloids Surf. B Biointerfaces* **2014**, *122*, 270–276. [CrossRef] [PubMed]
78. Cai, J.; Wang, J.; Ye, K.; Li, D.; Ai, C.; Sheng, D.; Jin, W.; Liu, X.; Zhi, Y.; Jiang, J. Dual-layer aligned-random nanofibrous scaffolds for improving gradient microstructure of tendon-to-bone healing in a rabbit extra-articular model. *Int. J. Nanomed.* **2018**, *13*, 3481–3492. [CrossRef] [PubMed]
79. Xu, Y.; Dong, S.; Zhou, Q.; Mo, X.; Song, L.; Hou, T.; Wu, J.; Li, S.; Li, Y.; Li, P. The effect of mechanical stimulation on the maturation of TDSCs-poly(L-lactide-*co*-ε-caprolactone)/collagen scaffold constructs for tendon tissue engineering. *Biomaterials* **2014**, *35*, 2760–2772. [CrossRef] [PubMed]
80. Sahoo, S.; Ang, L.T.; Goh, J.C.H.; Toh, S.-L. Growth factor delivery through electrospun nanofibers in scaffolds for tissue engineering applications. *J. Biomed. Mater. Res. A* **2010**, *93A*, 1539–1550.
81. Ye, Y.J.; Zhou, Y.Q.; Jing, Z.Y.; Liu, Y.Y.; Yin, D.C. Electrospun heparin-loaded core-shell nanofiber sutures for achilles tendon regeneration in vivo. *Macromol. Biosci.* **2018**, *18*, 1800041. [CrossRef] [PubMed]
82. Xu, Y.; Wu, J.; Wang, H.; Li, H.; Di, N.; Song, L.; Li, S.; Li, D.; Xiang, Y.; Liu, W. Fabrication of electrospun poly(L-lactide-*co*-ε-caprolactone)/collagen nanoyarn network as a novel, three-dimensional, macroporous, aligned scaffold for tendon tissue engineering. *Tissue Eng. Part C Methods* **2013**, *19*, 925–936. [CrossRef] [PubMed]
83. Riggin, C.N.; Qu, F.; Dong, H.K.; Huegel, J.; Steinberg, D.R.; Kuntz, A.F.; Soslowsky, L.J.; Mauck, R.L.; Bernstein, J. Electrospun PLGA nanofiber scaffolds release ibuprofen faster and degrade slower after in vivo implantation. *Ann. Biomed. Eng.* **2017**, *45*, 2348–2359. [CrossRef]
84. Tellado, S.F.; Balmayor, E.R.; Griensven, M.V. Strategies to engineer tendon/ligament-to-bone interface: Biomaterials, cells and growth factors. *Adv. Drug Deliv. Rev.* **2015**, *94*, 126–140. [CrossRef] [PubMed]
85. Sahoo, S.; Toh, S.L.; Goh, J.C.H. A bFGF-releasing silk/PLGA-based biohybrid scaffold for ligament/tendon tissue engineering using mesenchymal progenitor cells. *Biomaterials* **2010**, *31*, 2990–2998. [CrossRef]
86. Manning, C.N.; Schwartz, A.G.; Liu, W.; Xie, J.; Havlioglu, N.; Sakiyamaelbert, S.E.; Silva, M.J.; Xia, Y.; Gelberman, R.H.; Thomopoulos, S. Controlled delivery of mesenchymal stem cells and growth factors using a nanofiber scaffold for tendon repair. *Acta Biomater.* **2013**, *9*, 6905–6914. [CrossRef]
87. Ren, J.; Blackwood, K.; Doustgani, A.; Poh, P.; Steck, R.M.; Stevens, M.; Woodruff, M. Melt-electrospun polycaprolactone strontium-substituted bioactive glass scaffolds for bone regeneration. *J. Biomed. Mater. Res. A* **2014**, *102*, 3140–3153. [CrossRef]
88. Yao, Q.; Cosme, J.G.; Xu, T.; Miszuk, J.M.; Picciani, P.H.; Fong, H.; Sun, H. Three dimensional electrospun PCL/PLA blend nanofibrous scaffolds with significantly improved stem cells osteogenic differentiation and cranial bone formation. *Biomaterials* **2016**, *115*, 115–127. [CrossRef] [PubMed]
89. Poologasundarampillai, G.; Wang, D.; Li, S.; Nakamura, J.; Bradley, R.; Lee, P.D.; Stevens, M.M.; McPhail, D.S.; Kasuga, T.; Jones, J.R. Cotton-wool-like bioactive glasses for bone regeneration. *Acta Biomater.* **2014**, *10*, 3733–3746. [CrossRef]

90. Xu, T.; Miszuk, J.M.; Zhao, Y.; Sun, H.; Fong, H. Electrospun polycaprolactone 3D nanofibrous scaffold with interconnected and hierarchically structured pores for bone tissue engineering. *Adv. Healthc. Mater.* **2015**, *4*, 2238–2246. [CrossRef] [PubMed]
91. Chen, W.; Chen, S.; Morsi, Y.; Elhamshary, H.; El-newehy, M.; Fan, C.; Mo, X. Superabsorbent 3D scaffold based on electrospun nanofibers for cartilage tissue engineering. *ACS Appl. Mater. Interfaces* **2016**, *8*, 24415–24425. [CrossRef]
92. Si, Y.; Yu, J.; Tang, X.; Ge, J.; Ding, B. Ultralight nanofibre-assembled cellular aerogels with superelasticity and multifunctionality. *Nat. Commun.* **2014**, *5*, 5802. [CrossRef]
93. Rose, F.R.; Hou, Q.; Oreffo, R.O. Delivery systems for bone growth factors—The new players in skeletal regeneration. *J. Pharm. Pharmacol.* **2004**, *56*, 415–427. [CrossRef]
94. Lieberman, J.R.; Daluiski, A.; Einhorn, T.A. The role of growth factors in the repair of bone. Biology and clinical applications. *JBJS* **2002**, *84-A*, 1032–1044. [CrossRef]
95. Su, Y.; Su, Q.; Liu, W.; Lim, M.; Venugopal, J.R.; Mo, X.; Ramakrishna, S.; Al-Deyab, S.S.; El-Newehy, M. Controlled release of bone morphogenetic protein 2 and dexamethasone loaded in core–shell PLLACL–collagen fibers for use in bone tissue engineering. *Acta Biomater.* **2012**, *8*, 763–771. [CrossRef]
96. Shimer, A.L.; Öner, F.C.; Vaccaro, A.R. Spinal reconstruction and bone morphogenetic proteins: Open questions. *Injury* **2009**, *40*, S32–S38. [CrossRef]
97. Lin, Z.Y.; Duan, Z.X.; Guo, X.D.; Li, J.F.; Lu, H.W.; Zheng, Q.X.; Quan, D.P.; Yang, S.H. Bone induction by biomimetic PLGA-(PEG-ASP)$_n$ copolymer loaded with a novel synthetic BMP-2-related peptide in vitro and in vivo. *J. Control. Release* **2010**, *144*, 190–195. [CrossRef] [PubMed]
98. Suzuki, Y.; Tanihara, M.; Suzuki, K.; Saitou, A.; Sufan, W.; Nishimura, Y. Alginate hydrogel linked with synthetic oligopeptide derived from BMP-2 allows ectopic osteoinduction in vivo. *J. Biomed. Mater. Res. Part B Appl. Biomater.* **2015**, *50*, 405–409. [CrossRef]
99. Weng, L.; Boda, S.K.; Wang, H.; Teusink, M.J.; Shuler, F.D.; Xie, J. Novel 3D hybrid nanofiber aerogels coupled with BMP-2 peptides for cranial bone regeneration. *Adv. Healthc. Mater.* **2018**, *7*, 1701415. [CrossRef]
100. Zhou, X.; Feng, W.; Qiu, K.; Chen, L.; Wang, W.; Nie, W.; Mo, X.; He, C. BMP-2 derived peptide and dexamethasone incorporated mesoporous silica nanoparticles for enhanced osteogenic differentiation of bone mesenchymal stem cells. *ACS Appl. Mater. Interfaces* **2015**, *7*, 15777–15789. [CrossRef] [PubMed]

8

Penetration Enhancers in Ocular Drug Delivery

Roman V. Moiseev [1], Peter W. J. Morrison [1], Fraser Steele [2] and Vitaliy V. Khutoryanskiy [1,*]

[1] Reading School of Pharmacy, University of Reading, Whiteknights, P.O. Box 224, Reading RG66AD, UK
[2] MC2 Therapeutics, James House, Emlyn Lane, Leatherhead KT22 7EP, UK
* Correspondence: v.khutoryanskiy@reading.ac.uk

Abstract: There are more than 100 recognized disorders of the eye. This makes the development of advanced ocular formulations an important topic in pharmaceutical science. One of the ways to improve drug delivery to the eye is the use of penetration enhancers. These are defined as compounds capable of enhancing drug permeability across ocular membranes. This review paper provides an overview of anatomical and physiological features of the eye and discusses some common ophthalmological conditions and permeability of ocular membranes. The review also presents the analysis of literature on the use of penetration-enhancing compounds (cyclodextrins, chelating agents, crown ethers, bile acids and bile salts, cell-penetrating peptides, and other amphiphilic compounds) in ocular drug delivery, describing their properties and modes of action.

Keywords: ocular drug delivery; cornea; penetration enhancers; ocular conditions; ophthalmology

---

1. Introduction

According to the World Health Organization, the number of people who live with some form of distance or near vision impairment is about 1.3 billion worldwide [1]. This problem is very important because approximately 80% of external input of information delivered to the brain is processed by the visual pathway [2]. There were many methods and improvements of ocular drug delivery developed over the last decades exploring more effective treatments for different ocular diseases. Nevertheless, this field of medicine remains one of the most challenging.

The preferred method of ocular drug delivery is via topical application due to ease of access to the eye and the non-invasive nature of this administration route [3]. Self-medication by this means is achievable by most people that are not limited by dexterity issues or conditions affecting mental ability. Administration by a helper eliminates these potential difficulties. Ocular drug penetration is possible via the transcellular pathway, i.e., into and through cells, or the paracellular route, i.e., between cells, or a combination of both pathways [4].

Drug penetration enhancement can be achieved by inclusion of agents capable of modifying the tear film, mucous layer, and ocular membranes in a drug formulation [5]. A further strategy for enhancing drug penetration into the eye can be achieved by energy-driven means, where a small electrical current is used (iontophoresis) [6] or ultrasound is employed to drive the drug to enter the ocular tissues [7–9]. The use of microneedles for enhanced ocular drug delivery is another emerging area of research; however, this could be considered somewhat invasive and inconvenient [10–12].

Penetration enhancers are compounds that are able to enhance drug delivery across otherwise impermeable or limited permeability membranes such as the cornea, acting predominantly on the epithelia [5]. The use of penetration enhancers in transdermal applications is a well-established approach to facilitate drug delivery across the skin and this topic was covered in a number of excellent reviews [13,14]. Ocular drug delivery is still lacking good understanding and analysis of the effects of various penetration enhancers. It is, however, already established that penetration enhancers in ocular drug delivery facilitate delivery of active pharmaceutical ingredients through three main mechanisms or their combination [15,16]:

1. Altering tear film stability and the mucous layer at the ocular surface [17,18];
2. Modifying membrane components such as lipid bilayers of associated epithelial cells [19];
3. Loosening epithelial tight junctions [4,17].

Penetration-enhancing excipients for use in ocular formulations should ideally have the following characteristics: they should be non-toxic and non-irritating, efficacious at low concentrations, fast-acting, and their effect should be reversible [20,21].

This paper provides an overview of anatomy and physiology of the eye, discusses some common ophthalmological conditions, and presents an analysis of literature on the use of penetration enhancers in ocular drug delivery.

2. Ocular Anatomy and Physiology

The visual system is a sensory unit helping us to understand our environment, comprising a receptor (retina), sensory pathway (optic tract), and brain center (primary visual cortex). Each eyeball is embedded within the orbit, which is a pear-shaped cavity physically protecting the eye [1,22]. Adipose tissue surrounds the eye within the orbital cavity and helps to cushion the eye. Other accessory organs include lacrimal glands, eyebrows, eyelids, eyelashes, and muscles of the eye. The human eye is a complex organ comprising three different coats or layers, enclosing various anatomical structures as shown in Figure 1. Below, we briefly consider some specific tissues in the eye.

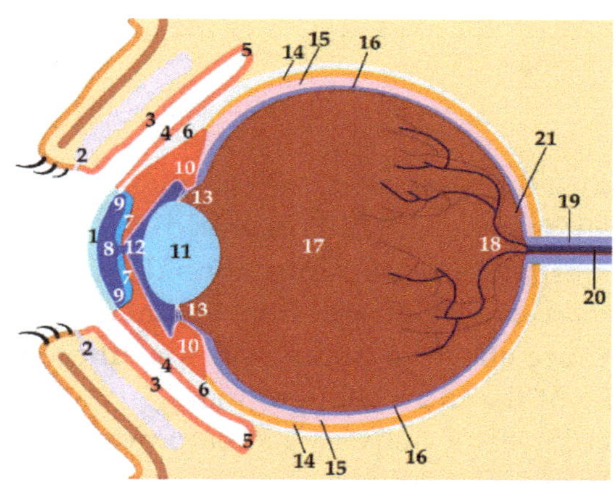

Figure 1. Anatomy of the human eye: 1—cornea; 2—meibomian glands; 3—palpebral conjunctiva; 4—bulbar conjunctiva; 5—conjunctival fornix; 6—sclera; 7—iris; 8—anterior chamber; 9—iridocorneal angle; 10—ciliary body; 11—lens; 12—posterior chamber; 13—suspensory ligament; 14—choroid; 15—retinal pigmented epithelium; 16—retina; 17—vitreous body; 18—optic disc; 19—optic nerve; 20—central artery and vein of the retina; 21—fovea.

2.1. The Outermost Layer (Tunica Fibrosa Oculi)

The fibrous tunic helps maintain the spherical shape of the eyeball and consists of the cornea and sclera. It is well known that less than 5% of the topically applied drug penetrates through the cornea [23]. However, the most accessible regions for drug application are the conjunctiva, sclera, and cornea. The cornea is an avascular, transparent, highly innervated structure, whose average diameter is ~11.5 mm vertically and ~12 mm horizontally. The average thickness of this structure is ~540 μm in the central part, and it is thicker toward the periphery [22]. The refractive power of this structure in the eye is roughly 42 diopters. The cornea is covered with the tear fluid, forming a film that protects its surface from dust and other particles. This film consists of three layers as shown in Figure 2: the outer lipid layer (delivered to the lid margins from the meibomian glands located within the tarsal plate) [24], middle aqueous layer (produced by the lacrimal gland, containing free lipid and soluble mucin), and mucous layer (which is mainly secreted by the goblet cells located within the conjunctiva as single cells with the highest density of those in the conjunctiva of the inferior eyelid) [25].

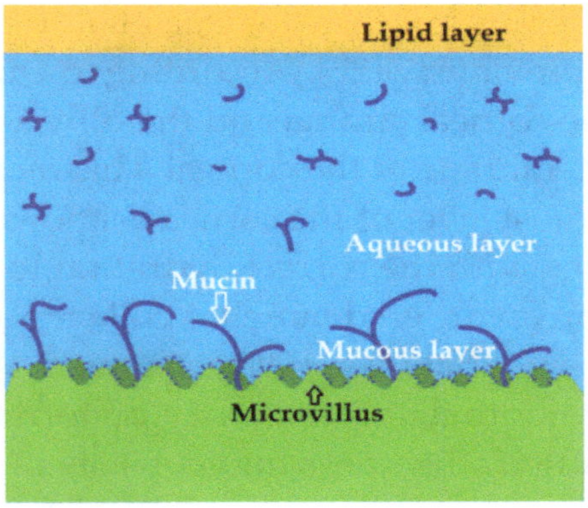

Figure 2. The tear film consists of the outer lipid layer, middle aqueous layer, and mucous layer.

The mucous layer is in contact with the corneal epithelium and is anchored via microvilli of the superficial epithelium cells. Apart from the tear film, there is another factor hampering ocular drug delivery—the structure of the cornea (Figure 3). The cornea consists of six different layers (epithelium, Bowman's membrane, stroma, Dua's layer, Descemet's membrane, and endothelium). The external layer of the cornea is the epithelium. It is relatively thin and is about 100 μm in the periphery of the cornea and approximately 50 μm in its center.

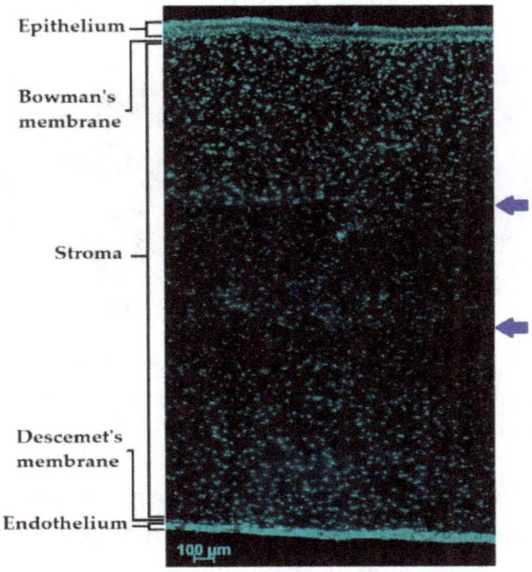

Figure 3. Micrograph demonstrating a cross-section of the multilayered structure of porcine cornea. Scale bar = 100 μm. Please note that this micrograph is a combination of three images stitched together using Inkscape 0.92.4 software due to the restrictions of the microscope camera field of view posing restrictions to the image in view. The arrows indicate stitches between images.

The main feature of this layer is the ability to regenerate non-keratinized stratified squamous epithelium. The high lipophilicity of the epithelium allows permeability to up to 90% of lipophilic small drug molecules and only about 10% of hydrophilic molecules. The cells of this layer have Ca^{2+}-dependent membrane adherent regions; tight junctions are formed between the zonula occludens, zonula adherens, and desmosomes [5]. The epithelium protects the eye against ultraviolet radiation (UVR) by means of a high concentration of tryptophan residues and ascorbate that absorb UVR [26]. The next layer that is placed right underneath the epithelium is the Bowman's membrane that is also called the anterior limiting membrane. Bowman's layer is acellular and composed primarily of collagen. The anterior limiting membrane reaches from 8 μm to 14 μm in thickness. The middle corneal layer is the stroma, also known as substantia propria due to the fact that it makes up to 90% of the total thickness of the cornea. It is composed of about 80% of water and collagen, proteins, mucopolysaccharides, and proteoglycans [5]. In 2013, Dua et al. reported a discovery of an additional corneal layer that was not detected previously [27]. According to Dua et al., this layer is about 15 μm in thickness and is located between the corneal stroma and the fifth corneal layer, Descemet's membrane. This is also the posterior limiting membrane of the cornea. This membrane is a ~6-μm-thick basement of the endothelium cells. The innermost layer of the cornea is known as the endothelium and plays the role of a pump, providing the cornea with the correct hydration to ensure transparency of this tissue. The clarity of the cornea depends on an ordered lamellar collagen structure and relative dehydration which requires endothelial cell density of at least 1000 cells/mm^2. According to the literature, there is a loss of the human cornea mean endothelial cell density in normal eye by approximately 0.6% per year [28]. The endothelium is ~5 μm in thickness and consists of a monolayer of squamous or low cuboidal cells [5].

Another layer providing the eyeball with protection is called the conjunctiva, of which all three portions are shown in Figure 4. The palpebral conjunctiva has blood vessels and covers the posterior surface of the upper and lower lids. The conjunctiva comprises two or more layers of isoprismatic to highly prismatic epithelial cells. The bulbar conjunctiva is an avascular slightly mobile layer that starts from the upper and lower fornices and lies over the sclera up to the cornea region. This anatomical coat consists of stratified non-keratinized epithelial cells [29]. The superior and inferior fornices form the conjunctival sac, which can act as a reservoir for instilled medicine or the placement of a drug-loaded ocular insert [30,31]. According to the literature, the estimated total area of the human conjunctival sac is approximately 16 cm^2 [24]. Figure 4 clearly demonstrates all three portions of the conjunctiva.

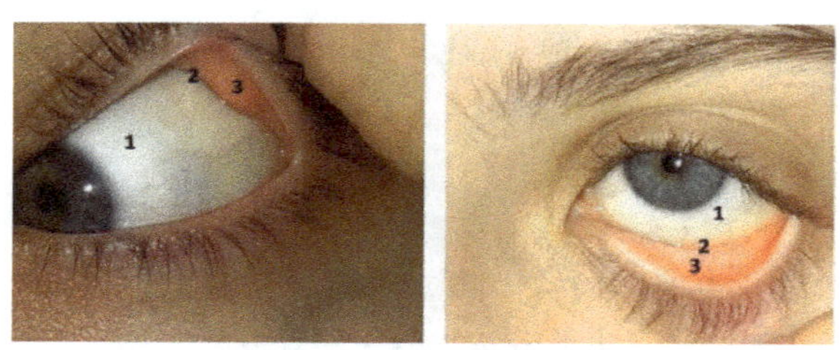

(a) (b)

Figure 4. Three portions of conjunctiva: (**a**) 1—bulbar conjunctiva; 2—superior conjunctival fornix; 3—palpebral conjunctiva of the upper lid; (**b**) 1—bulbar conjunctiva; 2—inferior conjunctival fornix; 3—palpebral conjunctiva of the lower lid.

The tough outer layer of the eye globe is called the sclera. This is covered by the episcleral, a loose connective tissue layer. In the anterior part of the eye, the sclera lies up to the corneal limbus, and posteriorly to the optic nerve. This layer comprises collagen, proteoglycans, elastin, and glycoproteins. These collagen bundles are not uniformly oriented, which results in the opaque but mechanically strong nature of the sclera. The sclera itself is pierced by a number of blood vessels, while being effectively avascular itself [32].

2.2. *Eye Chambers, Iris, Ciliary Body, and Lens*

One of the first intraocular structures that can be partially seen, due to the corneal transparency, is the anterior chamber of the eye. This is a space between the cornea's endothelium and anterior surface of the iris that is filled with aqueous humor. The latter is an optically clear fluid resembling blood plasma. The aqueous humor helps maintain appropriate intraocular pressure (IOP), and provides the cornea, trabecular meshwork, and lens with nutrition and oxygen, while removing metabolic wastes, as well as delivering molecules of neurotransmitters [33].

This fluid is formed and delivered to the posterior chamber by nonpigmented cells of the epithelia via ciliary processes [34]. Then, it flows through the pupil into the anterior chamber where two ways of outflow are found (Figure 5): (1) the conventional route is the primary outflow, where the aqueous humor is drained through the trabecular meshwork located at the anterior chamber angle (iridocorneal angle) to the Schlemm's canal (circular tube located in the limbus, 1-mm-wide region of merging epithelium of cornea and sclera), which delivers it directly into aqueous veins [35]; (2) uveoscleral outflow is provided by means of the iris root and the ciliary body face, where the aqueous humor crosses between fibers of the muscle into the supraciliary and suprachoroidal spaces and is collected by the choroidal blood circulation. The proportion of aqueous outflow via each route could be different according to the age and disease [36]. The aqueous humor consists of inorganic and organic ions, carbohydrates, glutathione, urea, amino acids, proteins, oxygen, carbon dioxide, and water. According to the literature, the concentration of Na^+ in the aqueous humor is almost the same as in the blood plasma, while the concentration of proteins is 200 times lower compared to plasma levels, and ascorbate's concentration is 20 to 50 times higher [33].

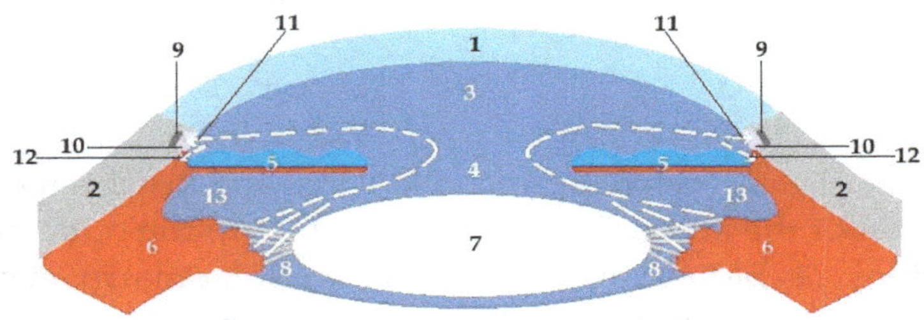

Figure 5. Pathways of aqueous humor outflow are indicated with arrows. 1—cornea; 2—sclera; 3—anterior chamber; 4—pupil; 5—iris; 6—ciliary body; 7—lens; 8—suspensory ligament; 9—Schlemm's canal; 10—trabecular meshwork; 11—trabecular route; 12—uveoscleral route; 13—posterior chamber.

The anterior chamber houses the iris, which separates anterior and posterior segments. Being attached to the anterior part of the ciliary body from the periphery, this anatomical structure has an aperture in its center that is called the pupil, the diameter of which can be regulated by the sphincter and dilator muscles located within the iris stroma (vascular connective tissue) to control the amount of light transmitting into the eye. At the posterior part of the iris, there are two epithelial layers—the anterior layer is slightly pigmented, while the posterior one has a high density of pigmentation and faces the posterior chamber. Just behind the iris lies another part of the uveal tract called the ciliary body. As already mentioned, production of the aqueous humor and uveoscleral outflow are among its functions. Additionally, the ciliary body is responsible for hyaluronate production and its release into the vitreous body, as well as for being a part of the accommodation mechanism due to the circular muscle fibers within the ciliary body. Also, this structure of the eye plays an important role in maintaining the blood–aqueous barrier [37].

The capsular bag is situated between the iris and the vitreous body and encapsulates the crystalline lens, which is a transparent biconvex avascular structure enclosed in the elastic capsule composed of collagen and that is attached to the ciliary body with the help of zonular fibers (the zonule of Zinn). Interestingly, the thickness of the anterior part of the capsular bag grows from 12–15 μm to 21 μm throughout life. Conversely, the thickness of the posterior part remains at about 2 μm. It is well known that the lens is the second most powerful refractive structure of the eye (after the cornea). It helps refract incoming light and focuses it onto the retina. When light is focused at a short focal distance, the suspensory ligaments are not under tension due to contraction of the ciliary muscle; thus, the lens thickens and results in higher refractive power. At the same time, distance vision requires the ciliary muscle to relax and, hence, to tense the lens-supportive apparatus which flattens the lens. Regarding the microscopic structure of the lens, it is composed of two types of cells. The cuboidal lens epithelial cells form a single layer that lines the anterior hemisphere, enlarging in the equator region and forming the lens "bow". The cells in this region function as stem cells for the lens. The bulk of the lens consists of lens fibers that differentiate to the point where no lens nucleus remains. These fiber cells extend in concentric layers from the anterior lens pole to the posterior one, where junctions at the terminus of the cells form the lens sutures [38]. The transparency and refractive properties of the lens are due to the uniform concentration gradient of the crystallins (α-, β-, γ-crystallins) that represent about 90% of the water-soluble proteins [39].

The third chamber of the eye is called the vitreous body, which is positioned at the back of the eyeball between the lens and the retina. It is a clear, gel-like substance occupying the main volume of the eye and is composed of long fine collagen fibers, proteins (over 80% of those are albumin and immunoglobulins), fibrillins, fibulins, agrin, opticin, pigment epithelium-derived factor, leucine-rich alpha-2 glycoprotein, thrombospondins, hyaluronic acid, polysaccharides, ascorbic acid, and water (about 98% of the whole volume). The vitreous body has no circulatory flow; hence, molecular movements are driven mostly by diffusion. Although the vitreous body is a remarkably stable structure, there is a gradual tendency for the gel to collapse in the course of a lifetime. This is commonly believed to be a result of degradation or alteration of the collagen fiber network. Moreover, the volume of the vitreous gel is about 4 mL at the age of 20 years, starting to gradually decrease after 40 years to less than 2.5 mL at 80 years [40–42].

2.3. Choroidea and Retina

The choroid is a vascular layer located between the sclera and Bruch's membrane (BM) extending from the ora serrata (region of the anterior edge of the retina) to the optic nerve. The choroid coat includes five distinct regions: (1) BM—thin, acellular extracellular matrix positioned right under the retina which acts like a filter to the retina; (2) the choriocapillaris (provides the outer retina with oxygen and nutrients); (3) layer with small and medium-sized vessels; (4) layer with large vessels; and (5) the suprachoroid. Apart from BM and the layer with choriocapillaris, the remainder of the choroidea, the stroma, is populated with melanocytes, connective tissue elements (including fibroblasts, mastocytes, elastic, and collagen fibrils), blood vessels, macrophages, dendritic cells, lymphocytes, nonvascular smooth muscle cells, intrinsic neurons, and nerve fibers associated with vessels [43–45].

The retina is a complex transparent tissue of ~0.55 mm at the edges of the fovea and of ~0.13 mm at the center (umbo). This innermost layer of the eye includes a nonsensory part and an optic part that are divided by the ora serrata. The anterior part does not provide any sensory function and covers the ciliary body and iris with bilaminar epithelium. The posterior portion of the retina lies from the ora serrata to the optic disc being attached only at these two locations. Interestingly, there is an area on the optic retina, roughly 5.5 mm in diameter, which is centered about 4 mm temporal to and 0.8 mm inferior to the center of the optic disc that is called macula (macula lutea or central retina) and which has xanthophyll and two or more layers of ganglion cells. Moreover, few regions can be distinguished within this part of the retina: (1) the fovea (fovea centralis) is a depression in the center of the macular area (~1.5 mm in diameter); (2) the foveola is a central floor of the fovea, which is approximately 0.35 mm in diameter; and (3) the umbo (central depression of the foveola). The optic part of the retina is composed of the retinal pigmented epithelium (RPE; the outer layer) and the cerebral layer (inner). RPE supplies the neurosensory layer with nutrition, as well as removes metabolic products. Additionally, it plays a key role in maintaining the blood–retina barrier (BRB) separating the neurosensory retina from the circulating blood. The inner retina comprises photoreceptors (approximately 120 million rods and 6–7 million cones that constitute the first neuron), bipolar cells (the second neuron), and multipolar ganglion cells (the third neuron), along with horizontal and amacrine cells. Interestingly, rod cells are responsible for peripheral vision acting at low light levels using the photosensitive molecule (rhodopsin) in visual phototransduction. In contrast, three types of cone cells (according to the color perception: red, blue, and green) are located only within the fovea area and are 30- to 100-fold less sensitive compared to rod cells, requiring the simultaneous activation of tens to hundreds of visual pigment molecules (that are homologous or even identical to those found in rods) to generate a detectable response resulting in their activity at relatively high light levels, thereby providing central vision and the ability to distinguish colors. Therefore, the retina is the site of transformation of light energy into a neural signal that is transmitted via the optic nerve to the visual cortex to be analyzed by the brain helping to "see" the environment [29,46,47].

3. Ocular Conditions

There are more than 100 recognized disorders of the eye [22]. Therefore, only some of the most common disorders or the conditions that could potentially benefit from the development of advanced topical formulations with enhanced drug permeability are briefly discussed here. Most frequent diseases of the cornea include keratitis, keratoconus, and dry eye syndrome.

Keratitis is a condition when the patient's cornea becomes inflamed. A wide range of germs could lead to this inflammatory condition, but the most common are *Staphylococcus aureus*, *Staphylococcus epidermidis*, *Streptococcus pneumoniae*, *Pseudomonas aeruginosa*, *Neisseria gonorrhoeae*, *Haemophilus*, herpes simplex and varicella zoster viruses, *Fusarium*, *Aspergillus*, *Candida*, and acanthamoeba. Patients typically complain of pain, foreign body sensation, photophobia, redness of the eye, tearing, discharge (sometimes purulent), and decreased visual acuity. Although this condition is mostly quite painful for the patient and requires urgent treatment, sometimes it can be almost asymptomatic (for instance, if caused by acanthamoeba).

Antibacterial drops combined with subconjunctival injections in severe cases are the choices of therapy in patients with keratitis. According to the most recent clinical recommendations [48], two main schemes are used to treat bacterial keratitis depending on the pathogen and the response to its therapy. The monotherapy includes the use of antibacterial eye drops consisting of fluoroquinolones (levofloxacin, moxifloxacin, gatifloxacin, besifloxacin, ofloxacin, or ciprofloxacin) that cover both Gram-positive (*Staphylococcus aureus, Staphylococcus epidermidis, Streptococcus pneumoniae*) and Gram-negative (*Pseudomonas aeruginosa, Neisseria gonorrhoeae, Haemophilus*) bacteria. However, these medications should be used with caution due to the possible resistance of some organisms, which can be noticed by controlling the clinical response. Therefore, there is a second treatment scheme, which combines fluoroquinolone eye drops and solutions for a topical or subconjunctival route that comprise other groups of antibiotics including cephalosporin (cefazolin, ceftazidime), aminoglycosides (gentamicin or tobramycin), penicillins (penicillin G, methicillin, or piperacillin), and glycopeptide antibiotics (vancomycin). For instance, cefazolin is commonly used for *Pseudomonas aeruginosa* infection. On the other hand, ceftazidime is effective against resistant forms of *Pseudomonas aeruginosa*. Vancomycin has efficacy against methicillin-resistant staphylococci, as well as against other Gram-positives. Additionally, corticosteroids (dexamethasone, prednisolone) can be used topically in terms of reducing pain and inflammation in bacterial keratitis but with caution, keeping in mind they inhibit re-epithelialization of the cornea [49,50]. Treatment with steroids should be avoided, when keratitis is induced by fungi or acanthamoeba, as well as in cases of any doubts regarding the effectiveness of the antimicrobial regimen.

Nonsteroidal anti-inflammatory drugs (NSAIDs) also may be recommended for reducing symptoms of inflammation only in the case of efficient antimicrobial therapy. In addition, preservative-free lubricants may be used for promoting healing and cycloplegic agents (cyclopentolate) to reduce discomfort associated with spasm of the ciliary body, as well as for decreasing formation of synechiae [48].

Topical usage of antiviral eye drops (acyclovir) is the core of treatment in cases of herpes simplex keratitis. Eye drops with trifluorothymidine or ganciclovir can be prescribed instead of acyclovir in cases of resistance to therapy. Also, prednisolone acetate- or dexamethasone-including eye drops are used to reduce the inflammation, albeit with the caveat regarding epithelial damage discussed above. In terms of preventing virus reactivation, the administration of oral antiviral agents is preferred. Conversely, in patients with keratitis induced by varicella zoster virus (herpes zoster ophthalmicus), Dworkin et al. [51] reported that topical antiviral therapy is ineffective. Hence, systemic usage of antiviral drugs is the choice of treatment. Additionally, cycloplegic eye drops (cyclopentolate) are used for preventing ciliary spasm that can be associated with this pathological condition. Topical preservative-free lubricants such as hydroxypropyl methylcellulose (and others) can also be added to the treatment [48].

Fungal keratitis should be generally treated with topical antifungal formulations that can be divided into a few groups depending on their mode of action: polyenes (amphotericin B, natamycin), imidazoles (clotrimazole, miconazole, econazole, ketoconazole), triazoles (itraconazole, fluconazole, voriconazole), pyrimidines (flucytosine), and echinocandins (micafungin, caspofungin) [49]. Systemic antifungal drugs can be recommended in severe cases involving deep stromal layers with a high risk of perforation of the cornea. Additionally, topical cycloplegic drugs can be used. The keratitis caused by acanthamoeba should be treated with topical anti-amoebic formulations [48]. Of note, the aim of this treatment is to eradicate amoebic cysts from the cornea. The first-line therapy includes biguanide agents (polyhexamethylene biguanide (PHMB), chlorhexidine) that are cystidical (active against cysts). The aromatic diamidines (propamidine, hexamidine) belong to the second-line medications providing more variable activity, along with being cystidical. In contrast, aminoglycosides (neomycin, paromomycin) or azole agents (clotrimazole, fluconazole, ketoconazole, miconazole) are almost not cystidical, being active against trophozoites [49]. However, they can be used in addition to first- or second-line therapy. According to the literature, adenylate cyclase can be administered topically to promote the conversion of cysts into a protozoal state [48].

Keratoconus is defined by Kanski and Bowling as a progressive disorder in which thinning of the central or paracentral stroma of the cornea occurs, accompanied by apical protrusion and irregular astigmatism [22]. It affects 0.05–5% of the population [48]. Patient complaints include blurred vision, mild photophobia, and increased vision impairment due to progressive myopia and astigmatism. The cause of this condition is still unknown, but some authors refer to such factors as combination of repeated trauma and existing abnormalities of the stroma. Additionally, in some cases, keratoconus presents in patients with other ocular and systemic conditions including, for example, disorders of the connective tissue. One widely used method for treatment of this condition is a corneal collagen cross-linking, which leads to stabilization of ectasia by using riboflavin eye drops and subsequent exposure to ultraviolet-A light. Also, implantation of the ring segment within the cornea can be used as an addition to the cross-linking procedure. In severe cases, keratoplasty (corneal transplantation) is a choice of treatment [22].

Dry eye disease (keratoconjunctivitis sicca) occurs in cases of inadequate tear volume or function, which results in an unstable tear film with disease of the surface of the eye. The prevalence of dry eye syndrome in American and Australian population is estimated to be around 5–16%, while in Asia it is higher and could reach up to 27–33% [49]. Severity of the symptoms may highly vary from patient to patient, but they mostly include a feeling of burning and blurred vision. Pathologies affecting the lacrimal gland and dysfunction of the Meibomian glands, as well as neurological diseases, can lead to the keratoconjunctivitis sicca [22,32]. The aim of therapy is to restore the normal surface of the eye by using tear supplementation along with inhibiting the aberrant inflammation observed in patients with chronic dry eye syndrome. Treatment of this condition is complex, but only the most common topical ocular formulations are discussed in this paper. The following groups of medicines are recommended: lubricants (carboxymethylcellulose, hydroxypropyl methylcellulose, and carbomer gels), hydroxypropyl guar/sodium hyaluronate or combinations (carboxymethylcellulose, polysaccharides or disaccharide), xanthan gum, phospholipids and soybean), artificial tears (with various electrolyte compositions, viscosity, and presence of preservatives), and eye drops with cyclosporine A (increasing tear production by reducing the inflammation of the lacrimal gland). However, lifitegrast is a topical anti-inflammatory medicine which is, at the moment, the only drug approved by the Food and Drug Administration for treating both symptoms and signs in patients with dry eye disease [48,49].

Cataract is a condition in which opacification of the crystalline lens occurs principally as a result of protein aggregation. According to some studies, the number of people in the world who become blind due to cataract is estimated as 20 million [52]. The Vision Loss Expert Group funded by the Bill and Melinda Gates Foundation, Fight for Sight, and others calculated that cataracts led to blindness in 10.6 million people and moderate to severe visual impairment in 34.4 million people [49]. A few classifications are used (depending on morphology, etiology, and maturity) but, in general, all cataracts can be divided into two groups: congenital and acquired. Among the latter group, one of the common types is the age-related cataract induced by metabolic processes of aging (including oxidative stress) of the human lens. Clinicians can hear from patients such symptoms as decreased visual acuity, changing of the contrast sensitivity, color perception, glare, monocular diplopia, and ghosting [48]. Surgical removal of the natural lens and its replacement with an intraocular lens (IOL) is currently the only solution for patients with this condition. However, scientists are actively searching for a potential topical treatment. Thus, it was found that pyruvate eye drops can effectively penetrate ocular membranes and potentially provide protection against oxidative stress [53], while Zhao et al. reported that using lanosterol-loaded nanoparticles can reverse protein aggregation in the lens [54].

Glaucoma is a progressive optic neuropathy that is accompanied by the excavation of the optic nerve head and a loss of visual sensitivity in the sequence beginning in the mid-peripheral visual field. Types of glaucoma are classified as open-angle, angle-closure, glaucoma due to another disease, and childhood onset glaucoma [55,56]. It is worth noting that the leading cause of irreversible blindness worldwide is glaucoma. The following indicators are considered as risk factors for developing glaucoma: increasing age (mostly after 40 years), race, family history, and using steroids. One of the major risks for the development and progression of glaucoma is intraocular pressure (IOP). The prevalence of this condition is 3.54% for people aged 40–80 years worldwide [56]. Even in normal-tension glaucoma with IOP not exceeding 21 mmHg, IOP remains a risk factor for progressive damage of the optic nerve [49]. One of the reasons why patients may not ask for medical help until developed stages of the disease occur is that it is usually asymptomatic. In some cases, patients may complain of halos, pain in the eye, headache, precipitants, and subjective loss of vision field [32]. Pharmacological treatment of glaucoma includes five main groups of topical formulations (prostaglandin analogues, beta-blockers, sympathomimetics (alpha-2-agonists), carbonic anhydrase inhibitors, and miotics). Eye drops with prostaglandin analogues (latanoprost, travoprost, bimatoprost, tafluprost) are considered to be a first-line therapy in open-angle glaucoma patients to reduce the IOP primarily by increasing uveoscleral outflow. A number of side effects (conjunctival hyperemia, irreversible hyperpigmentation of iris, reversible increasing pigmentation of the lid skin, lengthening along with thickening of eyelashes, and orbital fat loss), as well as limitations of using these therapies in inflamed eyes and in patients with herpetic keratitis in their anamnesis, may lead to replacing prostaglandin derivatives with beta-blockers. The latter IOP-lowering class of drugs reduces aqueous production and can be divided into two kinds of beta-blockers depending on the involved receptors: non-selective (timolol, carteolol, levobunolol) and β1-selective (betaxolol). However, the use of beta-blockers is relatively restricted in patients with asthma and cardiovascular diseases due to the potential bronchospasm, hypotension, heart block, and bradycardia. The carbonic anhydrase inhibitors (brinzolamide, dorzolamide) represent another type of topical formulations, which also lower levels of aqueous humor production, being contraindicated in patients with an allergy to sulfonamide antibiotics and patients with renal or liver failure. The mode of action of sympathomimetics (brimonidine and apraclonidine) is based on the stimulation of alpha-2-receptors, resulting in both the decrease of the aqueous secretion and enhancement of the uveoscleral outflow. On the other hand, bradycardia and heart block are among the contraindications for the use of these sympathomimetics. Alpha-2 agonists are mostly prescribed for short-term use (for instance, after laser iridotomy). The treatment of angle-closure glaucoma includes the use of miotics (pilocarpine and carbachol) that increase the outflow through the trabecular meshwork. Currently, numerous combined preparations are commercially available on the market (timolol and dorzolamide/brinzolamide/travoprost/bimatoprost/brimonidine/pilocarpine or brimonidine and brinzolamide). Regardless of the number of available options for topical treatment of glaucoma, there is still a demand of using systemic drugs, and laser and surgical procedures in some clinical cases [22,48].

Age-related macular degeneration (AMD) is a degenerative disorder affecting people over the age of 50 years. An estimated number of people affected by AMD is approximately 30–50 million worldwide [49]. There are two known forms of AMD. The majority of patients have so-called "dry" AMD that is usually asymptomatic, except for gradual central visual loss of night vision. Also, it may be accompanied by metamorphopsia and prolonged afterimages [57]. This stage is defined by formation of drusen (amorphous deposits located between the retinal pigmented epithelium (RPE) and the Bruch's membrane) and abnormalities of RPE including hyperpigmentation and atrophy. In a relatively small share of patients, this form progresses to the neovascular ("exudative" or "wet") AMD. This condition is characterized by the growth of new abnormal capillaries from the choriocapillaris (choroidal neovascularization) that penetrate the Bruch's membrane, resulting in hemorrhages or exudation, producing scar, retina, or RPE detachment. At this stage, patients complain of a rapid onset of visual loss, a central blind spot, or metamorphopsia. The treatment of "dry" AMD is mostly based on changing lifestyle and using oral vitamin supplements (ascorbic acid, vitamin E, alpha-carotene, and zinc), which are thought to delay its progression. On the other hand, the treatment of the neovascular ("wet") AMD should be started with intravitreal injections of anti-vascular endothelial growth factor agents (anti-vascular endothelial growth factor (VEGF) treatment: ranibizumab, aflibercept, pegaptanib, bevacizumab), which is an invasive procedure posing concern and discomfort for the patient. Moreover, there are some potential vision-threatening complications associated with intravitreal injections: infectious endophthalmitis, retinal tears, sterile inflammation, vitreous hemorrhage, cataract, elevation of the IOP, etc. [49]. The intravitreal injection still remains a primary delivery route of anti-VEGF agents. A serious limitation of this therapy is a relatively short half-life of VEGF following intravitreous injections [58], which implies the need for frequent administrations. Some approaches were recently reported to develop less invasive methods of delivery, for example, subconjunctival administration of lyophilized matrices containing bevacizumab [59].

The development of formulations capable of delivering anti-VEGF agents into the eye, when administered topically, will be of great advantage and could revolutionize the therapy of this condition. Davis et al. [60] reported the successful topical delivery of Avastin using annexin A5-associated liposomal formulations to the posterior segment of the eye in vivo (rats and rabbits) at physiologically significant levels. This could be considered as a major advancement that should attract further research and perhaps some studies into the use of penetration enhancers. Some advances in the development of topical formulations to the delivery of biopharmaceuticals to the posterior segment of the eye were recently discussed in several reviews [61].

Photodynamic therapy (PDT) is an option if patients have any contraindications for anti-VEGF therapy. Focal laser photocoagulation is the third solution that can be offered to a patient, which is uncommon due to common recurrence and presence of localized scotoma after the procedure [48].

Diabetic retinopathy (DR) also belongs to one of the leading causes of vision impairment, as prevalence of diabetes mellitus is increasing dramatically worldwide [62]. In fact, this is the most frequent microvascular complication of diabetes. According to Duh et al. [63], almost 100 million individuals were diagnosed with diabetic retinopathy. DR is divided into two groups: (1) the earlier stage of non-proliferative diabetic retinopathy (NPDR), which is characterized by microaneurysms, retinal hemorrhages, intraretinal microvascular abnormalities, and venous caliber changes; and (2) proliferative diabetic retinopathy (PDR) with pathologic pre-retinal neovascularization. Additionally, diabetic macular edema may occur during both NPDR and PDR, representing the most common cause of vision loss in patients with DR. This edema arises from diabetes-induced breakdown of the blood–retinal barrier, with consequent leakage of fluid and circulating proteins from the vessels into the neurosensory retina [63]. As a matter of priority, assessment of patients with DR relies on the control of glucose concentration in the patient's blood. The treatment of this condition involves laser photocoagulation (panretinal, focal, and grid), intravitreal anti-VEGF agents (aflibercept and ranibizumab), corticosteroids (dexamethasone and fluocinolone acetonide intravitreal implants), and vitrectomy in the case of vitreous hemorrhage [48]. Some of these therapeutic approaches could potentially benefit from the development of formulations that could deliver drugs to the eye topically.

4. Permeability of Ocular Membranes

The analysis of the physicochemical properties of various chemical compounds that cross membranes in the eye could be key in understanding the opportunities and obstacles in ocular drug delivery. Thus, according to Prausnitz and Noonan [64], the octanol–water partitioning coefficient (logP), which helps characterize the drug's hydrophilic–lipophilic properties, determines the ability of molecules to pass through cells of the epithelial and endothelial layers of the cornea and conjunctiva. The epithelium permeability accounts up to 90% for the lipophilic substances as a result of the high dependence on logP, while almost totally excluding macromolecules (with radius larger than 10 Å) [64]. Hence, the epithelium is the main limitation for intracorneal drug delivery. In contrast, stromal drug permeability is less dependent on logP but highly dependent on the radius of the molecules, providing a great barrier for lipophilic compounds of a small size (radius < 10 Å). Interestingly, the permeation across the endothelium layer relies on both logP and the size of the molecule (paracellular penetration route) and is slightly more impermeable for lipophilic small molecules in comparison to the corneal stroma. However, macromolecules cross the endothelium more easily than the stroma. The permeability of another ocular membrane, sclera, is relatively close to that of the corneal stroma. The data on conjunctival permeation are limited; however, according to some reports, it demonstrates a higher permeability compared to the cornea [64].

Edwards and Prausnitz [65] reported the development of a theoretical model that can help in predicting the permeability of the cornea for different solutes, which can be calculated using only two parameters: radius of the molecule and logP. This could be a very useful model in ocular drug delivery, but there are a few factors that were not taken into account by the authors: simplification of the structure of openings between the cells, as well as tight junctions in epithelial and endothelial layers, various permeability of cells within the epithelium layer, possible intracorneal binding of compounds, and different shape of molecules (assuming all of them to be solid spheres).

Recently, a few in vitro and ex vivo models were used to evaluate permeability and drug absorption by the cornea. Thus, according to Agarwal and Rupenthal [66], cell-based models are commonly used for studies of penetration. Advantages of these models include relatively lower cost compared to the use of laboratory animals, as well as minimizing the number of animal studies. However, this type of model is more suitable to evaluate the cytotoxicity of the compounds rather than their permeability and absorption by the cornea. This is because cell-based models are, in simple terms, five to six layers of the epithelial cells of the cornea (usually, corneal culture of the rabbit) but not the entire structure of the cornea. Additionally, these cell cultures neither have transporter molecules nor enzymes responsible for drugs metabolism. One of the closest models to the real cornea involves reconstructed tissue cultures which comprise different types of cells that help mimic the three-layer structure including the epithelium, stroma, and endothelium. For example, Kaluzhny et al. [67] recently developed an in vitro human three-dimensional corneal epithelial tissue model and demonstrated the applicability of this membrane for studies of drug permeability using several fluorescent markers, as well as latanoprost and bimatoprost.

Ex vivo corneas of various animals (rabbit, porcine, bovine) are also commonly used for evaluating corneal permeability and absorption; however, this model is not ideal due to the differences in the anatomical structure compared to the human cornea, as well as potentially different enzymes and molecules of active transporters. Thus, rabbit eyes are commonly used as ex vivo models, but the rabbit cornea does not have Bowman's layer, which results in higher penetration of substances in comparison with the human cornea. The eyeball size, thickness of the cornea, ratio of length of the cornea to eye-globe diameter, and histological structure (including Bowman's membrane) in porcine eyes are the closest to the human eye. Bovine eyes are also used in the studies of ocular tissue drug permeability despite the fact that these are larger than human eyes and their corneal epithelium is almost twice the thickness [66]. Loch et al. [21] conducted a comparative study of the permeation of three different drugs (ciprofloxacin hydrochloride, lidocaine hydrochloride, and timolol maleate) through porcine, rabbit, and bovine ocular tissues. They observed substantial differences between the apparent permeability coefficients (P_{app}) for different animal species.

$$P_{app} = \frac{Q}{A \times C_0}, \tag{1}$$

where Q is the steady-state appearance rate of the investigated substance on the acceptor side of the tissue (mol/s), C_0 is the initial concentration of the drug in the donor chamber (mol/L), and A is the surface area of the tissue (cm^2). In order to take into account the differences in the thicknesses of porcine, rabbit, and bovine tissues, they calculated effective diffusion coefficients using the following equation:

$$D_{eff} = P_{app} \times l, \tag{2}$$

where l is the tissue thickness (cm). The results of D_{eff} determination are presented in Figure 6. These results clearly show that the chemical nature of the drug has great influence on the tissue permeability. The authors also hypothesized that protein binding, tissue hydration, or transporters may play some role in the differences between different species.

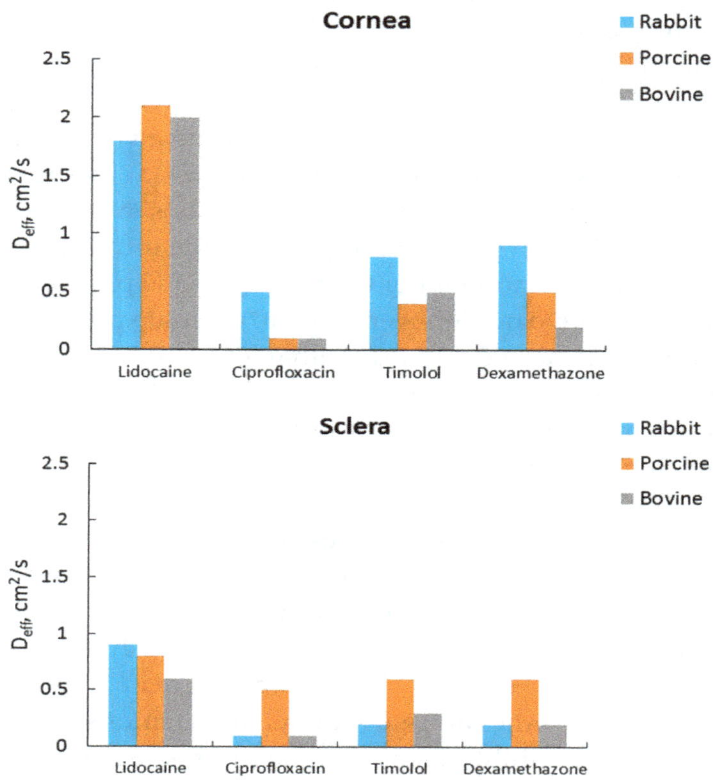

Figure 6. Effective diffusion coefficients D_{eff} (cm^2/s) of several drugs for rabbit, porcine, and bovine cornea and sclera. Data taken from Reference [21] with permission from Elsevier, 2012.

5. Penetration Enhancers

Anatomical and physiological features of the eye, ocular conditions, and permeability of ocular membranes were discussed above, and the review now moves to consider some of the different classes of penetration-enhancing compounds, describing their properties and modes of action.

5.1. Cyclodextrins

Cyclodextrins (CD) are water-soluble cyclic oligosaccharides shaped like a truncated cone. Native cyclodextrins include α-CD, β-CD, and γ-CD, which differ in the number of α-(1-4)-linked glucopyranose subunits (six, seven, and eight, respectively, Figure 7) [68]. There were many derivatives of CDs developed over the last decades, each bringing some improved properties such as enhanced aqueous solubility. The most common derivatives of CDs include hydroxypropyl-β- and γ-CD, the randomly methylated β-CD, and sulfobutylether β-CD [69]. Cyclodextrins have lipophilic cavities and hydrophilic hydroxyl groups associated with the external surfaces of their molecule [70]. They are capable of forming guest–host inclusion complexes, whereby lipophilic drugs with poor aqueous solubility reside within the hydrophobic cavity, where they are protected, but not covalently bound. The drug–CD complexes usually have improved aqueous solubility due to the hydrophilic properties of the external surface of the cyclodextrin molecule [71]. It is generally established that only free drug molecules from topical formulations with cyclodextrins are able to penetrate ocular membranes [72]. Since cyclodextrins are relatively large molecules, they are unable to permeate through intact lipophilic membranes, for example, the corneal epithelium; however, they allow drugs to interact with the epithelial surface. They have uses in pharmaceutical applications due to their drug solubility-enhancing properties, improved bioavailability, and improved formulation stability, capable of masking a drug's irritation effects; they are generally regarded as safe (GRAS) [73]. Drug–CD inclusion complex formation/dissociation is a dynamic process, where drug molecules are released and taken up spontaneously in the aqueous environment [74,75]. Lipophilic compounds are able to reside within the cyclodextrin molecule cavity through weak hydrophobic interactions. In the aqueous environment of the tear film, drugs can be released from drug–CD complexes by preferential take-up of cell-membrane lipids, such as cholesterol and phospholipids, and simultaneous ejection of the drug guest. There remains an opportunity for the drug to enter the epithelium membrane via the temporary disruption caused by lipid extraction during membrane–cyclodextrin interaction [68,76].

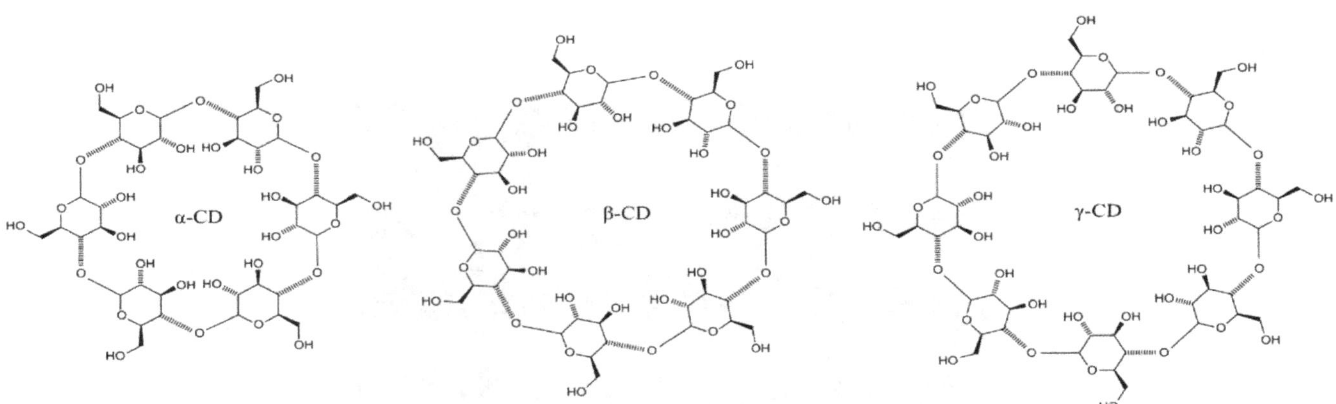

Figure 7. Structures of α-cyclodextrin, β-cyclodextrin, and γ-cyclodextrin. The image was reproduced under the Creative Commons Attribution Share Alike 3.0 Unported license [77].

The ability of α-CD to enhance corneal penetration for cysteamine (β-mercaptoethylamine; medication used to treat cystinosis, which is a rare, genetic disorder with abnormal accumulation of cystine within the corneal stroma resulting in photophobia) [78] was established by Pescina et al. [79] in ex vivo experiments with freshly excised pig corneas. The researchers also demonstrated lack of irritation caused by a 5.5% α-CD solution employing the Hen's Egg Test on the Chorioallantoic Membrane. Moreover, the addition of ethylenediamine-*N,N,N′,N′*-tetraacetic acid (EDTA) to α-CD established a good stability profile of cysteamine. According to Aktaş et al. [80], the eye drops consisting of pilocarpine nitrate and hydroxypropyl β-cyclodextrin (HP-β-CD) demonstrated a four-fold increase in transcorneal penetration compared to a drug formulation without CD. The researchers used side-by-side diffusion cells and corneas harvested from rabbits. In addition, the pupillary-response pattern was monitored in rabbits in vivo. The constriction of the pupil was remarkably increased due to the addition of the HP-β-CD-containing formulation of pilocarpine nitrate. Loftsson and Stefansson [81] designed low-viscosity eye-drop formulations with drug/γ-CD complexes which were then tested in vivo in rabbits and clinically in patients. The first aqueous eye-drop formulation included dorzolamide/γ-CD complexes and demonstrated high levels of the drug in the aqueous humor of rabbit eyes more than 24 h after a single application. The IOP-lowering effect of this solution in patients was observed after daily use compared to conventional eye drops with dorzolamide that should be given three times a day to provide the same effect. Other eye drops consisted of dexamethasone/γ-CD complexes and showed the ability to deliver dexamethasone to the posterior segment of the rabbit eye. Moreover, there were significant clinical improvements in patients with diabetic macular edema (DME) and intermediate uveitis patients with cystoid macular edema after the topical use of eye drops with dexamethasone/γ-CD. The results for DME patients were clinically similar to those after the intravitreal corticosteroid injection.

Morrison and co-workers [68] studied the penetration of riboflavin through freshly excised bovine corneas using formulations containing various cyclodextrins. They established that β-CD and HP-β-CD facilitate the permeation of riboflavin through the cornea; however, they do not affect the lag time of approximately 90–120 min, where the first portions of the drug begin crossing the cornea. The microscopic examination of the corneas treated with cyclodextrins indicated that these permeability enhancers cause some disruption of the epithelial structure. Further analysis of this disruption allowed the authors to establish the mechanism of permeability enhancement related to the extraction of cholesterol from corneal tissue observed in the case of formulations with β-CD and HP-β-CD. This resulted in a partial disruption of the corneal epithelia, which was evidenced from histological examination of the bovine corneal membranes exposed to solutions of cyclodextrins for different contact times. Figure 8 shows exemplary micrographs of corneas exposed to 30 mg·mL^{-1} solutions of β-CD compared to control non-exposed tissues. Samples of the cornea treated with β-cyclodextrin showed some epithelial disruption, which became more noticeable with longer exposure time. However, no extraction of cholesterol was observed when the corneas were exposed to water or α-CD and γ-CD.

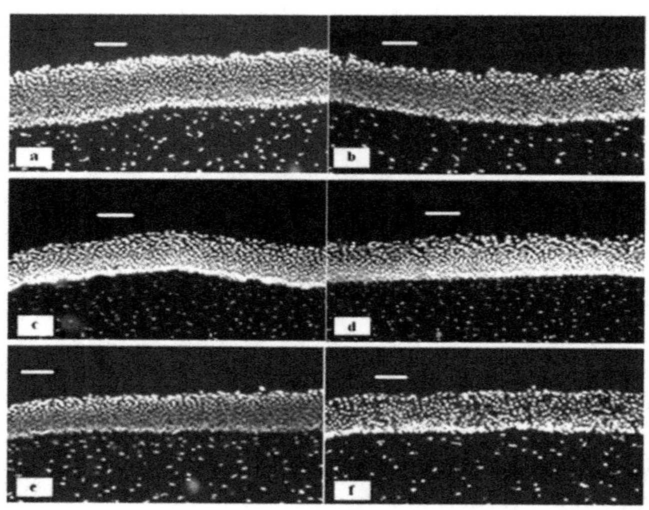

Figure 8. Micrographs of bovine cornea exposed to 1 mL of β-cyclodextrin (30 mg·mL^{-1}) (**b**,**d**,**f**) against non-exposed regions (**a**,**c**,**e**). Exposure time: 15 (**a**,**b**), 45 (**c**,**d**), and 75 min (**e**,**f**). Scale bar = 100 μm. Reproduced from Reference [68] with permission from American Chemical Society, 2013.

5.2. Chelating Agents

The corneal epithelium offers a highly resistant barrier against alien matter due to its lipophilic characteristics, preventing the transcellular transport of many drugs, and the existence of tight junctions, i.e., tightly adherent regions between cells, maintaining intimate cell contact, effectively preventing drug transport via the paracellular route. Tight junction functionality of the superficial epithelial cells depends on an undetermined availability of Ca^{2+} ions [4,82]. Calcium chelating agents are often included in topical ocular drug formulations as stabilizers. They were shown to offer temporary and reversible action when used for enhancement of ocular drug delivery. However, there is evidence that ethylenediamine-*N,N,N′,N′*-tetraacetic acid (EDTA) in topical ocular formulations can bring side effects due to accumulation within the iris and ciliary body, and can affect endothelial cells and capillaries associated with the uveal tract. Caution should be exercised due to toxicity implications, especially when medication is required in the long term [83]. Calcium chelators, a class of polyaminocarboxylic acids, for example, EDTA, ethylene glycol-bis(beta-aminoethyl)-*N,N,N′,N′*-tetraacetic acid (EGTA), 1,2-bis(o-aminophenoxy)ethane-*N,N,N′,N′*-tetraacetic acid (BAPTA) [84], and ethylenediamine-*N,N′*-disuccinic acid (EDDS) (Figure 9), are capable of reversibly enhancing drug penetration across otherwise penetration-resistant barriers such as the corneal epithelium [17].

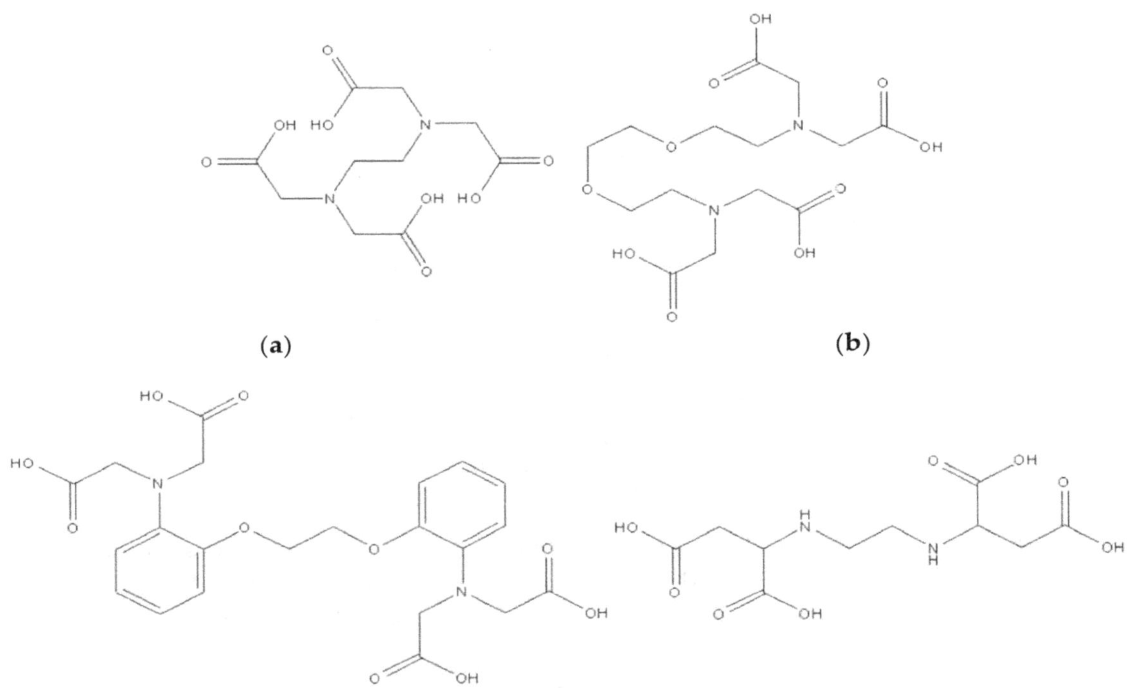

(a) (b) (c) (d)

Figure 9. Structures of ethylenediamine-*N,N,N′,N′*-tetraacetic acid (EDTA) (**a**), ethylene glycol-bis(beta-aminoethyl)-*N,N,N′,N′*-tetraacetic acid (EGTA) (**b**), 1,2-bis(o-aminophenoxy)ethane-*N,N,N′,N′*-tetraacetic acid (BAPTA) (**c**), and ethylenediamine-*N,N′*-disuccinic acid (EDDS) (**d**).

Their mode of action is achieved via disruption of tight junctions and adherens junctions by sequestration of interstitial Ca^{2+} ions, on which the barrier function is dependent. Research carried out by Morrison and Khutoryanskiy [17] showed that low-concentration aqueous solutions of EDTA, EGTA, and EDDS at 1 $mg{\cdot}mL^{-1}$ were capable of extracting Ca^{2+} ions from bovine corneas in vitro (Figure 10). The three formulations studied enhanced Ca^{2+} extraction and corneal penetration of riboflavin compared with phosphate-buffered saline. The same researchers investigated permeability enhancement of bovine corneas in vitro using transepithelial electrical resistance analysis (TEER), finding that all polyaminocarboxylic acid formulations investigated lowered TEER values, correlating with enhanced penetration of riboflavin across bovine epithelia into the corneal stroma. EGTA showed the best performance for Ca^{2+} extraction and penetration enhancement from the formulations explored.

Kikuchi et al. [85] investigated a synergistic relationship for enhancing ocular drug penetration when using a combination of EDTA and boric acid in various proportions. The researchers found that the co-formulation brought an improvement in drug penetration across the highly resistant epithelial membrane, but no enhancement to the already efficient permeation across de-epithelialized rabbit corneas. They concluded that the synergistic effects observed were due to improved transcellular permeability when compared to formulations with either EDTA or boric acid alone [85]. Topical aqueous ocular drug formulations incorporating polyaminocarboxylic acid penetration-enhancing agents induce disruption to the corneal epithelium, even at concentrations as low as 1 mg·mL^{-1}. Although this enhances corneal permeability to drugs, it can also introduce undesirable side effects such as ocular irritation. The use of topical ocular drug formulations incorporating mucoadhesive polymers, i.e., hyaluronic acid, chitosan, and alginate, together with polyaminocarboxylic acid penetration-enhancing agents, gives the benefits from these chelating agents whilst moderating the epithelial disruptive effects, allowing them to give moderate enhancement to ocular drug penetration without inducing irritation. The use of mucoadhesive polymers potentially offers a means to give improved drug efficacy, low dose, and sustained delivery with reduced issues of toxicity and minimal undesired side effects [86,87]. However, Rodriguez et al. [86] demonstrated that the combination of mucoadhesive polymers with permeability enhancers leads to the inhibition of permeability-enhancing effects.

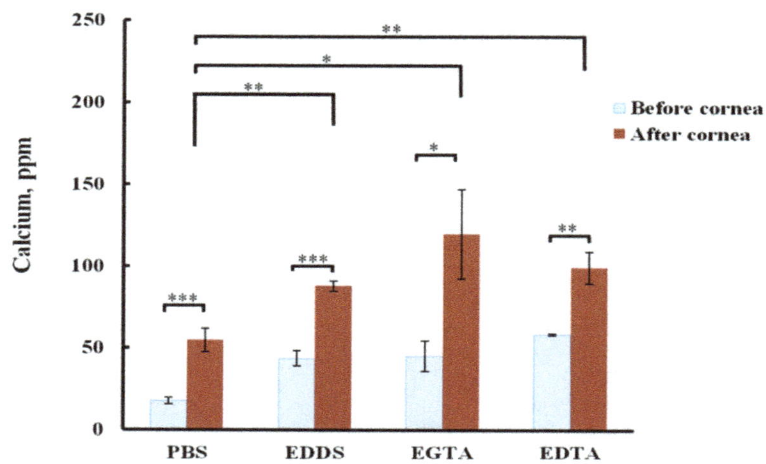

Figure 10. Calcium concentration in solutions containing phosphate-buffered saline (PBS), EDDS, EGTA, and EDTA (1 mg·mL^{-1}) before and after 3 h of exposure to bovine cornea. * $p < 0.05$, ** $p < 0.01$, *** $p < 0.001$; one-way ANOVA; $n = 3$. Reproduced from Reference [17] under the terms of the Creative Commons Attribution License (CC BY).

5.3. Crown Ethers

Crown ethers are synthetic cyclic oligomers of ethylene oxide consisting of linked ether groups; they are named this way because the shape of their molecules resembles that of a crown when its structure is viewed at its side elevation. Naming convention follows numbers divided by the letter "C" for "crown", whereby the larger number represents the number of atoms contained in the molecule, and the smaller number represents the number of oxygen atoms. The most common members are 12C4, 15C5, and 18C6, namely, the tetramer ($n = 4$), pentamer ($n = 5$), and hexamer ($n = 6$) (Figure 11).

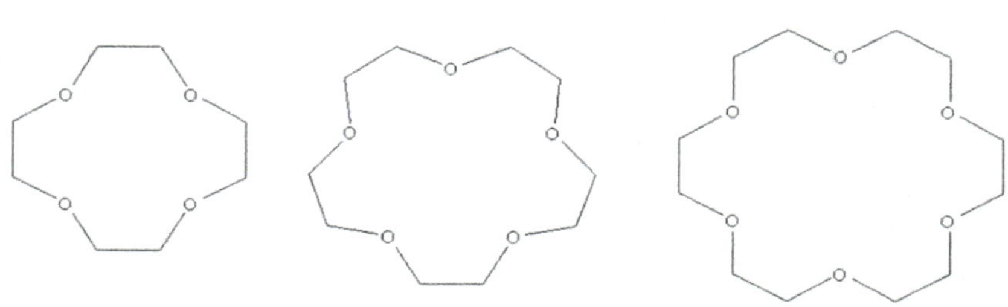

(a) (b) (c)

Figure 11. Structures of 12-crown-4 (**a**), 15-crown-5 (**b**), and 18-crown-6 (**c**).

Crown ethers were discovered accidentally by Pedersen whilst researching the development of complexing agents for divalent cations in the 1960s. During his research, Pedersen realized that the cyclic polyether by-products were capable of forming complexes with alkali metals [88]. Since Pedersen's pioneering work, many derivatives were developed [89–91], and these found uses in various fields of science, industry, and pharmacology. Crown ethers are able to form complexes with metal ions, as well as neutral and ionic organic molecules, and their complexes have the ability to traverse biological membranes [92–94]. They are employed for the treatment of tumors [95,96] and drug-loaded vesicular preparations [97,98]. Crown ethers are flexible molecules, allowing them to adapt to the environment they are exposed to. In aqueous solutions, they interact with this medium by exposing their hydrophilic oxygen atoms to water molecules; however, when these molecules encounter a lipophilic solvent, they interact via their lipophilic ethylenic groups [91]. These properties, together with their ionophoric qualities, make them ideal compounds for use in ocular drug delivery, where the formulation has to interact with both aqueous and lipophilic phases. At the time of writing of this review, there was only one published study investigating the use of crown ethers for enhanced ocular drug delivery [99]; Morrison et al. [100] investigated 12C4, 15C5, and 18C6 for use in ocular drug delivery, and they were able to show enhanced aqueous solubility of riboflavin up to 46%, potentially improving bioavailability (Table 1). Furthermore, all crown ether variants studied were capable of significantly enhancing Ca^{2+} extraction from bovine corneas in vitro compared with phosphate-buffered saline. In the same study the researchers were able to show enhanced corneal delivery of riboflavin to bovine corneal stroma in vitro with crown ether concentrations as low as 1 mg·mL^{-1}.

Table 1. Steady-state flux and apparent permeability of riboflavin through bovine cornea in phosphate-buffered saline (PBS) with and without crown ether. Reproduced from Reference [100] with permission from American Chemical Society, 2017.

Solution	Steady-State Flux (µmol·min^{-1})	P_{app} (cm·s^{-1} × 10^{-3})
PBS	0.0478	1.945
12C4 (1 mg·mL^{-1})	0.1208	6.138
15C5 (1 mg·mL^{-1})	0.1074	5.457
18C6 (1 mg·mL^{-1})	0.0753	3.826
12C4 (30 mg·mL^{-1})	0.3410	17.326
15C5 (30 mg·mL^{-1})	0.1961	9.964
18C6 (30 mg·mL^{-1})	0.1811	9.202

Morrison et al. [100] also carried out a toxicological investigation and in vivo penetration studies using the rat model. The toxicological investigation was able to show that crown ethers were no more toxic to ocular tissue than benzalkonium chloride, an excipient often used at low concentrations as a preservative in ocular drug formulations. The in vivo drug penetration study failed to show any statistically significant permeability enhancement compared to enhancer-free formulations, the most probable reason being due to natural clearance mechanisms that protect the eye from foreign material. However, their in vivo study was conducted using a very limited number of animals ($n = 3$) to achieve good levels of statistical significance. They concluded that further in vitro and in vivo investigations are required to better understand crown ethers as penetration enhancers for ocular drug formulations [100].

5.4. Surfactants

Surface active compounds (surfactants) are compounds that have lipophilic and hydrophilic moieties. Acting on a surface, or between aqueous and non-aqueous media interfaces, surfactants are able to reduce interfacial surface tension [101]. In pharmaceutical applications, surfactants are commonly used as excipients to solubilize formulation components, or in the case of permeability enhancement, they alter membrane properties by disrupting tear film and mucin, removing their protective properties, disrupting the integrity of the epithelia by loosening tight junctions or modifying epithelial cell membranes. These compounds are included in formulations in a wide range of pharmaceutical applications including oral, injectable, nasal, ocular, and transdermal, amongst others. The polar group determines the specific properties of surfactants, and they can be classified into four main groups: cationic, anionic, zwitterionic, and non-ionic. Cationic surfactants have a positive charge on the polar head group, anionic surfactants have a negative charge, zwitterionic surfactants have positive and negative charges depending on which environment they are exposed to, and non-ionic surfactants are neutral [102]. Non-ionic surfactants are the compounds of choice for many drug delivery scenarios including ocular drug delivery, bringing enhanced drug solubility, formulation stability, biocompatibility, and low toxicity compared with their anionic, amphoteric, and cationic counterparts [103,104]. Polyoxyethylene-9-lauryl ether, Tween-80 and Span-60 are non-ionic surfactants, and their mode of action is via phospholipid acyl chain perturbation. According to Marsh et al. [105], the 1% solutions of Tween-20 and Brij-35 showed a relatively high effectiveness in enhancing permeability of the cornea by a five-fold increase in penetration of fluorescein through the cornea without detected irritation of the eye. Saettone et al. [106] reported improved permeability of the rabbit cornea for the β-blockers (atenolol, timolol, levobunolol, and betaxolol) combined with Brij-35, -78, and -98. The increased penetration was greater for atenolol and timolol, which are hydrophilic, than for hydrophobic β-blockers (levobunolol and betaxolol), which can be due to the hydrophilic properties of the corneal stroma. The non-ionic surfactant D-alpha-tocopheryl poly(ethylene glycol) 1000 succinate is also a potential permeability enhancer for ocular drug delivery. Ostacolo et al. [107] showed that this penetration enhancer effectively increased the permeation of riboflavin through porcine corneas. Pharmasolve® (*N*-methyl-2-pyrrolidone) is another permeation enhancer that was studied by Li et al. [108] for transcorneal drug delivery using rabbit eyes. Interestingly, this penetration enhancer increased the apparent corneal permeability coefficients for ribavirin, enoxacin, puerarin, and ibuprofen by 4.04-, 2.76-, 2.67-, and 1.47-fold, respectively. Also, no ocular irritation was observed for formulations with less than 10% *N*-methyl-2-pyrrolidone. Montenegro et al. [109] demonstrated a significant improvement in penetration of acyclovir through the rabbit corneas in the presence of 5% *N*-methyl-2-pyrrolidone, positively charged phospholipid mixture, and sodium taurocholate after 90 min since the drug was administered on the ocular surface; however, after 180 min, only the phospholipid mixture was still effective. The taurocholate, Brij-78, and phospholipid mixture enhanced the permeation of timolol maleate across the cornea after 90 min, but only Brij-78 showed the ability to retain this effect after 180 min.

These are also natural surfactants produced by some plants that could be potentially useful as penetration enhancers. Saponins are a class of amphiphilic glycosides abundantly found in different plants that exhibit good penetration-enhancement properties. For instance, digitonin is a steroidal saponin (Figure 12) isolated from the *Digitalis purpurea* plant; it is capable of solubilizing cellular membrane lipids and cholesterol. Shih and Lee demonstrated that digitonin caused ocular epithelial exfoliation [110–112].

Benzalkonium chloride (BAC) is a cationic surfactant that is commonly used in many formulations for ocular drugs in low concentrations as a preservative. BAC is a known irritant even at low concentration (<0.01%); nevertheless, it acts as a penetration enhancer, which destabilizes the tear film and the protection offered by the mucous layer at the cornea surface. BAC also initiates changes within phospholipid bilayers of cellular membranes [113]. Recently, Johannsdottir et al. [114] reported an in vivo study of benzalkonium chloride's effect on the ocular penetration of dexamethasone in pigmented rabbits. They compared two eye-drop formulations of dexamethasone, where the drug formed a microsuspension with γ-CD in a vehicle containing poloxamer, NaCl, and EDTA with and without 0.02% (*w*/*v*) benzalkonium chloride. The analysis of the drug concentrations in different ocular tissues 2 h following the eye-drop administration indicated no statistically significant effects of benzalkonium chloride. The authors related the absence of permeability enhancement to the quick removal of benzalkonium chloride with tear fluid and its inability to penetrate into the cornea/conjunctiva and sclera to cause disruption of barrier function.

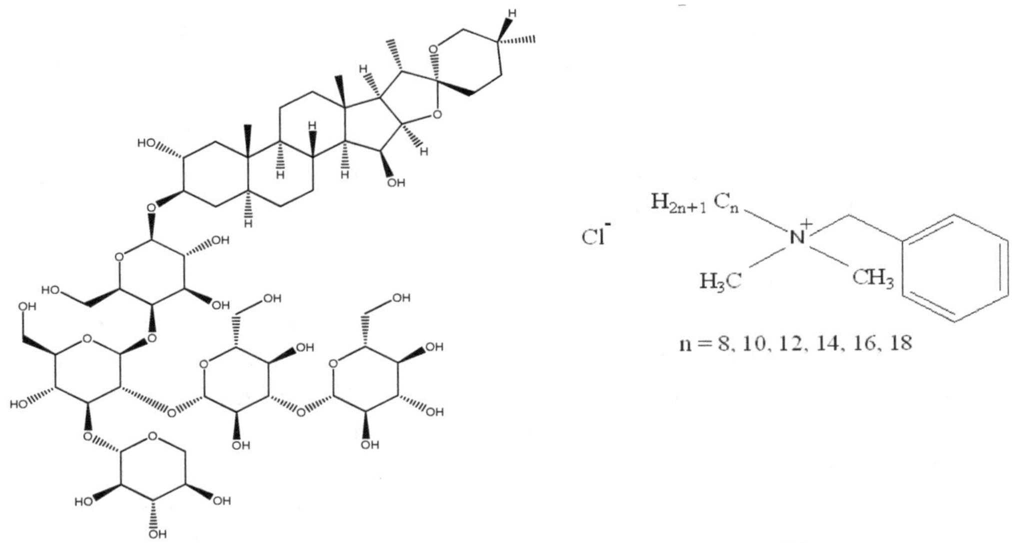

(a) (b)

Figure 12. Structures of digitonin (**a**) and benzalkonium chloride (**b**).

Sasaki et al. [115] compared the influence of a few penetration enhancers (saponin, EDTA, benzalkonium chloride, and paraben) on improving ocular absorption of thyrotropin-releasing hormone and luteinizing hormone-releasing hormone using diffusion cells with rabbit conjunctiva and cornea. The researchers showed that penetration of both hormones through the conjunctiva was improved by 0.5% saponin, 0.05% benzalkonium chloride, and 0.01% benzalkonium chloride. The permeability coefficient of conjunctiva was significantly improved for luteinizing hormone-releasing hormone using EDTA and paraben. The observed effects of permeation enhancers for conjunctiva were smaller compared to those on corneal penetration with luteinizing hormone-releasing hormone with paraben as the exception. EDTA and saponin increased the ratios of corneal to conjunctival permeation of both hormones. According to van der Bijl et al. [116], 0.01% benzalkonium chloride enhanced the permeation of cyclosporin A through frozen/thawed rabbit cornea.

Transcutol® P is another solubilizer mostly used as a transdermal penetration enhancer. Liu et al. [117] demonstrated that 0.005–0.03% Transcutol® P increased the apparent permeability coefficient by 1.5-, 1.5-, 3.0-, and 3.3-fold for ribavirin, gatifloxacin, levofloxacin hydrochloride, and enoxacin, respectively. Permeation for oxaprozin was inhibited with a maximum decrease by 2.8-fold for 0.03% Transcutol® P. In addition, no irritation was observed with Transcutol® P at concentrations of 0.005–0.03%, with the presence of slight irritation for 0.05% Transcutol® P. A non-ionic oil-in-water surfactant, Labrasol®, is also a potential excipient as a corneal penetration enhancer. It is composed of well-characterized polyethylene glycol (PEG) esters, a small glyceride fraction, and free PEG. Liu et al. [118] observed no ocular surface irritation for 0.5–3.0% Labrasol® and slight irritation for 5.0% Labrasol®. The penetration of baicalin solution through the rabbit cornea was enhanced by 1.69-, 3.14-, and 2.23-fold in the presence of 1.5%, 2.0%, and 3.0% Labrasol®, respectively.

5.5. Bile Acids and Bile Salts

Bile acids are steroid acids, all forms of cholic acid, and their sodium or potassium salts, and there are a number of derivatives that result from cholesterol metabolism in the liver which then undergo further transformations in the intestinal tract. They are soluble in water and are involved in the solubilization of dietary lipids within the gut. In the intestinal tract, they become conjugated with taurine and glycine, where the sodium and potassium salts of these conjugates are termed bile salts [119,120]. Bile acids are amphiphilic compounds naturally produced in the human digestive system; they are able to promote drug penetration across biological membranes. They are employed in drug formulations for enhancement of drug penetration via many mucosal routes including nasal, oral, buccal, ocular, pulmonary, and rectal mucosa. They are capable of forming vesicular drug-carrying systems which are able to promote epithelial drug transport via transcellular and paracellular routes [121]. Bile acids and bile salts have surfactant properties with an ability to form micelles or liposomes in the aqueous environment, otherwise known as "bilosomes"; these vesicular entities offer some interesting and novel properties in drug delivery [122]. Examples of many bile acid/bile salt derivatives include deoxycholate, glycocholate, and taurodeoxycholate (Figure 13). They are able to alter the rheological properties of ocular mucosal membranes [123], and the mucolytic properties of bile salts alter the protective mucus barrier, inducing changes in membrane characteristics allowing for enhanced drug transit into ocular tissue [4,124]. Dai et al. [125] investigated liposomes with bile salts for the ocular delivery of tacrolimus FK506, a calcineurin inhibitor, as a model drug. The liposomes they developed contained cholesterol (control) or bile salts (sodium taurocholate, sodium deoxycholate, and sodium glycocholate), prepared using a thin-membrane dispersion technique, achieving uniform particle size and drug entrapment. These liposomes exhibited controlled release of <5% over 24 h, thus avoiding a "burst release" often seen with some ocular drug delivery systems. They conducted ex vivo corneal permeability and in vivo corneal uptake experiments and demonstrated that liposomes with bile salts offered enhanced transcorneal drug permeability compared to the cholesterol-containing liposomes, enhancing the permeation of tacrolimus across the cornea up to four-fold. Furthermore, cytotoxicity studies showed that the liposomes with sodium taurocholate or sodium glycocholate were well tolerated, whereas those with deoxycholate showed evidence of corneal toxicity to spontaneously derived human corneal epithelial cells and in the rabbit model. The researchers concluded that liposomes incorporating sodium taurocholate and sodium glycocholate offer potential as ocular drug delivery systems for drugs of low aqueous solubility such as tacrolimus, due to their low toxicity and improved ocular permeability [125]. A cautious approach is generally required when employing bile acids and bile salts for enhanced ocular drug delivery; however, given the right choice of cholic acid variant or a derivative therewith, and the right choice of delivery vehicle, bile acids and their salts offer much potential for future ocular drug delivery systems.

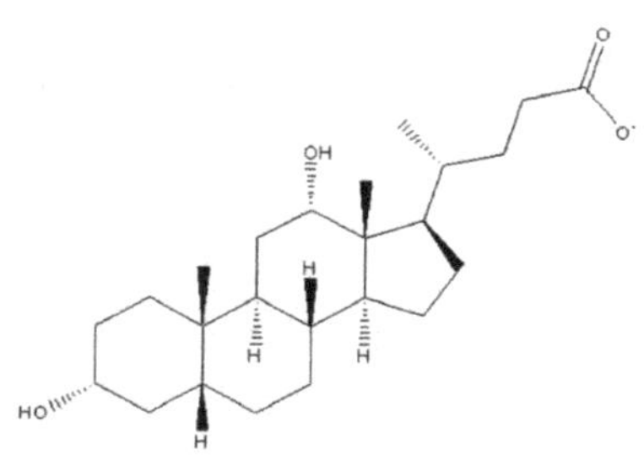

(a)

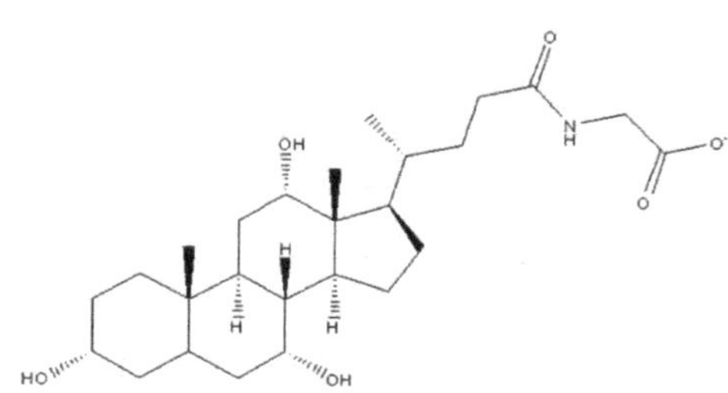

(b)

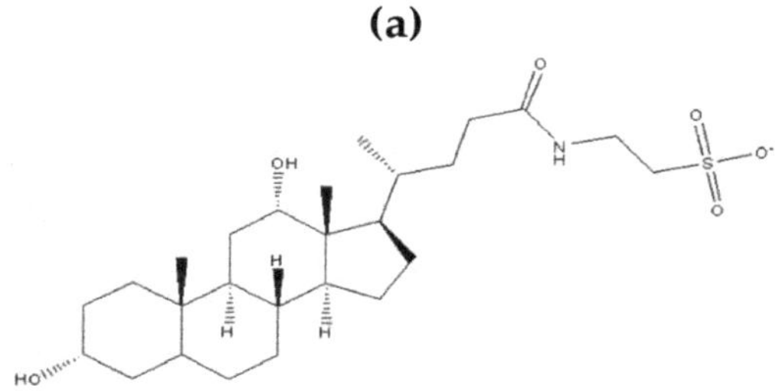

(c)

Figure 13. Structures of deoxycholate (**a**), glycocholate (**b**), and taurodeoxycholate (**c**).

Mahaling and Katti [126] recently investigated the effect of different enhancers (benzalkonium chloride, capric acid, EDTA, sodium glycocholate, and sodium taurocholate) on the penetration of polymeric nanoparticles in vivo in pigmented mice. It was established that sodium glycocholate and sodium taurocholate enhanced the permeability of nanoparticles in the conjunctiva. Benzalkonium chloride, sodium glycocholate, and sodium taurocholate enhanced bioavailability of nanoparticles in the iris and ciliary body. They also observed some inhibition effects; the use of EDTA decreased the bioavailability of nanoparticles in the lens and choroid, whereas sodium glycocholate showed a reduction in their presence in the choroid and retina. The authors concluded that a combination of penetration enhancers with a hydrophilic mucoadhesive coating on nanoparticles is a promising approach to enhance their bioavailability.

5.6. Cell-Penetrating Peptides

Cell-penetrating peptides (CPPs) are short chains of amino acids connected by amide bonds (peptide bonds); they form a diverse group of compounds derived from variable combinations of many different natural amino acid residues [127]. CPPs are capable of penetrating cellular membranes and have the ability to transport internalized hydrophilic cargo into cells, for example, drugs [128]. Liu et al. [129] investigated a number of fluorophore-labeled cell-penetrating peptides, namely, trans-activating transcriptional activator (TAT), penetratin, poly(arginine), low-molecular-weight protamine, and poly(serine), for their ocular permeability using side-by-side diffusion cells, ex vivo in a rabbit model. Protamine is a small arginine-rich protein; TAT and penetratin are complex polypeptides consisting of specific sequences of different amino acids, whereas poly(arginine) and poly(serine) represent homopolymers of corresponding amino acids. The structures of poly(arginine) and poly(serine) are shown in Figure 14. They also used human conjunctival epithelial cells to determine cytotoxicity and cellular uptake of CPPs. The researchers found penetratin to have excellent performance in enhancing drug permeability, whilst also showing the lowest cytotoxicity. Penetratin showed cellular uptake more than 25-fold compared with the control peptide poly(serine). This peptide also showed an increased permeation of 87.5 times using the rabbit excised corneas. When fluorophore-labeled penetratin was instilled into the cul-de-sac of rat eyes, it was widely distributed in the anterior and posterior segments and could be measured in the corneal epithelium and retina for at least 6 h. They concluded that penetratin could be a potential permeability enhancer for ophthalmic use; this peptide can be conjugated with bioactive compounds for topical delivery into the eye reaching as far as the retina. Further research on the design and synthesis of new cell-penetrating peptides for topical delivery into different layers of the cornea, with potential application as absorption enhancers for metabolic sensitive ophthalmic drugs, was recently conducted by Pescina et al. [130]. The researchers labeled the synthesized CPPs with 5-carboxyfluorescein and measured their diffusion and distribution within the cornea using an ex vivo porcine model and confocal microscopy. The synthesized peptides were also shown to be safe and well tolerated when tested on human conjunctival cell line. They concluded that the tested CPPs could provide useful ocular therapies, especially when used as transcorneal transporters for some drugs with unfavorable molecular characteristics, examples being the aminoglycoside antibiotic, cysteamine, and antiviral agents. Interestingly, in 2017, de Cogan et al. [131] reported a promising approach for topical delivery of an anti-VEGF agent (bevacizumab) linked to the CPP (5(6)-carboxyfluorescein–RRRRRR–COOH) to the posterior segment of the eye. The toxicity of CPP, assessed using cell cultures, was found to be low. This complex study was done in vivo and included optical coherence tomography (OCT) imaging of the CPP tagged with fluorescent dye passing into the rat's eye anterior segment, as well as assessment of topical delivery of the complex CPP–bevacizumab into the vitreous body with subsequent fixation of the time course of bevacizumab clearance from the vitreous body and retina. Moreover, the in vivo effectiveness of eye drops comprising a complex formulation of CPP with anti-VEGF agent was evaluated in a mouse model with choroidal neovascularization (CNV) which, as mentioned above, is common in patients with neovascular AMD. Mice received different treatment, which included intravitreal injection of the anti-VEGF agent, topical application of CPP with anti-VEGF (twice a day), or dexamethasone gavage (every day) for 10 days. Additionally, ex vivo experiments with topical delivery of anti-VEGF agents (ranibizumab and bevacizumab) into pig eyes were also conducted. As a result, CPP was observed within 6 min in the anterior chamber of the eye in rats. A single application of CPP–bevacizumab complex on the rat's cornea showed drug levels in the posterior segment that could be relevant to clinical concentrations. CPP–ranibizumab and CPP–bevacizumab complex concentrations in the posterior chamber of porcine eyes were also found to be clinically relevant. There was a significant decrease in CNV area in all mice that received intravitreal injection, eye drops with CPP with anti-VEGF drug, and dexamethasone gavage compared to the eyes treated with a laser only.

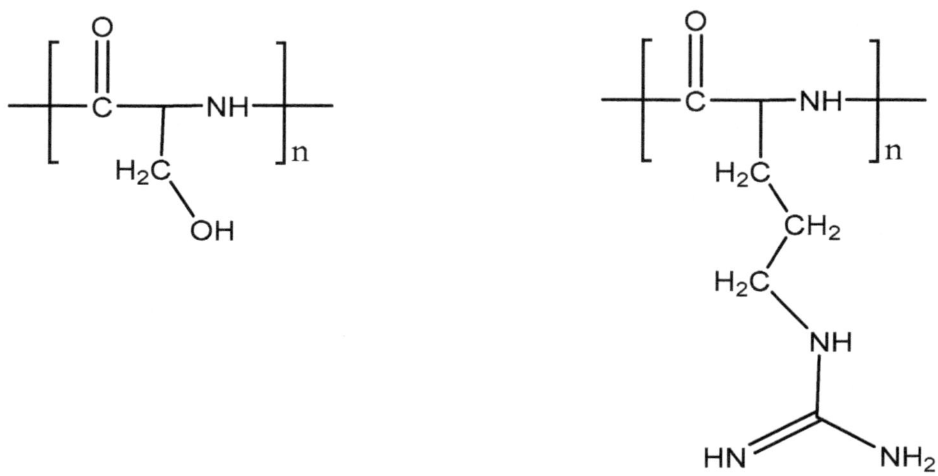

(**a**) (**b**)

Figure 14. Structures of poly-L-serine (**a**) and poly-L-arginine hydrochloride (**b**).

Nemoto et al. [132] demonstrated the permeability-enhancing features of poly-L-arginine hydrochloride for hydrophilic molecules (fluorescein isothiocyanate (FITC)-labeled dextran and pyridoxamine), across ocular membranes taken from Japanese white rabbits. The increase in P_{app} of FITC-labeled dextran in the cornea, conjunctiva, and conjunctiva/sclera composite was observed in the presence of poly-L-arginine (0.1 mg/mL) by 6.81-, 9.78-, and 7.91-fold, respectively. The permeation of pyridoxamine was also improved by adding poly-L-arginine by 7.98-, 4.67-, and 8.31-fold, respectively. The authors suggested that the mechanism of this permeability enhancement lies in the ability of poly-L-arginine to disassemble tight junction-associated proteins present in the cornea and conjunctiva. Thus, this compound can be used as a permeability enhancer for lipophobic compounds without producing significant damage to the epithelium.

Some progress in the application of cell-penetrating peptides in ocular drug delivery was recently reviewed by Pescina et al. [133]. The authors highlighted this topic as an emerging area in ocular therapeutics, which has great potential for the delivery of drugs and biopharmaceuticals both to the anterior and posterior segments of the eye.

5.7. Other Amphiphilic Compounds

Fatty acids facilitate ocular drug permeation by altering cell-membrane properties and loosening tight junctions. These compounds can also induce ion–pair complexation when formulated with cationic drugs. Caprylic acid and capric acid are examples of fatty acids (Figure 15). The former interacts with proteins, whilst the latter can affect both proteins and lipid components of cellular membranes [111]. Capric acid was shown to enhance ocular penetration of β-blockers, bringing moderate enhancement to the penetration of hydrophilic β-blockers, whilst only offering slight enhancement for lipophilic β-blockers [123]. Kato and Iwata attributed the penetration-enhancing effects of fatty acids for bunazosin to ion–pair interactions [134,135].

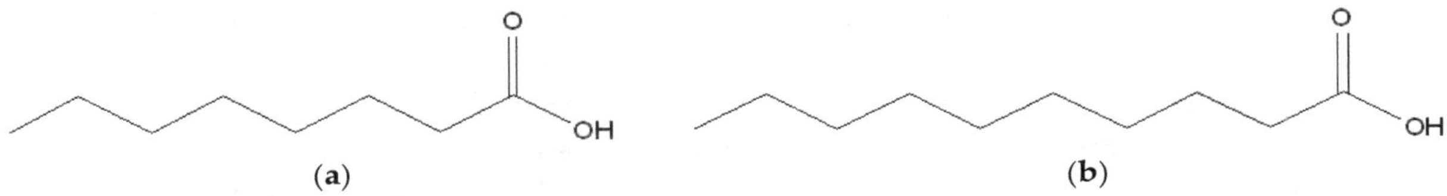

Figure 15. Structures of caprylic acid (**a**) and capric acid (**b**).

Gelucires are glyceride-based compounds with amphiphilic surfactant properties. Gelucires comprise mono-, di-, and triglycerides with mono- and diesters of polyethylene glycol [136]. The numbers 44 and 14 in the name of Gelucire 44/14 indicate the melting temperature of 44 °C and a hydrophilic–lipophilic balance of 14. Known for their drug absorption-enhancing performance, Gelucires have a good safety profile for pharmaceutical formulations and are "generally regarded as safe" (GRAS). Gelucire 44/14 was evaluated as a potential permeability enhancer in vitro and in vivo using different ophthalmic drugs and was shown to enhance transcorneal permeability of drugs with a range of hydrophilicity/lipophilicity whilst remaining safe to use and non-irritating [5,20]. Another potential corneal permeability enhancer is Azone™ (1-dodecylazacycloheptan-2-one), which is currently used mostly for transdermal drug delivery. This formulation is thought to act by partitioning into lipid bilayers of the bio-membrane and, as a result, disrupting its structure. Tang-Liu et al. [137] compared effects of four permeation enhancers (Azone™, hexamethylenelauramide, hexamethyleneoctanamide, and decylmethylsulfoxide (Figure 16)) with lipophobic (acetazolamide, cimetidine, guanethidine, and sulfacetamide), moderately hydrophobic (bunolol and prednisolone), and hydrophobic (flurbiprofen and its amide analogue) drugs through the rabbit cornea.

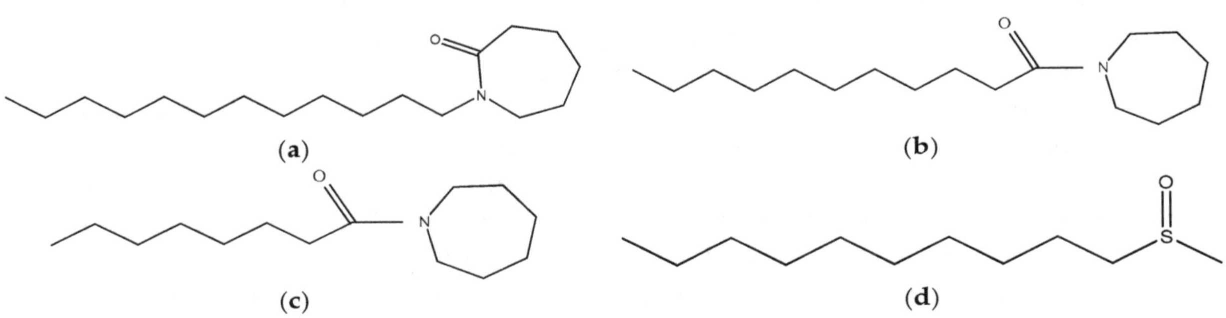

Figure 16. Structures of Azone™ (**a**), hexamethylenelauramide (**b**), hexamethyleneoctanamide (**c**), and decylmethylsulfoxide (**d**).

The researchers demonstrated that 0.1% Azone™ enhanced the permeability of lipophobic formulations 20-fold, while permeation of moderately hydrophobic compounds was enhanced at 0.025–0.1% Azone™ by two- to five-fold. Interestingly, there was inhibition instead of promotion of corneal permeability for flurbiprofen and its amide analogue in the presence of Azone™. Also, all four penetration enhancers used in this study showed similar ability to promote penetration through the cornea for cimetidine. Additionally, the researchers noticed a parabolic relationship between the rate of drug penetration and the lipophilicity of this compound. Afouna et al. [138] also tested gel formulations with Azone™ as a permeability enhancer, Carbopol-974® as a mucoadhesive, and *s*-timolol maleate as a model drug using rabbits. It was demonstrated that in vivo reduction of intraocular pressure for these formulations lasted roughly 3–4 times longer in comparison with the conventional timolol maleate eye drops. In 2016, Afouna et al. [139] reported the extension of in vitro parameters including release, onset, magnitude, and action duration up to two days for the gel formulations containing Azone™, Carbopol-974®, and latanoprost acid.

Borneol is a terpene derivative that can also be used as ocular penetration enhancer (Figure 17). According to Yang et al. [140], 0.1% synthetic borneol improved the permeability of two hydrophobic compounds (indomethacin and dexamethasone) through rabbit corneas by 1.23-and 2.40-fold, respectively, while the permeation of more hydrophilic drugs (ofloxacin, ribavirin, and tobramycin) was increased by 1.87-, 2.80-, and 3.89-fold, respectively. Natural borneol also enhanced the permeability with the following levels: 1.67, 2.00, 2.15, 2.18, and 3.39, respectively. It was also established that 0.1% borneol did not produce any damage to the cornea. The authors suggested that borneol's ability of promoting corneal permeability might be due to the changes in the arrangement of lipid molecules in the cell membrane of corneal epitheliocytes, increasing the orderliness of the molecular chains of lecithin.

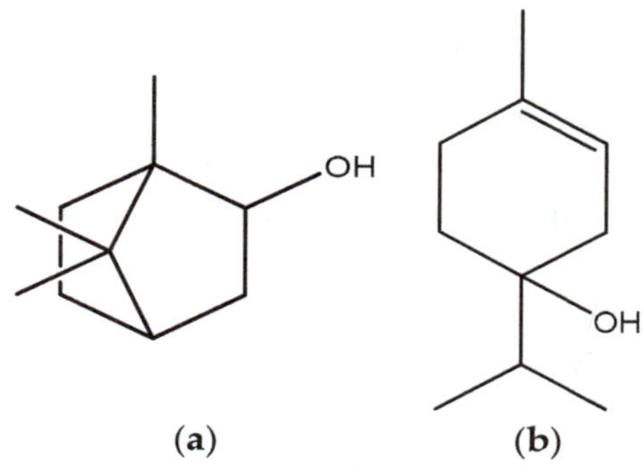

Figure 17. Structures of borneol (**a**) and terpinen-4-ol (**b**).

At the same time, terpinen-4-ol (Figure 17) can also be used as an ocular drug permeability enhancer. Afouna et al. [141] prepared and tested ophthalmic gel formulations with different concentrations of terpinen-4-ol as a penetration enhancer, Carbopol-934 as a mucoadhesive, and dorzolamide hydrochloride as a model drug. They demonstrated that permeation of this IOP-lowering drug across the excised rabbit's cornea was increased significantly with the concentration of terpinen-4-ol. It was shown that the highest concentration of this penetration enhancer (0.5%) demonstrated the best permeation features among tested formulations. The authors suggested that this permeability improvement may result from the thermodynamic activity increase, as well as from the change in the ratio between ionized and unionized dorzolamide hydrochloride species in favor of the latter. The cumulative amount of dorzolamide hydrochloride in the receiver chamber of a vertical Franz diffusion cell from ophthalmic gel formulations with different terpinen-4-ol concentrations and fixed concentration of Carbopol-934 through the excised rabbit's cornea is shown in Figure 18.

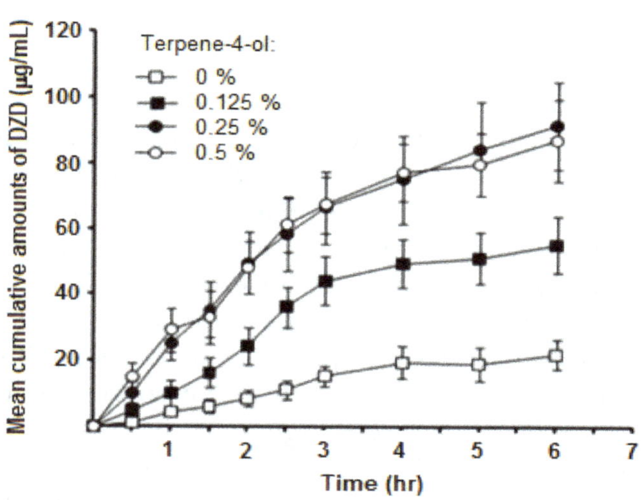

Figure 18. The cumulative amount of dorzolamide hydrochloride in the receiver chamber of a vertical Franz diffusion cell from ophthalmic gel formulations with various terpinen-4-ol concentrations and a fixed concentration of Carbopol-934 through the excised rabbit's cornea ($n = 3$). Reproduced from Reference [141] with permission from Elsevier, 2010.

Semifluorinated alkanes (SFAs) belong to the group of amphiphilic liquids that can dissolve lipophilic compounds forming clear solutions. Agarwal et al. [142] assessed the potential of two different SFAs for topical ocular drug delivery. Cyclosporin A (CsA) was dissolved in perfluorobutylpentane (F4H5) or perfluorohexyloctane (F6H8) and was compared with commercially available CsA ophthalmic emulsions, Restasis® and Ikervis®, in terms of corneal availability. The penetration of CsA through the cornea was evaluated by plotting the concentration of the corneal CsA per g of cornea (ng/g) against time and determining the mean area under curve of each formulation tested over 4 h (AUC (0–4 h)) (Figure 19). The permeability of the cornea was significantly enhanced for CsA after a single dose of 0.05% CsA in F4H5 and F6H8 was applied when compared to Restasis with the area under the curve over 4 h (AUC (0–4 h)) being at least eight-fold higher for both SFAs. Interestingly, the AUC (0–4 h) of 0.1% CsA in F4H5 was almost five-fold higher than with Ikervis. Thus, semifluorinated alkane-based CsA formulations may improve the therapeutic efficacy.

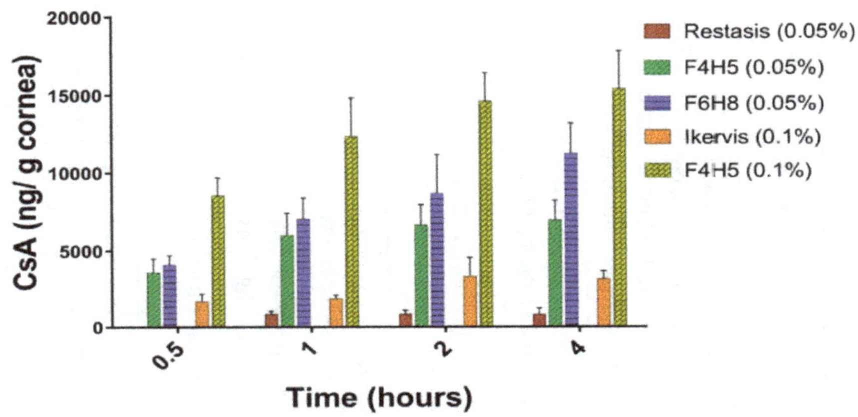

Figure 19. Corneal penetration of cyclosporin A (CsA) from the test formulations. The amount of CsA recovered (ng) per g of cornea after application of a single 50-μL dose was plotted against time (n = 5; mean ± standard error of the mean (SEM)). Reproduced from Reference [142] with permission from Elsevier, 2018.

6. Comparison of Different Penetration Enhancers

Different classes of penetration enhancers considered in this review are summarized in Table 2. Some of these compounds, such as EDTA and benzalkonium chloride, are already commonly used in ophthalmic formulations with different roles, e.g., as a buffering agent and antimicrobial preservative, respectively. However, these compounds may provide some permeability enhancement as an extra benefit. Cyclodextrins are used in some pharmaceutical formulations to facilitate the solubility of poorly soluble drugs; additionally, they could provide permeability-enhancing properties. Other amphiphilic molecules such as bile acids and Azone™ have established safety profiles but are not yet used in commercial ocular formulations. Crown ethers represent a relatively new class of permeability enhancers that will require more research into their efficiency and toxicological profile. Cell-penetrating peptides are highly promising permeability enhancers that received a lot of interest in the recent decade; more research is expected with these materials as they could potentially provide opportunities for formulating topical products for the delivery of biologicals.

Table 2. Different classes of penetration enhancers, their commercial applications, and possible mechanisms of action. EDTA—ethylenediamine-*N*,*N*,*N*′,*N*′-tetraacetic acid; TAT—trans-activating transcriptional activator; FDA—Food and Drug Administration.

Class of Enhancers	Examples of Compounds	Commercial Applications in Drug Delivery	Possible Mechanism of Penetration Enhancement
Cyclodextrins	α-, β-, γ-cyclodextrins	Some cyclodextrins are already used in commercial ocular formulations, e.g., Vitaseptol eye drops (Novartis). They are often used as enhancers of drug solubility.	Extraction of cholesterol and lipids from ocular membranes [68].
Chelating agents	EDTA	Disodium-EDTA is commonly used in ocular formulations as a buffering agent [143].	Extraction of Ca^{2+} from tight junctions [17].
Crown ethers	12-crown-4, 15-crown-5, 18-crown-6	None of these are currently used in commercial formulations for drug delivery.	Extraction of Ca^{2+} from tight junctions [100].
Surfactants	Benzalkonium chloride	Around 74% of ophthalmic preparations have benzalkonium chloride as a preservative [144].	Morphological changes in the epithelium [145].
Bile acids and salts	Deoxycholate, glycocholate, taurodeoxycholate	None of these are currently used in commercial formulations for drug delivery.	Different mechanisms leading to modification of the integrity of the corneal epithelium [121].
Cell-penetrating peptides	TAT, penetratin, poly(arginine), and poly(serine)	None of these are currently used in commercial formulations for drug delivery.	Direct translocation and endocytosis [133].
Other amphiphilic compounds	Azone™	Designed and widely researched mostly as a skin penetration enhancer. No FDA-approved products containing Azone™ on the market yet. It is recorded in Chinese Pharmacopoeia and widely used in China [146,147].	Changes in the structure and fluidity of biological membranes; facilitation of water influx leading to a more hydrated barrier [137].

7. Conclusions

Topical drug application is the most widely used treatment in ophthalmology due to its simplicity. However, some obstacles including low permeability of the cornea, tear reflex, blinking, and nasolacrimal drainage hamper drug delivery in this way. The analysis of physicochemical properties of various chemical compounds that cross ocular membranes, coupled with the histological structure of cornea, sclera, and conjunctiva, could be key in understanding the opportunities and obstacles in the ocular drug delivery. Penetration enhancers facilitate delivery of active pharmaceutical compounds through three main mechanisms or their combination: altering tear film stability and the mucous layer at the ocular surface, modifying membrane components such as lipid bilayers of associated epithelial cells, and loosening epithelial tight junctions. The variety of penetration enhancers (cyclodextrins, chelating agents, crown ethers, bile acids and bile salts, cell-penetrating peptides, and other amphiphilic compounds) enables an increase in the permeability of ocular membranes. However, ocular drug delivery remains one of the toughest problems in ophthalmology, and new formulations still need to be developed to allow better control of drug delivery and improved performance, whilst also minimizing undesired side effects.

Different penetration enhancers were identified and mechanisms of their action were researched in the past several decades. Many of these enhancers were also evaluated for their potential harmful effects on the eye. However, these toxicological studies were often done to evaluate short-term exposure of the ocular tissues to enhancers. Very little is known on the longer-term exposure and potential chronic applications.

Acknowledgments: We thank Yurii A. Kriuchkov for providing images of the eye (Figures 1 and 2). The authors are also grateful to Nikolai Khutoryanskiy for proofreading the manuscript.

References

1. World Health Organization. Available online: https://www.who.int/news-room/fact-sheets/detail/blindness-and-visual-impairment (accessed on 12 December 2018).
2. Haupt, C.; Huber, A.B. How axons see their way-axonal guidance in the visual system. *Front. Biosci.* **2008**, *13*, 3136–3149. [CrossRef] [PubMed]
3. Morrison, P.W.J.; Khutoryanskiy, V.V. Anatomy of the Eye and the Role of Ocular Mucosa in Drug Delivery. In *Mucoadhesive Materials and Drug Delivery Systems*, 1st ed.; Khutoryanskiy, V.V., Ed.; John Wiley & Sons, Ltd.: Chichester, UK, 2014; pp. 39–60, ISBN 9781119941439.
4. Kaur, I.P.; Smitha, R. Penetration enhancers and ocular bioadhesives: Two new avenues for ophthalmic drug delivery. *Drug Dev. Ind. Pharm.* **2002**, *28*, 353–369. [CrossRef] [PubMed]
5. Morrison, P.W.; Khutoryanskiy, V.V. Advances in ophthalmic drug delivery. *Ther. Deliv.* **2014**, *5*, 1297–1315. [CrossRef] [PubMed]
6. Lopath, P.; TecLens, C.L. Available online: https://player.vimeo.com/video/198253544 (accessed on 2 September 2018).
7. Del Amo, E.M.; Urtti, A. Current and future ophthalmic drug delivery systems. A shift to the posterior segment. *Drug Discov. Today* **2008**, *13*, 135–143. [CrossRef]
8. Zderic, V.; Clark, J.I.; Martin, R.W.; Vaezy, S. Ultrasound-enhanced transcorneal drug delivery. *Cornea* **2004**, *23*, 804–811. [CrossRef]
9. Vaka, S.R.; Sammeta, S.M.; Day, L.B.; Murthy, S.N. Transcorneal iontophoresis for delivery of ciprofloxacin hydrochloride. *Curr. Eye Res.* **2008**, *33*, 661–667. [CrossRef]
10. Jiang, J.; Gill, H.S.; Ghate, D.; McCarey, B.E.; Patel, S.R.; Edelhauser, H.F.; Prausnitz, M.R. Coated Microneedles for Drug Delivery to the Eye. *Investig. Ophthalmol. Vis. Sci.* **2007**, *48*, 4038–4043. [CrossRef]

11. Jiang, J.; Moore, J.S.; Edelhauser, H.F.; Prausnitz, M.R. Intrascleral drug delivery to the eye using hollow microneedles. *Pharm. Res.* **2009**, *26*, 395–403. [CrossRef]
12. Chen, H.; Jin, Y.; Sun, L.; Li, X.; Nan, K.; Liu, H.; Zheng, Q.; Wang, B. Recent Developments in Ophthalmic Drug Delivery Systems for Therapy of Both Anterior and Posterior Segment Diseases. *Colloid Interface Sci. Commun.* **2018**, *24*, 54–61. [CrossRef]
13. Williams, A.C.; Barry, B.W. Penetration enhancers. *Adv. Drug Deliv. Rev.* **2012**, *64*, 128–137. [CrossRef]
14. Lane, M.E. Skin penetration enhancers. *Int. J. Pharm.* **2013**, *447*, 12–21. [CrossRef] [PubMed]
15. Junginger, H.E.; Verhoef, J.C. Macromolecules as safe penetration enhancers for hydrophilic drugs-a fiction? *Pharm. Sci. Technol. Today* **1998**, *1*, 370–376. [CrossRef]
16. Sultana, Y.; Jain, R.; Aqil, M.; Ali, A. Review of ocular drug delivery. *Curr. Drug Deliv.* **2006**, *3*, 207–217. [CrossRef] [PubMed]
17. Morrison, P.W.J.; Khutoryanskiy, V.V. Enhancement in corneal permeability of riboflavin using calcium sequestering compounds. *Int. J. Pharm.* **2014**, *472*, 56–64. [CrossRef] [PubMed]
18. Chung, S.H.; Lee, S.K.; Cristol, S.M.; Lee, E.S.; Lee, D.W.; Seo, K.Y.; Kim, E.K. Impact of short-term exposure of commercial eyedrops preserved with benzalkonium chloride on precorneal mucin. *Mol. Vis.* **2006**, *12*, 415–421. [PubMed]
19. Burgalassi, S.; Chetoni, P.; Monti, D.; Saettone, M.F. Cytotoxicity of potential ocular permeation enhancers evaluated on rabbit and human corneal epithelial cell lines. *Toxicol. Lett.* **2001**, *122*, 1–8. [CrossRef]
20. Liu, R.; Liu, Z.; Zhang, C.; Zhang, B. Gelucire44/14 as a novel absorption enhancer for drugs with different hydrophilicities: In vitro and in vivo improvement on transcorneal permeation. *J. Pharm. Sci.* **2011**, *100*, 3186–3195. [CrossRef]
21. Loch, C.; Zakelj, S.; Kristl, A.; Nagel, S.; Guthoff, R.; Weitschies, W.; Seidlitz, A. Determination of permeability coefficients of ophthalmic drugs through different layers of porcine, rabbit and bovine eyes. *Eur. J. Pharm. Sci.* **2012**, *47*, 131–138. [CrossRef]
22. Bowling, B. *Kanski's Clinical Ophthalmology: A Systematic Approach*, 8th ed.; Saunders Ltd.: Philadelphia, PA, USA, 2015; p. 928, ISBN 978-0-7020-5572-0.
23. Järvinen, T.; Järvinen, K. Prodrugs for improved ocular drug delivery. *Adv. Drug Deliv. Rev.* **1996**, *19*, 203–224. [CrossRef]
24. Geerling, G.; Brewitt, H. *Surgery for the Dry Eye: Scientific Evidence and Guidelines for the Clinical Management of Dry Eye Associated Ocular Surface Disease*, 1st ed.; Karger: Basel, Switzerland, 2008; p. 325, ISBN 978-3-8055-8376-3.
25. Hodges, R.R.; Dartt, D.A. Conjunctival goblet cells. In *Encyclopedia of the Eye*, 1st ed.; Dartt, D.A., Besharse, J.C., Dana, R., Eds.; Academic Press: Oxford, UK, 2010; pp. 369–376, ISBN 978-0-12-374203-2.
26. Wang, L.; Li, T.; Lu, L. UV-induced corneal epithelial cell death by activation of potassium channels. *Investig. Ophthalmol. Vis. Sci.* **2003**, *44*, 5095–5101. [CrossRef]
27. Dua, H.S.; Faraj, L.A.; Said, D.G.; Gray, T.; Lowe, J. Human corneal anatomy redefined: A novel pre-Descemet's layer (Dua's layer). *Ophthalmology* **2013**, *120*, 1778–1785. [CrossRef] [PubMed]
28. Smith, G.T.; Dart, J.K.G. Cornea. In *Moorfields Manual of Ophthalmology*, 1st ed.; Jackson, T.L., Ed.; Mosby: Edinburgh, UK, 2008; pp. 144–221, ISBN 9781416025726.
29. Schlote, T.; Rohrbach, J.; Grueb, M.; Mielke, J. *Pocket Atlas of Ophthalmology*, 1st ed.; Thieme: Wemding, Germany, 2006; pp. 2–8, ISBN 3-13-139821-3.
30. Washington, N.; Washington, C.; Wilson, C.G. *Physiological Pharmaceutics: Barriers to Drug Absorption*, 2nd ed.; Taylor and Francis: New York, NY, USA, 2001; pp. 249–270, ISBN 9780748406104.
31. Shaikh, R.; Raj Singh, T.R.; Garland, M.J.; Woolfson, A.D.; Donnelly, R.F. Mucoadhesive drug delivery systems. *J. Pharm. Bioallied Sci.* **2011**, *3*, 89–100. [CrossRef] [PubMed]
32. Tsai, J.C.; Denniston, A.K.O.; Murray, P.I.; Huang, J.J.; Aldad, T.S. *Oxford American Handbook of Ophthalmology*, 1st ed.; Oxford University Press Inc.: New York, NY, USA, 2011; p. 768, ISBN 978-0-19-539344-6.
33. Goel, M.; Picciani, R.G.; Lee, R.K.; Bhattacharya, S.K. Aqueous humor dynamics: A review. *Open Ophthalmol. J.* **2010**, *4*, 52–59. [CrossRef] [PubMed]
34. Lang, G.K. *Ophthalmology: A Short Textbook*, 1st ed.; Thieme: Wemding, Germany, 2000; p. 586, ISBN 0-86577-936-8.
35. Caretti, L.; Buratto, L. *Glaucoma Surgery: Treatment and Techniques*, 1st ed.; Springer International Publishing: Cham, Switzerland, 2017; p. 133, ISBN 978-3-319-64854-5.

36. Sundaram, V.; Barsam, A.; Barker, L.; Khaw, P.T. *Training in Ophthalmology*, 2nd ed.; Oxford University Press: Gosport, UK, 2016; p. 568, ISBN 978-0-19-967251-6.
37. American Academy of Ophthalmology. Available online: https://www.aao.org/disease-review/anatomy-of-angle (accessed on 10 January 2019).
38. Albert, D.M.; Miller, J.W.; Azar, D.T.; Blodi, B.A. *Principles and Practice of Ophthalmology*, 3rd ed.; Saunders: Philadelphia, PA, USA, 2008; Volume 3, p. 5502, ISBN 978-1-4160-0016-7.
39. Andley, U.P. Crystallins in the eye: Function and pathology. *Prog. Retin. Eye Res.* **2007**, *26*, 78–98. [CrossRef] [PubMed]
40. Petrash, J.M. Aging and age-related diseases of the ocular lens and vitreous body. *Investig. Ophthalmol. Vis. Sci.* **2013**, *54*, ORSF54–ORSF59. [CrossRef]
41. Murphy, W.; Black, J.; Hastings, G. *Handbook of Biomaterial Properties*, 2nd ed.; Springer: New York, NY, USA, 2016; p. 676, ISBN 978-1-4939-3303-7.
42. Sebag, J. *Vitreous: In Health and Disease*, 1st ed.; Springer: New York, NY, USA, 2014; p. 925, ISBN 978-1-4939-1085-4.
43. Straatsma, B.R.; Landers, M.B.; Kreiger, A.E. The ora serrata in the adult human eye. *Arch. Ophthalmol.* **1968**, *80*, 3–20. [CrossRef] [PubMed]
44. Nag, T.C.; Kumari, C. Electron microscopy of the human choroid. In *Choroidal Disorders*, 1st ed.; Chhablani, J., Ruiz-Medrano, J., Eds.; Academic Press: Cambridge, MA, USA, 2017; pp. 7–20, ISBN 978-0-12-805313-3.
45. Schachat, A.P.; Wilkinson, C.P.; Hinton, D.R.; Sadda, S.V.R.; Wiedemann, P. *Ryan's Retina*, 6th ed.; Elsevier Health Sciences: Amsterdam, The Netherlands, 2017; Volume 1, p. 2976, ISBN 978-0-323-40197-5.
46. Agarwal, A. *Gass' Atlas of Macular Diseases*, 5th ed.; Saunders: Philadelphia, PA, USA, 2012; Volume 1, p. 1378, ISBN 978-1-4377-1580-4.
47. Kefalov, V.J. Phototransduction: Phototransduction in cones. In *Encyclopedia of the Eye*, 1st ed.; Dartt, D.A., Besharse, J.C., Dana, R., Eds.; Academic Press: Oxford, UK, 2010; pp. 389–396, ISBN 978-0-12-374203-2.
48. Denniston, A.K.O.; Murray, P.I. *Oxford Handbook of Ophthalmology*, 4th ed.; Oxford University Press: Oxford, Oxfordshire, UK, 2018; p. 1204, ISBN 978-0-19-881675-1.
49. Yanoff, M.; Duker, J.S. *Ophthalmology*, 5th ed.; Elsevier: Amsterdam, The Netherlands, 2018; p. 1440, ISBN 9780323528191.
50. Petroutsos, G.; Guimaraes, R.; Giraud, J.P.; Pouliquen, Y. Corticosteroids and corneal epithelial wound healing. *Br. J. Ophthalmol.* **1982**, *66*, 705–708. [CrossRef] [PubMed]
51. Dworkin, R.H.; Johnson, R.W.; Breuer, J.; Gnann, J.W.; Levin, M.J.; Backonja, M.; Betts, R.F.; Gershon, A.A.; Haanpaa, M.L.; McKendrick, M.W.; et al. Recommendations for the management of herpes zoster. *Clin. Infect. Dis. Off. Publ. Infect. Dis. Soc. Am.* **2007**, *44* (Suppl. 1), S1–S26. [CrossRef] [PubMed]
52. World Health Organization. Available online: http://origin.who.int/blindness/causes/priority/en/index1.html (accessed on 18 December 2018).
53. Chandra, P.; Hegde, K.R.; Varma, S.D. Possibility of topical antioxidant treatment of cataracts: Corneal penetration of pyruvate in humans. *Ophthalmologica* **2009**, *223*, 136–138. [CrossRef] [PubMed]
54. Zhao, L.; Chen, X.-J.; Zhu, J.; Xi, Y.-B.; Yang, X.; Hu, L.-D.; Ouyang, H.; Patel, S.H.; Jin, X.; Lin, D.; et al. Lanosterol reverses protein aggregation in cataracts. *Nature* **2015**, *523*, 607–611. [CrossRef] [PubMed]
55. Quigley, H.A. Use of animal models and techniques in glaucoma research: Introduction. In *Glaucoma: Methods and Protocols*, 1st ed.; Jakobs, T.C., Ed.; Humana Press: New York, NY, USA, 2018; pp. 1–10, ISBN 978-1-4939-7407-8.
56. Tham, Y.-C.; Li, X.; Wong, T.Y.; Quigley, H.A.; Aung, T.; Cheng, C.-Y. Global prevalence of glaucoma and projections of glaucoma burden through 2040: A systematic review and meta-analysis. *Ophthalmology* **2014**, *121*, 2081–2090. [CrossRef] [PubMed]
57. Jackson, T.L.; Egan, C.; Bird, A.C. Medical retina. In *Moorfields Manual of Ophthalmology*, 1st ed.; Jackson, T.L., Ed.; Mosby: Edinburgh, UK, 2008; pp. 412–518, ISBN 9781416025726.
58. Joseph, M.; Trinh, H.M.; Cholkar, K.; Pal, D.; Mitra, A.K. Recent perspectives on the delivery of biologics to back of the eye. *Expert Opin. Drug Deliv.* **2017**, *14*, 631–645. [CrossRef] [PubMed]
59. Burgalassi, S.; Monti, D.; Nicosia, N.; Tampucci, S.; Terreni, E.; Vento, A.; Chetoni, P. Freeze-dried matrices for ocular administration of bevacizumab: A comparison between subconjunctival and intravitreal administration in rabbits. *Drug Deliv. Transl. Res.* **2018**, *8*, 461–472. [CrossRef] [PubMed]

60. Davis, B.M.; Normando, E.M.; Guo, L.; Turner, L.A.; Nizari, S.; O'Shea, P.; Moss, S.E.; Somavarapu, S.; Cordeiro, M.F. Topical delivery of Avastin to the posterior segment of the eye in vivo using annexin A5-associated liposomes. *Small* **2014**, *10*, 1575–1584. [CrossRef]
61. Nayak, K.; Misra, M. A review on recent drug delivery systems for posterior segment of eye. *Biomed. Pharmacother.* **2018**, *107*, 1564–1582. [CrossRef] [PubMed]
62. Inokuchi, Y.; Hironaka, K.; Fujisawa, T.; Tozuka, Y.; Tsuruma, K.; Shimazawa, M.; Takeuchi, H.; Hara, H. Physicochemical Properties Affecting Retinal Drug/Coumarin-6 Delivery from Nanocarrier Systems via Eyedrop Administration. *Investig. Ophthalmol. Vis. Sci.* **2010**, *51*, 3162–3170. [CrossRef]
63. Duh, E.J.; Sun, J.K.; Stitt, A.W. Diabetic retinopathy: Current understanding, mechanisms, and treatment strategies. *JCI Insight* **2017**, *2*, 1–13. [CrossRef]
64. Prausnitz, M.R.; Noonan, J.S. Permeability of cornea, sclera, and conjunctiva: A literature analysis for drug delivery to the eye. *J. Pharm. Sci.* **1998**, *87*, 1479–1488. [CrossRef]
65. Edward, A.; Prausnitz, M.R. Predicted permeability of the cornea to topical drugs. *Pharm. Res.* **2001**, *18*, 1497–1508. [CrossRef]
66. Agarwal, P.; Rupenthal, I.D. In vitro and ex vivo corneal penetration and absorption models. *Drug Deliv. Transl. Res.* **2016**, *6*, 634–647. [CrossRef]
67. Kaluzhny, Y.; Kinuthia, M.W.; Truong, T.; Lapointe, A.M.; Hayden, P.; Klausner, M. New Human Organotypic Corneal Tissue Model for Ophthalmic Drug Delivery Studies. *Investig. Ophthalmol. Vis. Sci.* **2018**, *59*, 2880–2898. [CrossRef] [PubMed]
68. Morrison, P.W.; Connon, C.J.; Khutoryanskiy, V.V. Cyclodextrin-mediated enhancement of riboflavin solubility and corneal permeability. *Mol. Pharm.* **2013**, *10*, 756–762. [CrossRef] [PubMed]
69. Stefánsson, E.; Loftsson, T. Microspheres and nanotechnology for drug delivery. In *Retinal Pharmacotherapeutics*, 1st ed.; Nguyen, Q.D., Rodrigues, E.B., Farah, M.E., Mieler, W.F., Eds.; W.B. Saunders: Edinburgh, UK, 2010; pp. 86–90, ISBN 978-3318055641.
70. Cal, K.; Centkowska, K. Use of cyclodextrins in topical formulations: Practical aspects. *Eur. J. Pharm. Biopharm.* **2008**, *68*, 467–478. [CrossRef] [PubMed]
71. Loftsson, T.; Stefansson, E. Cyclodextrins in eye drop formulations: Enhanced topical delivery of corticosteroids to the eye. *Acta Ophthalmol. Scand.* **2002**, *80*, 144–150. [CrossRef]
72. Jarho, P.; Urtti, A.; Pate, D.W.; Suhonen, P.; Järvinen, T. Increase in aqueous solubility, stability and in vitro corneal permeability of anandamide by hydroxypropyl-β-cyclodextrin. *Int. J. Pharm.* **1996**, *137*, 209–216. [CrossRef]
73. Chordiya, M.A.; Senthilkumaran, K. Cyclodextrin in drug delivery: A review. *Res. Rev. Pharm. Pharm. Sci.* **2012**, *1*, 19–29.
74. Stella, V.J.; Rajewski, R.A. Cyclodextrins: Their future in drug formulation and delivery. *Pharm. Res.* **1997**, *14*, 556–567. [CrossRef]
75. Loftsson, T.; Brewster, M.E.; Másson, M. Role of cyclodextrins in improving oral drug delivery. *Am. J. Drug Deliv.* **2004**, *2*, 261–275. [CrossRef]
76. Loftssona, T.; Jarvinen, T. Cyclodextrins in ophthalmic drug delivery. *Adv. Drug Deliv. Rev.* **1999**, *36*, 59–79. [CrossRef]
77. Skowron, S. Cyclodextrin. Available online: https://commons.wikimedia.org/wiki/File:Cyclodextrin.svg (accessed on 9 May 2019).
78. Lisch, W.; Seitz, B. *Corneal Dystrophies*, 1st ed.; Karger: Basel, Switzerland, 2011; Volume 48, p. 159, ISBN 978-3-8055-9720-3.
79. Pescina, S.; Carra, F.; Padula, C.; Santi, P.; Nicoli, S. Effect of pH and penetration enhancers on cysteamine stability and trans-corneal transport. *Eur. J. Pharm. Biopharm.* **2016**, *107*, 171–179. [CrossRef]
80. Aktas, Y.; Unlu, N.; Orhan, M.; Irkec, M.; Hincal, A.A. Influence of hydroxypropyl beta-cyclodextrin on the corneal permeation of pilocarpine. *Drug Dev. Ind. Pharm.* **2003**, *29*, 223–230. [CrossRef] [PubMed]
81. Loftsson, T.; Stefansson, E. Cyclodextrins and topical drug delivery to the anterior and posterior segments of the eye. *Int. J. Pharm.* **2017**, *531*, 413–423. [CrossRef] [PubMed]
82. Abdulrazik, M.; Beher-Cohen, F.; Benita, S. Drug Delivery Systems for Enhanced Ocular Absorption. In *Enhancement in Drug Delivery*, 1st ed.; Touitou, E., Barry, B.W., Eds.; CRC Press: Boca Raton, FL, USA, 2006; pp. 489–526, ISBN 978-0-8493-3203-6.

83. Grass, G.M.; Wood, R.W.; Robinson, J.R. Effects of calcium chelating agents on corneal permeability. *Investig. Ophthalmol. Vis. Sci.* **1985**, *26*, 110–113.
84. Deli, M.A. Potential use of tight junction modulators to reversibly open membranous barriers and improve drug delivery. *Biochim. Biophys. Acta* **2009**, *1788*, 892–910. [CrossRef] [PubMed]
85. Kikuchi, T.; Suzuki, M.; Kusai, A.; Iseki, K.; Sasaki, H. Synergistic effect of EDTA and boric acid on corneal penetration of CS-088. *Int. J. Pharm.* **2005**, *290*, 83–89. [CrossRef] [PubMed]
86. Rodriguez, I.; Vazquez, J.A.; Pastrana, L.; Khutoryanskiy, V.V. Enhancement and inhibition effects on the corneal permeability of timolol maleate: Polymers, cyclodextrins and chelating agents. *Int. J. Pharm.* **2017**, *529*, 168–177. [CrossRef] [PubMed]
87. Andrés-Guerrero, V.; Vicario-de-la-Torre, M.; Molina-Martínez, I.T.; Benítez-del-Castillo, J.M.; García-Feijoo, J.; Herrero-Vanrell, R. Comparison of the In Vitro Tolerance and In Vivo Efficacy of Traditional Timolol Maleate Eye Drops versus New Formulations with Bioadhesive Polymers. *Investig. Ophthalmol. Vis. Sci.* **2011**, *52*, 3548–3556. [CrossRef]
88. Pedersen, C.J. Cyclic polyethers and their complexes with metal salts. *J. Am. Chem. Soc.* **1967**, *89*, 7017–7036. [CrossRef]
89. Pedersen, C.J. Macrocyclic Polyethers: Dibenzo-18-crown-6 Polyether and Dicyclohexyl-18-crown-6 Polyether. In *Organic Synthesis*; John Wiley & Sons: Hoboken, NJ, USA, 2003; Volume 52, ISBN 9780471264224.
90. Ouchi, M.; Inoue, Y.; Kanzaki, T.; Hakushi, T. Molecular design of crown ethers. 1. Effects of methylene chain length: 15- to 17-crown-5 and 18- to 22-crown-6. *J. Org. Chem.* **1984**, *49*, 1408–1412. [CrossRef]
91. Steed, J. First- and second-sphere coordination chemistry of alkali metal crown ether complexes. *Coord. Chem. Rev.* **2001**, *215*, 171–221. [CrossRef]
92. Boojar, M.M.; Goodarzi, F. Cytotoxicity and the levels of oxidative stress parameters in WI38 cells following 2 macrocyclic crown ethers treatment. *Clin. Chim. Acta* **2006**, *364*, 321–327. [CrossRef] [PubMed]
93. Capel-Cuevas, S.; de Orbe-Payá, I.; Santoyo-González, F.; Capitan-Vallvey, L.F. Double-armed crown ethers for calcium optical sensors. *Talanta* **2009**, *78*, 1484–1488. [CrossRef] [PubMed]
94. Song, M.Z.; Zhu, L.Y.; Gao, X.K.; Dou, J.M.; Sun, D.Z. Microcalorimetric study on host-guest complexation of naphtho-15-crown-5 with four ions of alkaline earth metal. *J. Zhejiang Univ. Sci. B* **2005**, *6*, 69–73. [CrossRef] [PubMed]
95. Marjanovic, M.; Kralj, M.; Supek, F.; Frkanec, L.; Piantanida, I.; Smuc, T.; Tusek-Bozic, L. Antitumor potential of crown ethers: Structure-activity relationships, cell cycle disturbances, and cell death studies of a series of ionophores. *J. Med. Chem.* **2007**, *50*, 1007–1018. [CrossRef] [PubMed]
96. Kralj, M.; Tušek-Božić, L.; Frkanec, L. Biomedical potentials of crown ethers: Prospective antitumor agents. *ChemMedChem* **2008**, *3*, 1478–1492. [CrossRef] [PubMed]
97. Muzzalupo, R.; Nicoletta, F.P.; Trombino, S.; Cassano, R.; Iemma, F.; Picci, N. A new crown ether as vesicular carrier for 5-fluoruracil: Synthesis, characterization and drug delivery evaluation. *Colloids Surf. B Biointerfaces* **2007**, *58*, 197–202. [CrossRef] [PubMed]
98. Darwish, I.; Uchegbu, I. The evaluation of crown ether based niosomes as cation containing and cation sensitive drug delivery systems. *Int. J. Pharm.* **1997**, *159*, 207–213. [CrossRef]
99. Chehardoli, G.; Bahmani, A. The role of crown ethers in drug delivery. *Supramol. Chem.* **2019**, *31*, 221–238. [CrossRef]
100. Morrison, P.W.J.; Porfiryeva, N.N.; Chahal, S.; Salakhov, I.A.; Lacourt, C.; Semina, I.I.; Moustafine, R.I.; Khutoryanskiy, V.V. Crown Ethers: Novel Permeability Enhancers for Ocular Drug Delivery? *Mol. Pharm.* **2017**, *14*, 3528–3538. [CrossRef]
101. Hartman. Surface-Active Compounds. BODE Science Centre. Available online: https://www.bode-science-center.com/center/glossary/surface-active-compounds.html (accessed on 21 September 2018).
102. Sekhon, B. Surfactants: Pharmaceutical and Medicinal Aspects. *J. Pharm. Technol. Res. Manag.* **2013**, *1*, 11–36. [CrossRef]
103. Jiao, J. Polyoxyethylated nonionic surfactants and their application in topical ocular drug delivery. *Adv. Drug Deliv. Rev.* **2008**, *60*, 1663–1673. [CrossRef] [PubMed]
104. Kumar, G.P.; Rajeshwarrao, P. Nonionic surfactant vesicular systems for effective drug delivery—An overview. *Acta Pharm. Sin. B* **2011**, *1*, 208–219. [CrossRef]
105. Marsh, R.J.; Maurice, D.M. The influence of non-ionic detergents and other surfactants on human corneal permeability. *Exp. Eye Res.* **1971**, *11*, 43–48. [CrossRef]

106. Saettone, M.F.; Chetoni, P.; Cerbai, R.; Mazzanti, G.; Braghiroli, L. Evaluation of ocular permeation enhancers: In vitro effects on corneal transport of four β-blockers, and in vitro/in vivo toxic activity. *Int. J. Pharm.* **1996**, *142*, 103–113. [CrossRef]
107. Ostacolo, C.; Caruso, C.; Tronino, D.; Troisi, S.; Laneri, S.; Pacente, L.; Del Prete, A.; Sacchi, A. Enhancement of corneal permeation of riboflavin-5′-phosphate through vitamin E TPGS: A promising approach in corneal trans-epithelial cross linking treatment. *Int. J. Pharm.* **2013**, *440*, 148–153. [CrossRef]
108. Li, X.; Pan, W.; Ju, C.; Liu, Z.; Pan, H.; Zhang, H.; Nie, S. Evaluation of Pharmasolve corneal permeability enhancement and its irritation on rabbit eyes. *Drug Deliv.* **2009**, *16*, 224–229. [CrossRef]
109. Montenegro, L.; Bucolo, C.; Puglisi, G. Enhancer effects on in vitro corneal permeation of timolol and acyclovir. *Pharmazie* **2003**, *58*, 497–501.
110. Kaur, I.P. Ocular Penetration Enhancers. In *Enhancement in Drug Delivery*, 1st ed.; Touitou, E., Barry, B.W., Eds.; CRC Press: Boca Raton, FL, USA, 2006; pp. 527–548, ISBN 978-0-8493-3203-6.
111. Sahoo, S.K.; Dilnawaz, F.; Krishnakumar, S. Nanotechnology in ocular drug delivery. *Drug Discov. Today* **2008**, *13*, 144–151. [CrossRef]
112. Shih, R.L.; Lee, V.H. Rate Limiting Barrier to the Penetration of Ocular Hypotensive Beta Blockers Across the Corneal Epithelium in the Pigmented Rabbit. *J. Ocul. Pharmacol.* **1990**, *6*, 329–336. [CrossRef]
113. Wilson, W.S.; Duncan, A.J.; Jay, J.L. Effect of benzalconium chloride on the stability of the precorneal film in rabbit and man. *Br. J. Ophthalmol.* **1975**, *59*, 667–669. [CrossRef]
114. Johannsdottir, S.; Jansook, P.; Stefánsson, E.; Myrdal Kristinsdottir, I.; Marta Asgrimsdottir, G.; Loftsson, T. Topical drug delivery to the posterior segment of the eye: The effect of benzalkonium chloride on topical dexamethasone penetration into the eye in vivo. *J. Drug Deliv. Sci. Technol.* **2018**, *48*, 125–127. [CrossRef]
115. Sasaki, H.; Yamamura, K.; Mukai, T.; Nishida, K.; Nakamura, J.; Nakashima, M.; Ichikawa, M. Modification of ocular permeability of peptide drugs by absorption promoters. *Biol. Pharm. Bull.* **2000**, *23*, 1524–1527. [CrossRef] [PubMed]
116. Van Der Bijl, P.; Engelbrecht, A.H.; Van Eyk, A.D.; Meyer, D. Comparative permeability of human and rabbit corneas to cyclosporin and tritiated water. *J. Ocul. Pharmacol. Ther.* **2002**, *18*, 419–427. [CrossRef] [PubMed]
117. Liu, Z.; Li, J.; Nie, S.; Guo, H.; Pan, W. Effects of Transcutol P on the corneal permeability of drugs and evaluation of its ocular irritation of rabbit eyes. *J. Pharm. Pharmacol.* **2006**, *58*, 45–50. [CrossRef] [PubMed]
118. Liu, Z.; Zhang, X.; Li, J.; Liu, R.; Shu, L.; Jin, J. Effects of Labrasol on the corneal drug delivery of baicalin. *Drug Deliv.* **2009**, *16*, 399–404. [CrossRef] [PubMed]
119. Russell, D.W. The enzymes, regulation, and genetics of bile acid synthesis. *Annu. Rev. Biochem.* **2003**, *72*, 137–174. [CrossRef]
120. Chiang, J. Bile Acids: Bile acids: Regulation of synthesis. *J. Lipid Res.* **2009**, *50*, 1955–1966. [CrossRef]
121. Stojančević, M.; Pavlović, N.; Goločorbin-Kon, S.; Mikov, M. Application of bile acids in drug formulation and delivery. *Front. Life Sci.* **2013**, *7*, 112–122. [CrossRef]
122. Rajput, T.; Chauhan, M. Bilosome: A bile salt based novel carrier system gaining interest in pharmaceutical research. *J. Drug Deliv. Ther.* **2017**, *7*, 4–16. [CrossRef]
123. Sasaki, H.; Igarashi, Y.; Nagano, T.; Nishida, K.; Nakamura, J. Different Effects of Absorption Promoters on Corneal and Conjunctival Penetration of Ophthalmic Beta-Blockers. *Pharm. Res.* **1995**, *12*, 1146–1150. [CrossRef]
124. Morimoto, K.; Nakai, T.; Morisaka, K. Evaluation of permeability enhancement of hydrophilic compounds and macromolecular compounds by bile salts through rabbit corneas in-vitro. *J. Pharm. Pharmacol.* **1987**, *39*, 124–126. [CrossRef] [PubMed]
125. Dai, Y.; Zhou, R.; Liu, L.; Lu, Y.; Qi, J.; Wu, W. Liposomes containing bile salts as novel ocular delivery systems for tacrolimus (FK506): In vitro characterization and improved corneal permeation. *Int. J. Nanomed.* **2013**, *8*, 1921–1933. [CrossRef]
126. Mahaling, B.; Katti, D.S. Understanding the influence of surface properties of nanoparticles and penetration enhancers for improving bioavailability in eye tissues in vivo. *Int. J. Pharm.* **2016**, *501*, 1–9. [CrossRef] [PubMed]
127. González de Llano, D.; Polo Sánchez, C. Peptides. In *Encyclopedia of Food Sciences and Nutrition*, 2nd ed.; Caballero, B., Ed.; Academic Press: Oxford, UK, 2003; pp. 4468–4473, ISBN 978-0-12-227055-0.
128. Dupont, E.; Prochiantz, A.; Joliot, A. Penetratin story: An overview. *Methods Mol. Biol.* **2011**, *683*, 21–29. [CrossRef] [PubMed]

129. Liu, C.; Tai, L.; Zhang, W.; Wei, G.; Pan, W.; Lu, W. Penetratin, a potentially powerful absorption enhancer for noninvasive intraocular drug delivery. *Mol. Pharm.* **2014**, *11*, 1218–1227. [CrossRef]
130. Pescina, S.; Sala, M.; Padula, C.; Scala, M.C.; Spensiero, A.; Belletti, S.; Gatti, R.; Novellino, E.; Campiglia, P.; Santi, P.; et al. Design and Synthesis of New Cell Penetrating Peptides: Diffusion and Distribution Inside the Cornea. *Mol. Pharm.* **2016**, *13*, 3876–3883. [CrossRef]
131. De Cogan, F.; Hill, L.J.; Lynch, A.; Morgan-Warren, P.J.; Lechner, J.; Berwick, M.R.; Peacock, A.F.A.; Chen, M.; Scott, R.A.H.; Xu, H.; et al. Topical Delivery of Anti-VEGF Drugs to the Ocular Posterior Segment Using Cell-Penetrating Peptides. *Investig. Ophthalmol. Vis. Sci.* **2017**, *58*, 2578–2590. [CrossRef]
132. Nemoto, E.; Takahashi, H.; Kobayashi, D.; Ueda, H.; Morimoto, Y. Effects of poly-L-arginine on the permeation of hydrophilic compounds through surface ocular tissues. *Biol. Pharm. Bull.* **2006**, *29*, 155–160. [CrossRef]
133. Pescina, S.; Ostacolo, C.; Gomez-Monterrey, I.M.; Sala, M.; Bertamino, A.; Sonvico, F.; Padula, C.; Santi, P.; Bianchera, A.; Nicoli, S. Cell penetrating peptides in ocular drug delivery: State of the art. *J. Control. Release* **2018**, *284*, 84–102. [CrossRef]
134. Kato, A.; Iwata, S. In vitro study on corneal permeability to bunazosin. *J. Pharm.-Dyn.* **1988**, *11*, 115–120. [CrossRef]
135. Kato, A.; Iwata, S. Studies on improved corneal permeability to bunazosin. *J. Pharm.-Dyn.* **1988**, *11*, 330–334. [CrossRef]
136. Antunes, A.; De Geest, B.; Vervaet, C.; Remon, J. Gelucire 44/14 based immediate release formulations for poorly water-soluble drugs. *Drug Dev. Ind. Pharm.* **2012**, *39*, 791–798. [CrossRef] [PubMed]
137. Tang-Liu, D.D.; Richman, J.B.; Weinkam, R.J.; Takruri, H. Effects of four penetration enhancers on corneal permeability of drugs in vitro. *J. Pharm. Sci.* **1994**, *83*, 85–90. [CrossRef] [PubMed]
138. Afouna, M.; Hussein, A.; Ahmed, O. Influence of the Interplay between Azone™ as Permeation Enhancer a and Carbopol-974® as a Mucoadhesive upon the in vitro Transcorneal Release and the in vivo Antiglaucoma Effect of S-Timolol Maleate Ophthalmic Gel Formulations. *Int. J. PharmTech Res.* **2014**, *6*, 298–315.
139. Afouna, M.I. Maximization of the In Vitro transcorneal release and the In Vivo IOP-lowering effects of Latanoprost Ophthalmic gel formulations using Azone as a penetration enhancer and Carbopol-974 as a mucoadhesive. *J. Excip. Food Chem.* **2016**, *7*, 20–35.
140. Yang, H.; Xun, Y.; Li, Z.; Hang, T.; Zhang, X.; Cui, H. Influence of borneol on in vitro corneal permeability and on in vivo and in vitro corneal toxicity. *J. Int. Med. Res.* **2009**, *37*, 791–802. [CrossRef] [PubMed]
141. Afouna, M.I.; Khedr, A.; Abdel-Naim, A.B.; Al-Marzoqi, A. Influence of various concentrations of terpene-4-ol enhancer and carbopol-934 mucoadhesive upon the in vitro ocular transport and the in vivo intraocular pressure lowering effects of dorzolamide ophthalmic formulations using albino rabbits. *J. Pharm. Sci.* **2010**, *99*, 119–127. [CrossRef] [PubMed]
142. Agarwal, P.; Scherer, D.; Gunther, B.; Rupenthal, I.D. Semifluorinated alkane based systems for enhanced corneal penetration of poorly soluble drugs. *Int. J. Pharm.* **2018**, *538*, 119–129. [CrossRef] [PubMed]
143. Epstein, S.P.; Ahdoot, M.; Marcus, E.; Asbell, P.A. Comparative toxicity of preservatives on immortalized corneal and conjunctival epithelial cells. *J. Ocul. Pharmacol. Ther.* **2009**, *25*, 113–119. [CrossRef] [PubMed]
144. European Medicines Agency. Available online: https://www.ema.europa.eu/en/documents/report/benzalkonium-chloride-used-excipient-report-published-support-questions-answers-benzalkonium_en.pdf (accessed on 27 June 2019).
145. Green, K.; Tonjum, A.M. The effect of benzalkonium chloride on the electropotential of the rabbit cornea. *Acta Ophthalmol.* **1975**, *53*, 348–357. [CrossRef]
146. Chen, Y.; Quan, P.; Liu, X.; Wang, M.; Fang, L. Novel chemical permeation enhancers for transdermal drug delivery. *Asian J. Pharm. Sci.* **2014**, *9*, 51–64. [CrossRef]
147. Jampilek, J. Azone® and Its Analogues as Penetration Enhancers. In *Percutaneous Penetration Enhancers Chemical Methods in Penetration Enhancement*, 1st ed.; Dragicevic, N., Maibach, H.I., Eds.; Springer: Berlin/Heidelberg, Germany, 2015; pp. 69–105, ISBN 978-3-662-47038-1.

9

Biomedical Applications of Electrospun Nanofibers: Drug and Nanoparticle Delivery

Rajan Sharma Bhattarai [1], Rinda Devi Bachu [1], Sai H. S. Boddu [2,*] and Sarit Bhaduri [3,4]

1 College of Pharmacy and Pharmaceutical Sciences, The University of Toledo Health Science Campus, Toledo, OH 43614, USA; RajanSharma.Bhattarai@rockets.utoledo.edu (R.S.B.); RindaDevi.Bachu@rockets.utoledo.edu (R.D.B.)

2 Department of Pharmaceutical Sciences, College of Pharmacy and Health Sciences, Ajman University, Ajman 2758, UAE

3 Department of Mechanical, Industrial and Manufacturing Engineering, University of Toledo, Toledo, OH 43614, USA; Sarit.Bhaduri@utoledo.edu

4 Department of Surgery (Dentistry), University of Toledo, Toledo, OH 43614, USA

* Correspondence: s.boddu@ajman.ac.ae

Abstract: The electrospinning process has gained popularity due to its ease of use, simplicity and diverse applications. The properties of electrospun fibers can be controlled by modifying either process variables (e.g., applied voltage, solution flow rate, and distance between charged capillary and collector) or polymeric solution properties (e.g., concentration, molecular weight, viscosity, surface tension, solvent volatility, conductivity, and surface charge density). However, many variables affecting electrospinning are interdependent. An optimized electrospinning process is one in which these parameters remain constant and continuously produce nanofibers consistent in physicochemical properties. In addition, nozzle configurations, such as single nozzle, coaxial, multi-jet electrospinning, have an impact on the fiber characteristics. The polymeric solution could be aqueous, a polymeric melt or an emulsion, which in turn leads to different types of nanofiber formation. Nanofiber properties can also be modified by polarity inversion and by varying the collector design. The active moiety is incorporated into polymeric fibers by blending, surface modification or emulsion formation. The nanofibers can be further modified to deliver multiple drugs, and multilayer polymer coating allows sustained release of the incorporated active moiety. Electrospun nanofibers prepared from polymers are used to deliver antibiotic and anticancer agents, DNA, RNA, proteins and growth factors. This review provides a compilation of studies involving the use of electrospun fibers in biomedical applications with emphasis on nanoparticle-impregnated nanofibers.

Keywords: electrospinning; parameters; drug delivery; applications

---

1. Electrospinning and Its History

Electrospinning is a process of forming micro/nanometer-sized polymeric fibers, either hollow or solid, with the application of the electric force on the polymeric solution at the tip of a conducting tube. It is one of the most commonly used techniques to obtain continuous fibers in the nanometer size range [1–3]. Electrospinning, also known as electrostatic spinning, has been used extensively for over three decades, and its usefulness in the fields of science and technology is still on the increase. Bose et al. first described the aerosols generated by the application of electric potential to the fluids in 1745 [4]. Further, Lord Rayleigh studied the amount of charge needed by the fluid to overcome the surface tension of a drop. Cooley and Morton patented the first device to spray the liquids under the influence of electrical charge in 1902 and 1903, and the fabrication of artificial silk was undertaken by Kiyohito et al. in 1929 [4]. Studies in the 1940s, 1950s and 1960s were limited and mainly focused on obtaining uniform-sized particle/fibers, decreasing the size, understanding and optimizing parameters, and designing the instruments [5,6]. In the 1990s, the process was finally taken up by educational institutions and, since then, many studies have been carried out on the versatility of manufacturing and the applications of the electrospun particles [2].

1.1. Process of Electrospinning

The electrospinning process involves the use of a very high voltage source (of either positive or negative polarity) to charge the polymer solution or melt, a grounded collector, and a syringe pump (Figure 1). It is advisable to perform the electrospinning process in a closed hood with minimal atmospheric influence, which serves as a safety measure for fibers and for the personnel. When a sufficient repulsive charge is accumulated and the repulsive force is equal to the surface tension, the drop surface on the conducting tube starts to form a cone called a Taylor cone. The conducting polymer solution/melt can exist in an equilibrium cone form under the influence of the electric field at an angle of 49.3° [7]. If the electric field is increased further, the repulsive force overcomes the surface tension. This results in the formation of a liquid jet from the Taylor cone when there is sufficient attraction between the molecules in the solution/melt. If the solution does not have sufficient cohesive attraction, the jets break and the resulting particles are sprayed onto a collector plate. The fiber originating from the Taylor cone travels through the air towards the collector plate, and during the process, the solvent evaporates, leading to a solid fiber deposit onto the collector plate [6,7]. The jet starts to experience instability after traveling through the air for a short distance and then starts to whip, thus increasing the path distance to the collector. This process assists in fiber thinning and solvent evaporation. There are multiple theories proposed on the reason behind jet instability. Some of the prominent theories include: repulsive interaction of charges in the polymer jet [8]; increase in charge density during jet thinning, thus increasing radial charge repulsion to cause jet splitting at a critical charge density [9]; and, "whipping" instability (spiraling loops) [10], causing the fiber to turn, bend [11] and/or splay [12]. Shin et al. have suggested the whipping stability concept based on the results obtained using high-speed photography, where a single strand of jet whipped very fast to give a cone-like appearance [11]. The "inverted cone" appearance had long been misunderstood as a splitting of the jet midway through its travel in the air.

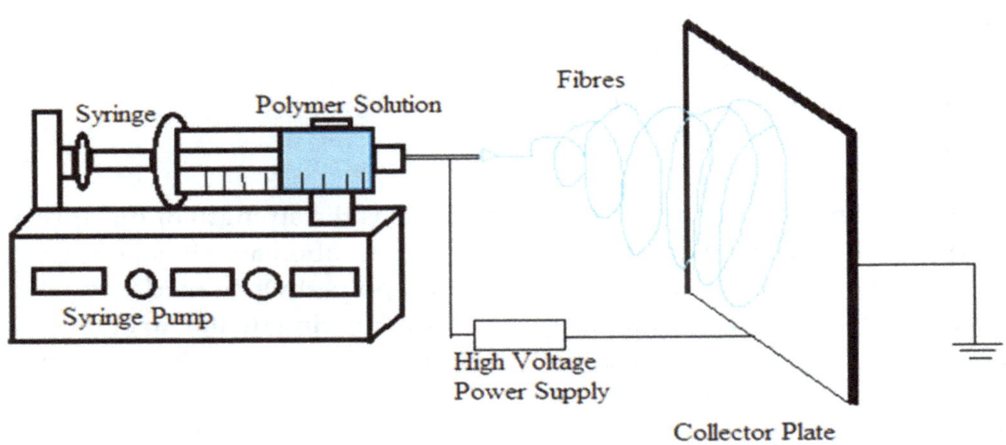

Figure 1. Schematic of electrospinning system. The system consists of polymer solution/melt in a syringe, mounted on a syringe pump, operating at a constant slow speed. High voltage direct current supply is connected to the needle of the syringe to charge the fluid. With sufficient voltage, the fluid forms a Taylor cone and then jet erupts from the cone towards the collector plate with whipping instability.

1.2. *Physics of Electrospinning*

When the electric field/voltage is increased gradually and the surface of the drop becomes convex at a certain voltage, V_c (critical voltage) is reached. At V_c, the jets (electrospinning) and sprays (electrospraying) begin, which are represented by Equation (1):

$$V_c = 4\frac{H^2}{L^2}\left(Ln\frac{2L}{R} - \frac{3}{2}\right)(0.117\pi\gamma R) \quad (1)$$

where H is the separation between capillary and the collector, L is the length of capillary, R is the radius of capillary and γ is the surface tension [7]. This relationship was identified by Taylor, and a similar relationship for the potential required for the electrospraying of charged pendant drops of solutions from the pendant in a capillary tube was established by Hendrick et al., in Equation (2) [13,14]:

$$V = 300\sqrt{20\pi\gamma \mathrm{r}} \quad (2)$$

where, V is the required voltage, γ is the surface tension and r is the radius of the pendant drop. Even though viscosity and conductivity are vital in the electrospinning process, they are missing from the equation. The use of applied voltage and the surface tension gives a representative equation for slightly conducting, medium- to low-conductivity solutions [14].

2. Parameters of Electrospinning

The electrospinning process is simple and does not involve heavy machinery. The processing parameters and solution parameters affect the size, porosity and uniformity of the fibers. These parameters have been discussed individually; however, the observations made in any particular study by a team of researchers are not universal. The modification of a parameter in one polymer may produce a totally different result with another polymer. In addition, none of the parameters act independently during the electrospinning process, and the final fibers are the result of a combination of several parameters.

2.1. *Process-Related Parameters of Electrospinning*

2.1.1. Applied Voltage

The primary factor influencing the formation of fibers is the strength of the applied DC voltage. The size of the fiber, formation of beads and absence of jet formation are all dependent on the applied DC voltage. With an increase in the applied voltage of a polyethylene oxide (PEO)/water system, the originating site for the jet changes from the tip of the pendant drop to the tip of the capillary, and the volume of the pendant drop decreases gradually (Figure 2). When the fiber is formed from within the capillary, the bead defects in the fiber increase [6,15]. A reduction in voltage up to some range moves the splaying (instability) point towards the tip of the capillary (i.e., the jet becomes unstable earlier) [12]. A study by Reneker and Chun reported no significant change in the fiber diameter with a change in the electric field with PEO solution [16]. On the other hand, electrospun polyvinyl alcohol (PVA)/water solution exhibited a broad diameter distribution above 10 kV [17,18]. In another study, Megelski et al. observed an increase in fiber size of polystyrene with a decrease in spinning voltage and with no significant change in the pore formation in fibers [19].

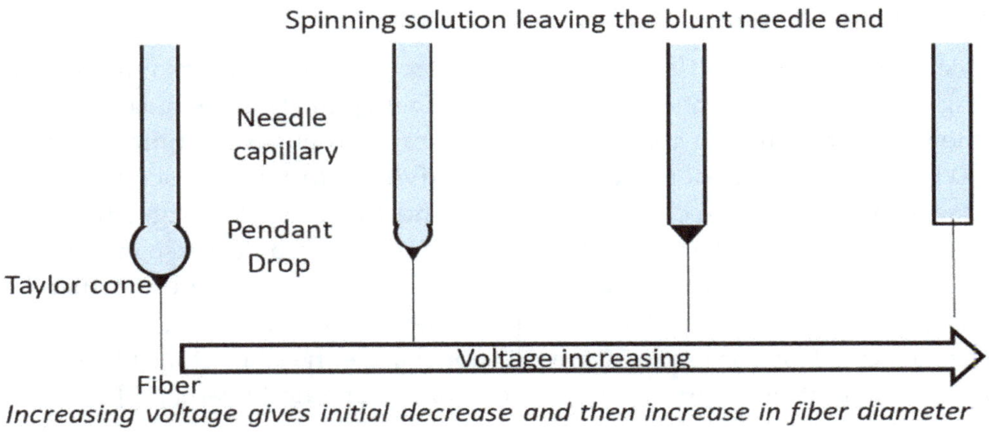

Figure 2. The effect of applied electric field on Taylor cone formation (dark colored tip). At low electric field, pendant drop is formed at the tip of the capillary and then a cone is formed on the tip. When the applied voltage is increased gradually, the drop size decreases until just a cone is formed at the tip of the capillary. If the voltage is further increased, fiber formation starts from within the needle without forming a visible Taylor cone on the blunt tip of the needle.

The fibers formed during the electrospinning process transport the charge to the grounded collector plate to close the circuit. This allows the electric current associated with the process to be measured; it is small (high voltage, 10–15 kV, high resistance and therefore very low current). When conductivity, dielectric constant and flow rate through the pump remain the same, an increase in current indicates an increase in the mass of the fibers formed. During the electrospinning process, the increase in current is gradual at first and then increases sharply from one voltage point, while sharp, steep increases are observed during electrospraying. The point of a sharp change in current could be indicative of the defect/change in the bead density [15].

Studies on the reversal of polarity obtained by grounding the solution in capillary and charging the collects resulted in inconsistent findings. Kilic et al. studied the effect of polarity on the electrospinning process of 7.5 wt% poly(vinyl alcohol)/water solution on production efficiency and nanofiber morphology. They concluded that due to the lack of columbic force acting on the polymer jet, the new reversed setup resulted in less nanofiber production. They also reported that the diameter and pore size of the web layer were much finer and more homogeneously distributed in the conventional setup [20]. On the other hand, Varesano et al. reported the production of good quality nanofibers with multi-jet electrospinning using both conventional and reverse polarity [21].

2.1.2. Flow Rate

The polymer flow rate has a direct impact on the size, shape and porosity of electrospun fibers. A study on polystyrene/tetrahydrofuran (THF) solutions by Megelski et al. reported an increased fiber diameter and pore size with flow rate. However, at high flow rates, bead defects and flat, ribbon-like structures were observed due to insufficient drying [19]. In a different study, a similar effect on fiber morphology was observed with a 20 wt% solution of nylon 6 in formic acid at a constant electric field of 20 kV at flow rates of 0.1, 0.5, 1 and 1.5 mL/h. An optimal flow rate of 0.5 mL/h resulted in fibers with the narrowest fiber diameter distribution and a stable Taylor cone. However, at a flow rate of 0.1 mL/h, the Taylor cone could not be maintained and reduced over time to obtain fiber from within the capillary tip. At flow rates of 1.0 mL/h and 1.5 mL/h, the electric field was not sufficient to spin all the solution, and only a few drops were sprayed as they broke off from the capillary due to the gravitational force [22].

2.1.3. Capillary–Collector Distance

The distance between the capillary and the collector is another factor which plays a significant role in controlling the size and morphology of the nanofibers [23]. This distance needs to be optimized as it might be the factor that distinguishes electrospraying and electrospinning. Typically a distance ranging from 10 to 20 cm is considered to be an effective spinning distance with the conventional method of electrospinning [24]. According to Doshi and Reneker, the larger the distance from the Taylor cone, the smaller the fiber diameter [9]. Jaeger et al. reported a decrease in fiber diameter (19 μm, 11 μm and 9 μm) with increasing distance (1 cm, 2 cm and 3.5 cm) from the orifice [12]. In another study investigating the electrospun polystyrene polymer fibers, decreasing the distance between the capillary and the collector from 35 cm to 30 cm did not change the diameter of the fibers significantly; however it led to the formation of non-homogeneous and elongated beads [19].

2.2. Solution-Related Parameters of Electrospinning

2.2.1. Concentration of Solution

Viscosity and surface tension, which determine the spinnability of a solution, should be taken into consideration in determining the concentration of solution/melt for electrospinning. Surface tension is a dominating factor in a low concentration solution (low viscosity, <1 poise), and at such concentration, drops will be formed instead of a continuous fiber. At a higher concentration (viscosity >20 poise), the flow of the solution cannot be controlled and maintained. In the PEO/water study discussed above in Section 2.1.1, a concentration range of 4–10 wt% with viscosity and surface tension ranging between 1–20 poise and 55–35 dynes/cm, respectively, were studied. At low concentrations of 4%, fibers were not sufficiently dry and formed fiber junctions and bundles. At higher concentrations, straight and cylindrical fibers with fewer fiber junctions and bundles were reported. The diameter of the electrospun PEO fibers increased with concentration, and a bimodal size distribution was observed above 7 wt% concentration. The average diameter of the fibers was reported to be related to solution concentration through the power law relationship, with an exponent of 0.5 [15]. A statistical study by Sukigara et al. on regenerated silk proved that the silk concentration was the most important parameter in producing uniform fibers of a diameter less than 100 nm [25]. Fong et al. investigated the effect of viscosity on morphology defects (bead formation) of electrospun nanofibers formed from PEO solutions. An increase in bead diameter and decrease in bead density was observed with solution viscosity. At higher viscosity, the shape of beads changed from spherical to spindle resulting in the formation of nanofibers with diminished morphology defects [26]. Solutions with low polymer concentration and high surface tension produced droplets as the viscoelastic forces could not overcome the repulsive forces of charge, resulting in the fragmentation of fiber jet into droplets. At higher concentrations, the viscoelastic forces are sufficient to prevent the fragmentation resulting in the formation of smooth nanofibers. Nanofibers of polyacrylonitrile solutions were formed in the viscosity range of 1.7 to 215 centipoise. With increase in viscosity, the fiber jet length and the nanofiber diameter increased and the drop at the capillary tip changed from hemispherical to conical shape [27]. In a different study, 15 and 20% w/v solutions of poly(desaminotyrosyl-tyrosine ethyl ester carbonate) (poly(DTE carbonate)) were electrospun at a voltage of 10 kV to 25 kV at 10 cm distance. Beaded fibers were observed during electrospinning at a lower concentration solution until the voltage reached 20 kV, and the density of beads decreased until the voltage reached 15 kV; average fiber diameter increased, while increasing the voltage from 20 kV to 25 kV. At higher solution concentrations, the smooth fibers obtained showed an increasing diameter and decreasing fiber density with the increase in the electric field from 10 kV to 25 kV [28].

2.2.2. Molecular Weight

The molecular weight of polymer influences the solution viscosity and thus has an important effect on fiber morphology. For example, decreasing the molecular weight of poly(vinyl alcohol) while maintaining other parameters constant resulted in the formation of bead-like structures. On the other hand, higher molecular weight resulted in smooth fibers initially followed by ribbon-like fibers upon further increase in molecular weight [29]. Ultra-high molecular weight polymers, such as polyacrylamide (molecular weight 9×10^6 g/mol), exhibited a variety of fiber morphologies even with a minute change in the concentration within the range 0.3–3.0 wt%. Beaded and smooth fibers were formed at concentrations between 0.3 to 0.7 wt%, whereas smooth fibers with ribbons coexisted at 0.7 to 2 wt%. Above 2.0 wt%, only ribbons were formed, which were either helical or zigzag with triangular beads on them [30]. Additionally, a study on the melts of polypropylene with varying molecular weights showed an increase in the fiber diameter with molecular weight. High molecular weight polymers show the highest degree of entanglement and pose difficulties for the electric field to pull on individual polymer chains to obtain a thin fiber [31].

2.2.3. Solution Viscosity

Viscosity determines the solution's ability to form fibers. Smooth continuous fibers can be obtained at optimum viscosity for a particular polymer solvent combination. The viscosity, molecular weight of the polymer and polymer concentration are interrelated, and one cannot be independently judged. Low viscosity fails to form the fibers, while high viscosity requires a higher electric field for electrospinning, making it hard to operate [25,32]. Baumgarten observed the formation of fine droplets at a lower viscosity and with incomplete drying. At higher viscosity, the droplets bumped into each other in mid-air due to incomplete drying with acrylic polymer [27]. When a solution has low viscosity, surface tension dominates the process of fiber formation, but at optimum concentration, it is the combined effect of both parameters [29,33–36]. Yang et al. suggested a mixed solvent system of dimethylformamide (DMF) and ethanol (50:50) for obtaining the best electrospun fibers of poly(vinyl pyrrolidone) and attributed the success to the combined effect of solution viscosity and charge density [10].

2.2.4. Surface Tension of the Solution

Surface tension is the measure of cohesive forces between the molecules in solution form and is dependent upon the solution composition, polymer and solvent(s) used. Yang et al. studied the influence of solvents on the formation of nanofibers with poly(vinyl pyrrolidone) and concluded that lower surface tension with high viscosity formed smooth nanofibers with ethanol as the solvent. They proposed the use of a multi-solvent system to obtain optimum surface tension and viscosity parameters for better electrospun fibers [10]. Like viscosity, surface tension can define the range of solvents and concentrations to be used in the electrospinning process [18].

2.2.5. Conductivity and Surface Charge Density

The impact of conductivity and surface charge density of solution also plays an important role in the process of electrospinning. It is important to have high conductivity for a greater charge-carrying capacity. A highly conductive solution experiences a stronger tensile force in an electric field compared to the less conductive solution, making the former preferable for electrospinning. An increase in the conductivity of the solution causes a substantial decrease in the diameter of the nanofibers. The radius of the fiber jet varies inversely as the cube root of the conductivity of solution [37]. For preparation of acrylic microfibers, Baumgarten reported that the jet radius is dependent on the inverse cube root of electric conductivity [27]. Natural polymers, being polyelectrolytic, have better charge-carrying ability and lead to poor fiber formation compared to synthetic polymers [38]. Hayati et al. observed that stable jets could be obtained by semi-conducting liquids by applying sufficient voltage. Due to insufficient free charges, the insulating liquids, such as paraffin oil, could not build an electrostatic charge on the surface, while highly conducting water produced an unstable stream and sparking at higher electric fields. Consequently, insulating liquids and semiconducting liquids could produce stable fibers [39]. Yet another study on poly(vinyl alcohol) solution showed that the addition of a small amount of sodium chloride drastically increased the conductivity and decreased the fiber diameter [17]. The addition of sodium chloride has an effect on decreasing the occurrence of beads in PEO solution [26]. Sodium phosphate [38], potassium phosphate [38], ammonium chloride [26], and lithium chloride [26] are also used to obtain better fibers by changing the conductivity of solutions. Huang et al. used compounds soluble in organic solvents, such as pyridine, that react with formic acid in solution to form a salt. Pyridine improves the conductivity and can easily be removed to obtain dry fibers. The addition of 0.4 wt% of pyridine doubled the electrical conductivity of 2% nylon-4,6 in formic acid [40].

2.2.6. Solvent Volatility

The distance between the tip of the capillary and the collector is only a few centimeters (typically 10–15 cm), and the path taken by the jet to reach the collector is a few folds more. The fibers formed during the process are porous and dry fast, depending on the choice of the solvent used for solubilization of the polymer. The insufficiently dried fiber may attach to itself mid-air [27], form ribbon-like fibers [19] or attach to itself after depositing on the collector. A study on polystyrene fibers showed that the use of more volatile tetrahydrofuran (THF) as a solvent produced high-density pores and increased the surface area of fibers by up to 40%. The same polymer in DMF lost the microtexture completely. A combination of these solvents in different ratios gave different morphology profiles as the volatility of the mixture varied [19].

3. Types of Electrospinning

The type of electrospinning process can have a significant impact on fiber formation in addition to the process and solution parameters. Two main aspects to deal with in the type of electrospinning are solution vs. melt electrospinning and nozzle configuration [6].

3.1. Solution vs. Melt vs. Emulsion Electrospinning

Electrospun fibers are generally obtained from polymer solutions or melts or emulsions. Melt spinning has high-throughput rate and process safety; solutions have the advantage of using a large variety of polymeric materials, lower energy consumption and superior mechanical, optical and electrical properties of prepared fibers. Emulsion electrospinning is needed for high melting polymers to prepare flame-retardant fibers. A comparison of different spinning methods using poly(lactic acid) (PLA) as a model polymer has been reported by Gupta et al. [41].

The melt of the polymer with other additives is extruded through the capillary, resulting in a thin fiber that cools and solidifies rapidly during its time in the air before depositing onto the collector [41]. Take-up speed, drawing temperature and draw ratio define the structural and tensile properties of the fiber. Draw ratio is the amount of stretching that the material undergoes during the drawing stage of electrospinning. The increase in draw ratio [42] and take-up speed [43] increases the molecular chain orientation along the fiber axis as well as the overall crystallinity of fibers formed from the melt. A higher entanglement of polymer fibers amongst themselves gives sub-par fibers compared to the solution of the same polymer.

The solution spinning method is ideal for polymers or blends of polymers that are thermally unstable or degrade upon melting. Based on how the solvent used for preparing the polymer solution is removed from the fibers, this method can be divided into two different types, namely, dry spinning and wet spinning. The dry spinning process uses hot air or inert gas on the polymer jet to facilitate the solvent's evaporation and fiber solidification. For example, Postema et al. used a solvent combination of chloroform and toluene to produce PLA fibers of high strength by using dry spinning and hot-drawing processes. They were able to obtain an optimal tensile strength of 2.2 GPa by electrospinning at 25 °C [44]. The wet-spinning process involves the use of a viscous coagulation bath containing the liquid, which is miscible with the spinning solvent but not with the polymer. The interaction between the polymer solvent and non-solvent leads to phase separation and then solvent removal from the jet.

This process is known to show fiber defects that can, to some extent, be limited by using 3–5 mm of air gap before the non-solvent, as this allows for stress relaxation of the polymeric chain [41].

In the emulsion electrospinning process, finely ground polymers, insoluble and non-melting, are mixed with another polymer solution with a catalyst and emulsifying agents. The formed emulsion is then electrospun by either the dry or the wet spinning method. This technique has been used in preparing fibers from fluorocarbons with high melting points, ceramics, and polymer blends with flame-retardant properties [45]. Persano et al. have discussed in detail the methods and their industrial application in their review [45].

3.2. Nozzle Configuration

Nozzle configuration relates to the number and the arrangement of capillary tubes from which the jets of fibers emerge. A single nozzle configuration is the simplest and most common configuration, wherein the charged solution flows through a single capillary (Figure 1). This particular configuration has been used to electrospin different polymeric fibers either singly [46,47] or in combination [48] or solvent systems [10]. Co-electrospinning of polymer blends in the same solvent or a mixture was the first and most common modification in the process. Zhou et al. mixed polyaniline with poly(ethylene oxide) in chloroform to obtain nanofibers of a size below 30 nm [49]. Sometimes polymer blends are used to obtain the final properties of fibers. If the polymers are not miscible in a common solvent, or when a homogeneous solution of polymers cannot be obtained, thermodynamic and kinetic aspects should be considered for electrospinning. One way around that problem is to modify the nozzle configuration, where different polymer solutions are electrospun from different capillaries, side-by-side. In this type of configuration, two polymer solutions pass through separate capillaries arranged side-by-side, which are connected to a high voltage supply and never come into contact until they reach the end of the capillary. A single Taylor cone is formed, which ejects the jet with a non-uniform mixture of both polymer solutions and, after drying, is deposited in the collector (Figure 3). The side-by-side technique yields Janus fibers having two different materials on either side of the fiber. The special morphology obtained provides combinational properties of two different polymers and allows several post electrospinning modifications [50]. For this type of configuration to work, it is necessary that both the polymeric solutions have similar conductivity for them to form a single Taylor cone and eject as a mixture. A bicomponent system consisting of poly(vinyl chloride)/segmented polyurethane and poly(vinyl chloride)/poly(vinyl fluoride) was studied [51].

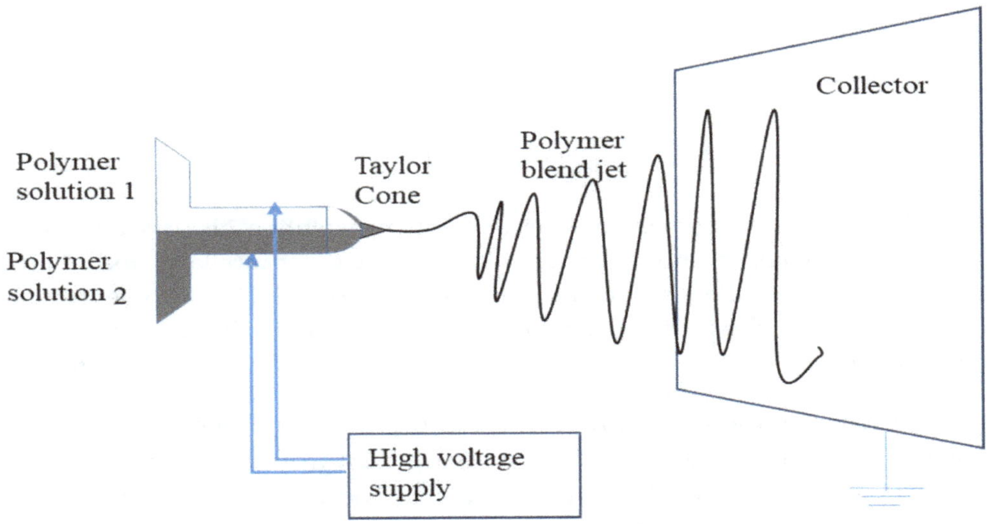

Figure 3. Side-by-side electrospinning schematic diagram: Polymer solutions 1 and 2 pass through separate capillaries, which are connected to the same high voltage supply, at either the same or different rates. A single Taylor cone is formed, which ejects the jet with non-uniform mixture of both the polymer solutions and, after drying, is deposited on the collector.

A second type of nozzle configuration that has recently been introduced is coaxial configuration. Two separate polymer solutions flow through two different capillaries, where the small capillary is within the larger capillary. This configuration can easily encapsulate a small fiber within a larger fiber, forming core-shell morphology (Figure 4). In one study, living cells were encapsulated in poly(dimethylsiloxane) fiber with high cell viability (67.6 ± 1.9%) compared to the control cells (70.6 ± 5.0%). Though the initial viability was comparable, over time, issues with cell morphology and growth rate were observed. This was the first study of its kind, and authors noted the need for further research to obtain the best possible results for encapsulation of living cells [52]. Encapsulation of a model protein, fluorescein isothiocyanate conjugated bovine serum albumin (BSA), with poly(ethylene glycol) in poly(epsilon-caprolactone), was able to sustain the release of the drug, defining its use in drug delivery. Coaxial fibers of proteins, such as fibrinogen [53], BSA, and lysozyme [54] and growth factors, such as bone morphogenetic protein2 (BMP-2) [55], bFGF [56], PDGF [57], VEGF [58], and EGF [59] have been reported. Apart from the regular parameters that affect the quality of fibers being produced by coaxial electrospinning, the relative flow rate of the core and the shell solutions (ratios between 5:1 and 6:1) is important in determining the encapsulation efficiency [60]. At a lower flow rate, the core phase is not continuous, which results in breaking up of the core, whereas a higher flow rate causes the formation of pendent droplets. Wang and co-workers reported that at an optimal flow rate, the core diameter could be easily controlled. Also, the flow rate is related to the core diameter by scaling laws of $d_f{\sim}Q_c^{0.18}$ where d_f represents the inner diameter of the fiber and Q_c represents the flow rate of core solution [61] This method is widely used in tissue engineering to achieve sustained, local and efficient gene and growth factor delivery to the cells [60,62,63]. Coaxial fibers of different non-steroidal anti-inflammatory drugs such as ketprofen [64], flurbiprofen axetil [65], and ibuprofen [64] and antibiotics such as levofloxacin, tetracycline hydrochloride, ciprofloxacin, moxifloxacin, and fusidic acid [66] were prepared and investigated. Though this method is now widely used, it still has the drawbacks of complexity of design and precise control of spinning parameters e.g., interfacial tension, viscoelasticity of the polymers or two different solutions used.

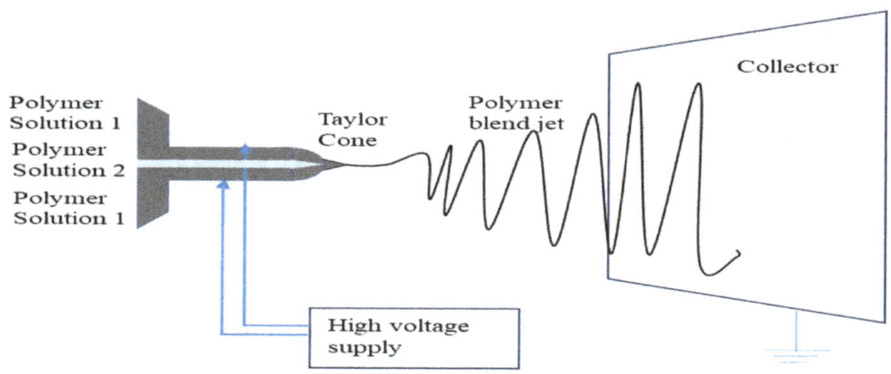

Figure 4. Coaxial electrospinning schematic diagram: Polymer solution 2 is passed through the inner capillary tube, while polymer solution 1 is passed through the outer capillary tube. The Taylor cone is formed where the inner solution (polymer solution 2) is surrounded by the outer solution. The jet erupts from the Taylor cone, and during that process, the polymer in the inner layer is coated with the polymer in the outer layer. The dried fiber with a core-shell design is then deposited on the collector.

The multi-jet electrospinning based on multiple capillaries arranged in circular geometry is yet another modification of the nozzle that can both increase the throughput and facilitate scale up and commercialization. This modification increases the mat thickness, deposits in a larger area and can mix fibers of different materials for better strength and versatility of use [21,67]. In the study by Varesano et al., the morphology of PEO fibers was found to be acceptable in both polarities applied in standard and reverse configuration [21]. The main drawback of the multi-capillary method is the alteration of the electric field due to the presence of other electrospinning jets in the vicinity [68].

This can be overcome by using an auxiliary electrode of any polarity [69] or by using a secondary electrode [70]. Hong et al. fabricated an elastic, fibrous, composite sheet with biodegradable poly(ester urethane) urea (PEUU) and poly(lactide-co-glycolide) (PLGA) using a two-stream electrospinning setup with a rotating metal rod as the collector [71]. Such composite sheets possessed better breaking strains, tensile strength and suture retention capacity. In a review article, Persano et al. discussed different multi-jet configurations and the further possibilities of syringe-free approaches to multi-jet electrospinning [45].

3.3. Collector Modification

The collector plate can be configured based on the application of polymeric fibers. Commercially, the most common collectors are stationary plates (or aluminum foil) and rotating plates. Both these types of collectors can be subdivided further into continual or patterned. A continual collector is simple and can be used to obtain fibers with a random internal structure on a stationary type, while some degree of directional control can be gained with the higher speed of a rotating collector. The patterned collectors have thin conductive wires separated from one another by an air gap. During the process, the fibers are deposited either between or perpendicular to the wires, individually, achieving some degree of alignment. Properly aligned polymer fibers are mostly useful in tissue engineering. In the rotating type of patterned collector, operation at lower speeds deposits fibers between the conductive wires, while deposits at the higher speed are dependent on electrostatic and mechanical forces increasing the degree of alignment. For research purposes, different designs of collectors have been used, including: mesh [72], pin [73], grids [74], liquid bath [75,76], rotating rods [77], rotating cylinder [78], parallel bars [77], rotating drum with wire wound on it [79], and disc [34,80].

4. Methods of Incorporating Drugs

Electrospinning is easy and cost effective, and it offers great flexibility in selecting materials, high loading capacity and high encapsulation efficiency, which makes it suitable for medical and drug-related research. There are various methods of drug loading in the polymeric solution for electrospinning.

4.1. Blending

Blending is the primary method for incorporating drugs into the polymer solution by dissolving or dispersing the drug and then subsequently electrospinning. Though this method is simple and easy, the physicochemical properties of the drug and the polymer need to be precisely considered, as these affect the encapsulation efficiency, the drug distribution in the fiber and the kinetics of the drug release. Lipophilic drugs (e.g., paclitaxel) should be dissolved in a lipophilic polymer and hydrophilic drugs (e.g., doxorubicin hydrochloride) in a hydrophilic polymer for better encapsulation. When the drug is not dissolved properly in the polymer solution, a dispersion is obtained, which might lead to burst release if the drug migrates to the fiber surface [81]. To obtain a sustained release of the drug from the electrospun fibers, in order to enhance the drug-loading efficiency and to reduce the burst release, different combinations of the mixtures of hydrophilic and hydrophobic polymers are used [82–84]. This process was modified by Ma et al. to obtain highly porous chitosan nanofibers by electrospinning chitosan/polyethylene oxide (PEO) blend solutions and then removing PEO with water [85]. They then soaked the porous nanofibers in 0.1 wt% paclitaxel solution to load the drug, and then into 4 wt% hyaluronic acid for encapsulation. Mickova et al. have compared electrospinning of a liposome by blending and by coaxial electrospinning and have reported that blend electrospinning could not conserve intact nanofibers [86].

4.2. Surface Modification

Surface modification is the technique in which the therapeutic agent is bound or conjugated to the fiber surface to make it structurally and biochemically similar to the tissue. The drug release in this case will be attenuated, and the functionality of the biomolecules will be protected [87]. The burst release and short-term release will be mitigated with this strategy, making it highly applicable for slow and prolonged delivery of gene or growth factors. Incorporation of DNA, growth factors and enzymes, conjugated to fibers, preserves their bioactivity and functionality [87–90]. The modulation of drug release can also be obtained if surface modification is done on blended electrospun fibers. Im et al. fluorinated the electrospun fibers to obtain controlled release of the drug by introducing a hydrophobic group onto the surface [91]. In one modification, Yun et al. oxyfluorinated the multi-walled carbon nanotubes (MWCNTs) to introduce the functional groups and improve the compatibility with the PVA/polyacrylic acid (PAA) polymer solution before electrospinning the composite mixture [92]. Kim et al. surface modified the fiber and loaded it with small-interfering RNA (siRNA) to obtain better results in gene silencing and wound healing [93]. Co-axial electrospinning encapsulates biomolecules like DNA into the fiber, in contrast to surface localization of DNA fibers with the blending process. Luu et al. reported that the transfection efficiency of electrospun DNA was significantly lower than Fugene 6, a commercially available transfection mediation agent [94]. To overcome the drawback, the electrospinning method was changed to coaxial to get a polymer coating around the biomolecules, which not only modified the release, but also protected the core against the direct exposure to the environment [60,62,95]. For additional benefits, the shell polymer can also be loaded with other bioactive molecules, such as non-viral gene-delivery vectors, for delivering the released DNA [62].

4.3. Emulsion

Another approach is the process of forming an emulsion for electrospinning, where the drug or the protein solution is emulsified within a polymer solution. The latter acts as an oil phase, and spinning such an emulsion produces a well-distributed fiber for a low molecular weight drug [96] and a core-shell for a high molecular weight drug [97–99]. The success of this process is mainly dependent on the ratio of the aqueous solution to the polymer solution. This governs the distribution behavior of the molecule in fiber, which in turn determines the release profile, structural stability and bioactivity of the encapsulated biomolecules [97]. As the drug and the polymers are dissolved in appropriate solvents, avoiding the need of a common solvent, various combinations of hydrophilic drugs and lipophilic polymer can be used. Unlike coaxial spinning, emulsion spinning might damage macromolecules, such as pDNA, due to shearing force and interfacial tension between the two phases. Such instances can be avoided by preventing denaturation by the condensation of pDNA [98,99].

4.4. Multi-Drug Delivery

Multi-drug delivery is a recent approach in which multiple drugs with or without similar therapeutic effects are combined and electrospun with suitable polymer(s) [100,101]. Wang et al. have used drug-loaded polymeric nanoparticles for the core and drug-loaded polymer for the sheath to obtain a chain-like structure with a distinct release behavior, enabling a program or temporality release of multiple agents [100]. Xu et al. have developed a hydrophilic model of bovine serum albumin (BSA) drug-loaded chitosan microspheres and suspended them in poly(l-lactic acid) (PLLA) solution with a hydrophobic model drug (benzoin) and polyvinylpyrrolidone (PVP) as a release tuner [101]. It is difficult to achieve independent release of the drugs in a multidrug system, as both drugs are held by the carrier, which provides the same diffusion pathways and matrix-degradation rate [95]. Okuda et al. have developed a multilayered drug-loaded electrospun nanofiber mesh fabricated for time-programmed dual release by sequential electrospinning. The formulation has four layers: the drug-loaded mesh (the top layer), the barrier mesh (blank polymer), the second drug-loaded mesh and the last basement mesh. This system provided for the development of electrospun fibers with controlled drug release and time of release by optimizing the fiber size, thickness of each layer and relative position of the layer. Though the authors have used two dyes as model drugs, this approach is significant for the biochemical modulation in chemotherapy with multiple-anti tumor drugs [102]. A graphical presentation of the same is shown in Figure 5.

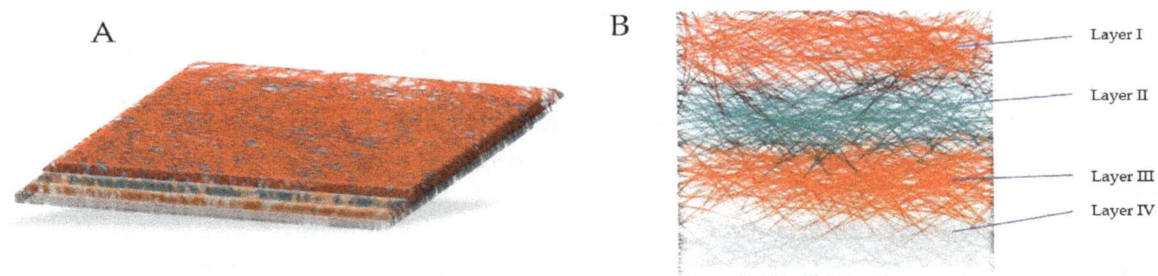

Figure 5. Graphical presentation of multi-drug delivery system: (**A**) overview; (**B**) cross sectional view of a tetra-layered sequential electrospun mesh. Cross-sectional view consists of drug loaded mesh (layer I), barrier mesh (layer II), second drug loaded mesh (layer III) and basement mesh (layer IV). Redrawn from [102].

4.5. Multilayer Coated

Yet another innovative method of incorporation and delivery of drug combines the large surface area of electrospun fibers with polyelectrolyte multilayer structures [95]. Such a multilayer uses either electrostatic or hydrogen bonding or acid-base pairing in layer-by-layer adsorption of polymers [103]. Chundar et al. have used two oppositely charged weak polyelectrolytes, polyacrylic acid (PAA) and poly allylamine hydrochloride (PAH), to produce nanofibers loaded with methylene blue as a model drug. In addition to polymers, a hydrophobic layer of perfluorosilane and PAA/poly(N-isopropylacrylamide) (PNIPAAM) was coated. The latter also provided temperature-controlled drug-release properties. Im et al. used alginate and chitosan to coat the lactobacillus-incorporated polyvinyl alcohol-based electrospun fibers. This formulation was designed to release lactobacillus in the large intestine after chitosan and alginate were dissolved in the acidic and then neutral environments of the GIT [104].

5. Electrospun Nanofibers in Drug Delivery

The electrospinning process has been used in drug delivery for treating various diseases. Electrospun fibers are administered mainly via oral and topical routes and as implantable systems.

5.1. Vitamins, NSAIDS and Natural Products

The transdermal drug delivery system (TDDS) delivers the drugs locally or systemically via the skin. This is mainly suitable for drugs that cannot be taken by the oral route, either because of extensive degradation in the GIT or because the drug undergoes extensive first pass metabolism [105]. Electrospun fibers of vitamins, anti-inflammatory and antioxidant drugs are mainly given by transdermal route [92,106–111]. Taepaiboon et al. have loaded vitamin A acid (all-*trans* retinoic acid) and vitamin E (α-tocopherol) in cellulose acetate polymer-based electrospun fibers and solvent cast films [110]. The results obtained revealed that the electrospun fiber mats showed a gradual and consistent increase in the cumulative vitamin release assayed using a total immersion technique over the test period of 24 h for vitamin E- and 6 h for vitamin A-loaded fiber. The corresponding solvent cast films showed a burst release of vitamins. A similar study performed by Nagwhirunpat et al. compared the electrospun and solvent cast film of polyvinyl alcohol loaded with meloxicam, an anti-arthritis drug [111]. They observed significantly higher skin permeation flux of the drug from electrospun fiber mats than with the solvent cast film, and the flux increased with an increase in drug concentration in both cases. Yun et al. developed an electro-responsive TDDS fiber by electrospinning poly(vinyl alcohol)/poly(acrylic acid)/multi-walled carbon nanotubes (PVA/PAA/MWCNT) with ketoprofen. The swelling, drug-release properties and conductivity of nanofibers were dependent upon the MWCNT, oxyfluorination and oxygen content during oxyfluorination [92]. The fibers were found to be non-toxic and biocompatible, with cell viability of more than 80%. In a similar study, Im et al. worked to understand the effect of MWCNT on ketoprofen delivery in an electro-sensitive

TDDS with polyethylene oxide and pentaerythritol triacrylate polymers [109]. This study supported the impact of MWCNT in influencing conductivity and drug-release behavior. Reda et al. formulated ketoprofen-loaded Eudragit® L and Eudragit® S electrospun nanofibers for treating oral mucositis. The rapid evaporation of solvent during electrospinning prevented the drug molecules from forming crystalline aggregates within the nanofibers. In addition, the amount of ketoprofen released from nanofibers was significantly higher than that released from corresponding solvent-casted films. Furthermore, a marked reduction in inflammatory infiltrate was seen in mucositis-induced rabbits with developed nanofibers [112]. Apart from the synthetic chemicals, a natural/herbal extract containing asiaticoside from *Centella asiatica* was incorporated into the electrospun fibers based on cellulose acetate polymer [106]. Suwantong et al. used two forms of the drug, pure asiaticoside and a crude extract from the plant. They observed a better release profile from the pure drug than from the extract assayed using the immersion method, while the release from both fiber mats was significantly low in the pigskin method. In addition, they checked the release profile of the solvent cast films, which were much lower. They further reported that the extract-loaded fibers and films were toxic to normal human dermal fibroblasts at the extraction concentrations of 5 and 10 mg/mL [106].

5.2. Antibiotics/Antibacterial Agents and Wound Dressing

In recent years, antibiotics and antibacterial agents have been the most common drug molecules that are encapsulated, using different polymers and their combinations as carriers. Different polymers, such as PLA, PLGA and PCL, are primarily used in the polymeric electrospun fibers for biodegradability, and other natural and synesthetic hydrophilic or hydrophobic polymers are used to control the release pattern of the drug. Kenaway et al. used tetracycline hydrochloride with poly(ethylene-co-vinyl acetate) (PEVA), PLA and their 50:50 blend to deliver the drug for treating periodontal disease [113]. They reported over five days of release with PEVA and the blend, suggesting their applicability in controlled-release technology. In another study by Alhusein et al., electrospun fibers of tetracycline HCl using PCL and PEVA were developed for potential application in wound healing and skin-structure infections. The developed three-layered electrospun matrix showed controlled release and also higher antibacterial efficacy when compared to the commercially available test disks of the drug [114]. The same group of researchers also reported high biological activity of the developed fiber matrices in complex models of biofilm formation. The fibers killed preformed biofilms and mature dense colonies of *Staphylococcus aureus* MRSA252 and also inhibited the formation of new biofilms [115]. Wang et al. have electrospun PVA nanofibers containing pleurocidin, a novel, broad-spectrum antimicrobial peptide, for food preservation applications [116]. Direct application of the active moiety is not possible because of the loss in its bioactivity. This study reported higher inhibition efficacy of the drug from nanofibers against *Escherichia coli* in apple cider.

Wound dressings protect the wound from external microorganisms and absorb/adsorb the exudate from the wound, providing an acceptable cosmetic appearance. The use of different components in the wound dressing prevents infection of the wound and accelerates the healing process [117]. The components added to the inert dressings are mainly bioactives in the form of films, hydrogels, foams and sponges [84]. With respect to wound healing, electrospun fiber mats have the advantage of high surface area for efficient absorption of exudates; in addition to adjusting the moisture of the wound and promoting scar-free regeneration of skin cells, these mats have porosity enough to supply oxygen for cell respiration, yet not enough for bacterial infections [58,117,118]. In one study by Jannesari et al., electrospun nanofibers of poly(vinyl alcohol) and poly(vinyl acetate) were prepared individually and in a 50:50 blend of the polymers. The nanofibers prepared using the polymer blend sustained the drug release and were found to be comfortable due to significant swelling [84]. In an in vitro microbial study, Said et al. have shown a faster bacterial colonization and biofilm formation in fusidic acid-loaded PLGA fibers, which in turn enhanced the release of the drug, eradicated planktonic bacteria and suppressed the biofilm [119]. Thakur et al. used the dual spinneret electrospinning apparatus to prepare a single scaffold of lidocaine and mupirocin [120]. Two drugs with varying lipophilicities were found to have different release profiles. Lidocaine showed a burst release, while mupirocin showed sustained release, providing action for over 72 h. Wang et al. have fabricated nanofibers of ethylene-co-vinyl alcohol (EVOH) with different antibacterial drugs and silver for wound dressings with superior germ killing capacity [121]. Silver nanoparticles have been used in many other studies for similar applications [66,122]. Recently, Chutipakdeevong et al. have utilized the hybridization method to combine the properties of *Bombyx mori* silk fibroin with poly(ε-caprolactone) (PCL) electrospun fibers [123]. The PCL fiber surfaces were coated with silk fibroin protein using the lyophilization technique and then surface modified with fibronectin to improve their biological function. The surface-modified hybrid showed significant proliferation of normal human dermal fibroblast (NHDF), followed by hybrid scaffold and then neat PCL fibers.

5.3. Delivery of Anticancer Agents

Anticancer agents, such as doxorubicin, paclitaxel, cisplatin and dichloroacetate, have been incorporated into electrospun fibers with polymers such as PLA, PLGA and PLLA for postoperative chemotherapy. A water-in-oil (*w/o*) emulsion, with water soluble drugs in aqueous phase and polymeric solutions of PEG-PLA in chloroform as oily phase, was prepared and electrospun to obtain fibers [124]. In a continuation study, hydrophobic paclitaxel and hydrophilic doxorubicin were simultaneously loaded in the emulsion based electrospinning process for multi-drug delivery [125]. The cytotoxicity study of rat Glioma C6 cells showed higher inhibition and apoptosis in combination therapy compared to the single-drug system. In another study, an in vitro cytotoxicity study of the same cells showed a sustained release of platinum-based cisplatin for more than 75 days without burst release and four times better cytotoxicity than the free drug [126]. Lee et al. have fabricated biodegradable PLGA fibers sheets for local delivery of epigallocatechin-3-O-gallate (EGCG) to reduce intimal hyperplasia in injured abdominal aorta [116]. The EGCG-loaded sheets exhibited initial burst release for 24 h, followed by sustained release for more than 30 days in phosphate buffer. In vivo studies showed promising results against intimal hyperplasia after application of the EGCG-loaded fibers, compared to PLGA control.

Recently, electrospun fibers have been used for local chemotherapy. Liu et al. encapsulated doxorubicin in PLLA polymer fiber and examined its efficacy for local chemotherapy against secondary hepatic carcinoma by wrapping the whole liver with carcinoma with the fiber-mat [127]. In the first 24 h, the drug was rapidly released from the fiber to localize in the liver tissue. It also significantly inhibited the tumor growth and increased the median survival time of the mice in the experiment. Luo et al. prepared fibers with core-loaded hydroxycamptothecin (HCPT) and 2-hydroxypropyl-β-cyclodextrin complexed HCPT, and observed that the inclusion complex showed superior antitumor activity and fewer side effects compared to the free drug [128]. Ma et al. loaded paclitaxel in the porous chitosan nanofiber and then encapsulated the fiber in polyanionic macromolecular hyaluronic acid (HA). The MTT assay in prostate cancer cells showed that the drug-loaded nanofiber mats were good at prohibiting cell attachment and proliferation [129]. The drawback of the fibers was an initial burst release of drug within the first 48 h. Chen et al. incorporated titanocene dichloride in PLLA polymer-based fibers [130]. The MTT assay in human lung tumor (SPCA-1) cells showed that drug contents of 40, 80, 160 and 240 mg/L had cell growth inhibition rates of 11.2%, 22.1%, 44.2% and 68.2%, respectively. Apart from the synthetic anticancer drug, natural products with anticancer properties and minimal side effects have been studied. Suwantong et al. electrospun curcumin in cellulose acetate solution and observed that curcumin is almost completely (~90 to ~95%) released in the total immersion method, while considerably low values were obtained for transdermal diffusion through pig skin [108]. In another study, Shao et al. fabricated green tea polyphenols (GTP) in poly(ε-caprolactone)/multi-walled carbon nanotube (PCL/MWCNTs) composite nanofibers by electrospinning. The cytotoxicity experiment showed a significant inhibitory effect in A549 and Hep G2 tumor cells [131]. Table 1 provides a compilation of studies involving the use of electrospun fibers in delivering antibiotics, anticancer agents and NSAIDS.

Table 1. Studies involving the use of electrospun fibers in drug delivery (partial listing).

Drug(s)	Polymer(s)	Solvent Composition	Spraying Type
	Antibacterial agents		
Tetracycline hydrochloride	PEUU and PLGA [71]; PLA, PEV, PLA/PEVA [113]; PLA/PCL [132] PLLA [133,134]; PCL, PEVA [114]	1,1,1,3,3,3-Hexafluoro-2-propanol [71]; Chloroform [113]; Chloroform, dimethylformamide [132]; Chloroform: acetone (2:1) [133,134]; chloroform:methanol (9:1) [114]	Single nozzle; Coaxial [133,134]
Gentamycin sulfate and Resveratrol (antioxidant)	PCL [133]	Chloroform: ethanol (3:1)	Coaxial
Ciprofloxacin Hydrochloride	PVA, Poly(vinyl acetate) [84]	Diluted acetic acid solution	Single nozzle
Fusidic acid and rifampicin	PLGA [135]	Tetrahydro Furan/Dimethylformamide	Single nozzle
Mefoxin	PLGA [83]	DMF	Single nozzle
Metronidazole benzoate	PCL [136]	Dichloromethane (DCM:DMF)	Single nozzle
Ciprofloxacin hydrochloride, Levofloxacin hemihydrate, Moxifloxacin hydrochloride	coPLA, coPLA/PEG [137]	DCM:DMSO (3:1)	Single nozzle
Lidocaine and mupirocin	PLLA [120]	Hexafluoroisopropanol	Dual spinneret
Ornidazole (Biteral®)	PCL	Chloroform and DMF (3:7)	Single nozzle
Potassium 5-nitro-8-quinolinolate	Chitosan/PEO [138]	2% (*w*/*v*) acetic acid	Single nozzle
Itraconazole and ketanserin	PU [139]	DMF, DMAc	Single nozzle
Pleurocidin	PVA [116]	Distilled water	Single nozzle
	NSAIDS		
Ketoprofen	PVA/PAA/MWCNT [92]; PEO/PETA/MWCNT [109]; EC and PVP [140]; PVP/Zein [141]	Deionized water [92,109] Ethanol-water [140,141]	Single nozzle Coaxial [141]
Ibuprofen	PLGA PEG-g-CHN [142]	DMF	Side-by-side
Fenbufen	PLGA/Gelatin [82]	2,2,2-trifluoroethanol	Single nozzle
Rhodamine B/Naproxen	Chitosan nanoparticles/PCL composite [100]	Acetic acid/chloroform: methanol (3:1)	Single nozzle yet core/sheath fiber
Meloxicam	PVA [111]	Water	Single nozzle

Table 1. *Cont.*

Drug(s)	Polymer(s)	Solvent Composition	Spraying Type
Anticancer agents			
Doxorubicin [127] Doxorubicin Hydrochloride	PLLA [127] PEG-PLA [124,143]	Chloroform-methano-DMSO [127] Chloroform [143] w/o emulsion [124]	Single nozzle Emulsion [124]
Hydroxycamptothecin	HPCD [128]	DMSO	Emulsion
Paclitaxel	Chitosan/PEO/HA [84] PLGA [144,145]	Acetic acid/distilled water [84] DCM and DMF	Single nozzle
Cisplatin	PLA/PLGA [126]	DCM	Single nozzle
Dichloroacetate	PLA [146]	Chloroform	Single nozzle
1,3-Bis(2-chloroethyl)-1-nitrosourea	PEO and PEG-PLLA [147]	Chloroform	Single nozzle/Emulsion
Curcumin	Cellulose acetate [108]	Acetone/dimethylacetamide (2:1)	Single nozzle
Green tea polyphenols (GTP)	PCL/MWCNT [131]	Dichloromethane	Single nozzle
Titanocene dichloride	PLLA [130]	Dichloromethane	Single nozzle

PLA: Poly(lactic acid); PEVA-Poly(ethylene-co-vinylacetate); PCL: poly(ε-caprolactone); PCL-co-PCLEEP: Copolymer of caprolactone and ethyl ethylene phosphate; PLGA: Poly(D,L-Lactic acid-co-glycolic acid); PEUU: poly(ester urethane) urea; EC: ethyl cellulose; PEO: Poly(ethylene oxide); PU: Polyurethane; DMAc: Dimethylacetamide; PETA: pentaerythritol triacrylate; PEI-HA: Poly(ethylenimine)-hyaluronic acid; PVP: polyvinylpyrrolidone; PEG-g-CHN: poly(ethylene glycol)-g-Chitosan; PEG-PLA: poly(ethylene glycol)-poly(lactic acid); PLLA: poly(L-lactic acid); HPCD: 2-hydroxypropyl-β-cyclodextrin; HA: Hyaluronic acid; MWCNT: multi-walled carbon nanotubes, PAA–Poly(acrylic acid); PECCL: poly(ethylene carbonate-ε-caprolactone); PDLLA: poly(D,L-lactic acid).

5.4. DNA, RNA, Protein and Growth Factor Delivery

The most commonly loaded bioactive materials in electrospun fibers include DNA, RNA, proteins and growth factors. The electrospinning process applied to the bioactive materials should be designed in such a way that the activity and functional efficacy of the material is preserved during and after electrospinning. Before coaxial electrospinning, few studies on bioactive materials had been done with the blending process. The stability of the growth factors is the limiting aspect in formulating them in tissue-engineered scaffolds. Human nerve growth factor (hNGF) was encapsulated with BSA as a carrier protein into the nanofibers of PCL and poly(ethyl ethylene phosphate) (PCLEEP). The protein released in a sustained manner for more than three months from the electrospun fibers and showed partial retention of bioactivity [148]. The same group also co-encapsulated small-interfering RNA (siRNA) and transfection reagent (TKO) complexes within a nanofiber of caprolactone and ethyl ethylene phosphate (PCLEEP, diameter ~400 nm) to obtain a sustained release of siRNA for up to 28 days [149]. The release of siRNA was enhanced and more significant gene knockdown was obtained when compared with electrospun fibers of PCL containing siRNA [150]. Schneider et al. demonstrated that biofunctionalized silk mats containing epidermal growth factor (EGF) are extremely promising in achieving bioactive wound dressings for the wound healing process [151]. Similarly, Zhang et al. showed that the poly(ethylene carbonate-ε-caprolactone) scaffolds with VEGF maintained good growth and spread morphology in human umbilical vein endothelial cells [152]. After the introduction of the coaxial electrospinning method, most biomolecules are preferentially encapsulated using this method, forming a core of biomolecule and shell of polymer in a core-shell structure. The polymeric shell protected and released biomolecules in a sustained manner. Saraf et al. prepared fiber scaffolds with plasmid DNA (pDNA) within the core of poly(ethylene glycol) and non-viral gene delivery vector poly(ethylenimine)-hyaluronic acid (PEI-HA) within the sheath polymer poly(ε-caprolactone) (PCL) by coaxial electrospinning [62]. They achieved variable transfection activity over extended periods of time upon the release of pDNA and non-viral gene delivery vectors from electrospun fiber scaffolds. Mickova et al. have proposed the use of liposomes in the core of polyvinyl alcohol (PVA) and shell of PCL for protecting the enzymatic activity of horseradish peroxidase [86]. The encapsulated enzyme retained its activity because of the shielding effect of the lipid sphere of liposome. Chen et al. encapsulated chitosan/siRNA nanoparticles in PLGA by electrospinning to control the release behavior at different pH conditions. In addition, the encapsulated siRNA showed up to 50% enhanced green fluorescent protein (EGFP) gene silencing activity after 48 h of transfection in H1299 cells [143]. Surface functionalization of nanofibers was performed for MMP-2-siRNA (Matrix metalloproteinase) in linear polyethyleneimine (LPEI) coated nanofibers with various nitrogen/phosphate (N/P) ratios [93]. In an animal study for seven days, it was observed that the siRNA in these fibers increased the MMP-2 gene silencing effect and neo-collagen accumulation at the wound site. Fabrication of surface modified electrospun fibers containing growth factors conjugated with heparin or polysaccharides is becoming common [87,89,153]. A burst release of nerve growth factor was observed from electrospun scaffolds conjugated with chitosan/poly(vinyl alcohol) [89]. Basic fibroblast growth factor was incorporated in heparin containing a polyelectrolyte nanoparticle, and that was electrostatically adsorbed on the chitosan matrix to overcome the problem of burst release [87]. Han et al. fabricated a composite design containing poly(ethylene glycol)-poly-(ε-caprolactone) diacrylate (PEGPCL) hydrogels coupled with electrospun mats of poly(ε-caprolactone) to control the burst release and to extend the release duration of nerve growth factor [154]. The bioactivity of the growth factor was demonstrated by PC-12 cells' neurite extension. Further, immobilization and delivery of the growth factor for the bone tissue engineering is discussed in the review by Chen and Lv [155]. In addition, electrospinning has extensively been used and reviewed for tissue scaffold engineering with or without any active moiety incorporated in the polymeric matrix. Table 2 provides a list of studies involving the use of electrospun fibers in delivering proteins, DNA, RNA and human factors.

5.5. Nanoparticle Impregnated Nanofibers

Electrospun nanofibers containing nanoparticles is another area of research that has been widely investigated for various applications, including surface-enhanced Raman scattering [156], antimicrobial packaging [157], dye-sensitized solar cells [158], food preservation [159], biowarfare decontamination [160], water treatment [161], high-performance gas sensing [162], and environmental remediation [163]. In drug delivery, these novel impregnated nanofibers are being explored in the areas of wound care, regenerative medicine, dental engineering, and for cancer treatment. In this section, we briefly summarized biomedical applications of nanoparticle impregnated nanofibers.

A study conducted by Lee et al. investigated the efficacy of chitosan (CTS) nanofibers containing silver nanoparticles for topical wound care. Silver nanoparticles were generated directly in the chitosan solution by chemical reduction using sodium borohydride. The nanoparticle solution obtained was then poured into sodium hydroxide resulting in the formation of CTS/AgNPs composite, which was further subjected to electrospinning to form nanofibers. The prepared fibers showed excellent antibacterial activity against *P. aeruginosa* and methicillin-resistant *S. aureus* when compared to the pure CTS nanofibers [164]. Similarly, Shi et al. prepared Ag/polyacrylonitrile (Ag/PAN) anti-bacterial nanofibers for use in implant scaffolds and biotextiles. Initially, PAN was dissolved in DMF and a known amount of $AgNO_3$ was added to form the pre-electrospinning solution. The solution was then treated using helium atmospheric plasma to reduce $AgNO_3$ into metallic silver nanoparticles. Finally, the solution obtained was electrospun to form nanofibers containing embedded Ag nanoparticles. SEM images revealed the smooth and continuous nature of the nanofibers. The nanofibers demonstrated a sustained release of silver ions and also showed higher antibacterial activity against Gram positive (*B. cereus*) and Gram negative bacteria (*E. coli*) when compared to the untreated nanofibers [165]. Another study conducted by Castro-Mayorga et al., investigated the antiviral properties of Ag nanoparticles in coated polyhydroxyalkonates. The films of poly(3-hydroxybutyrate-co-3-hydroxyvalerate) (PHBV) were developed by depositing a coat of electrospun fiber mat containing post-processed PHBV18/Ag nanoparticles over PHBV3 films formed by compression molding. Energy dispersive X-ray (EDX) analysis showed that Ag nanoparticles were homogeneously distributed into the coating and on the PHBV3/PHBV18 film. Moreover, cell culture analysis revealed no infectious feline calicivirus (FCV) recovery when treated with the prepared films, while murine norovirus (MNV) was decreased by 0.86 log [166].

Nie and Wang studied the complex of DNA and poly lactide-co-glycolide (PLGA)/hydroxyapatite (HAp) composite scaffolds fabricated by electrospinning for their use in bone tissue engineering. DNA was incorporated into the scaffolds in the form of naked DNA or DNA/chitosan nanoparticles before/after fiber fabrication. The results revealed that the scaffolds were non-woven and predominantly composed of PLGA with a dispersion of HAp nanoparticles. The addition of HAp nanoparticles showed an increase in the release rate of DNA from the scaffolds containing both naked and encapsulated DNA. Moreover, the scaffolds with encapsulated DNA/chitosan nanoparticles also showed a higher cell attachment, greater cell viability and desired transfection efficiency in human marrow stem cells (hMSCs) [167]. A similar study conducted by Tanaka and co-workers fabricated hydroxyapatite/PLA composite electrospun nanofibers for bone tissue engineering. The surface-modified HAp nanoparticles of stearic acid were dispersed uniformly in the PLA nanofibers and were evaluated for their mechanical strength. The authors concluded that the electrospun fibers showed higher strength when compared to the unmodified ones [168]. Table 3 provides a partial listing of studies involving the use of electrospun fibers in tissue engineering.

Table 2. Studies involving the use of electrospun fibers in delivery of proteins, DNA, RNA and human factors (partial listing).

Drug(s)	Polymer(s)	Solvent Composition	Spraying Type
plasmid DNA (pDNA)	PEI-HA [62]		Coaxial
siRNA	PCL [150]; PCLEEP [149] Chitosan/PLGA [169]	2,2,2-Trifluoroethanol (TFE) [150]; RNase-free water [149]; Hexafluoro-2-isopropanol/water [169]	Single nozzle
Human glial cell-derived neurotrophic factor	PCL-co-PCLEEP [170]	Dichloromethane	Single nozzle
Human β-nerve growth factor	PCL-co-PCLEEP [148]	Dichloromethane	Single nozzle
Endothelial growth factor VEGF	PECCL [152]	-	Single nozzle
Bovine Serum Albumin (BSA)	PEO [171]	Deionized water	Single nozzle
Lysozyme	PLA [97]	Chloroform	Emulsion
Human-nerve growth factor (NGF)	Poly(L-lactide-co-caprolactone) [172]	Chloroform	Emulsion
DNA	PLA-PEG and PLGA [94]	DMF	Single nozzle
Growth factors (VEGF, PDGF)	Poly(urethane) [63]	Chloroform: ethanol (75:25)	Coaxial
Horseradish peroxidase	PVA/PCL [86]	-	Coaxial

Table 3. Studies involving the use of electrospun fibers in tissue engineering (partial listing).

Drug(s)	Polymer(s)	Solvent Composition	Spraying Type
Wound healing, tissue engineering, hemostatic agent	Collagen-PEO [173,174]	Hydrochloric acid	Single nozzle
Adenovirus with gene for green fluorescent protein	Poly(ε-caprolactone) [60]	Chloroform: ethanol (75:25)	Coaxial
Guided tissue regeneration	PDLLA/PLGA [175]	Chloroform:DMF (9:1) and THF/DMF (3:1)	Single nozzle

Liposome-enriched nanofibers were investigated for delivering and preserving horseradish peroxidase (HRP) enzymatic activity. Liposomes were prepared using soybean derived L-α-phosphatidylcholine encapsulating horseradish peroxidase (HRP) by the extrusion technique. This study compared the activity of HRP in nanofibers developed by coaxial or blend electrospinning with and without liposomes. Blend nanofibers were prepared by electrospinning unilamellar liposomes dispersed in an aqueous solution of PVA and nanofibers, while the coaxial nanofibers were developed using PVA-core/PCL-shell with embedded liposomes. The results indicate that the blending of liposomes could not conserve the intact liposomes, while the nanofibers obtained by coaxial electrospinning retained liposomes. In addition, the core/shell nanofibers not only preserved the activity of encapsulated HRP enzyme but also enhanced the proliferation of mesenchymal stem cells (MSC) [86].

Poly (L-lactic acid-co-ε-caprolactone) (PLACL) nanofibers containing magnesium oxide (MgO) nanoparticles in synergy with aloe vera (AV), curcumin (CUR) and β-cyclodextrin (β-CD) were prepared and evaluated for treating breast cancer. In vitro toxicity of electrospun nanofibers composed of PLACL; PLACL with AV; PLACL with AV and MgO; PLACL with AV, MgO and CUR; and PLACL with AV, MgO, and β-CD was assessed in MCF-7 cells using the MTT assay. The results showed that PLACL nanofibers containing CUR showed the greatest cell death among all other nanofibrous scaffolds. However, PLACL nanofibers without MgO nanoparticles exhibited greatest tensile strength [176]. Sperm-shaped microrobots were studied for targeting breast cancer cells in vitro using fabricated nanoparticles. The microrobots were fabricated using electrospinning by a solution composed of polystyrene, dimethylformamide and nanoparticles of iron oxide. Under the influence of an oscillating magnetic field, the robotic sperm could controllably take S-shaped, U-shaped, square paths and selectively target the MCF-7 cells. Moreover, the cell membrane was not damaged after penetration of the robotic sperm into the cancerous cells [177].

Electrospun nanofibers composed of poly (ε-caprolactone) (PCL) and zero valent zinc nanoparticles were investigated by Sezer et al. to promote neuroglial cell proliferation. Chemical characterization studies indicated that the nanoparticles did not interact chemically with the PCL matrix. In addition, the nanofibers enhanced the tensile strength of the PCL matrix and promoted cell proliferation depending on the amount of zinc nanoparticles embedded inside the PCL matrix [178]. Another study investigated the efficiency of electrospun hybrid scaffolds composed of cyclosporine-loaded PLGA nanoparticles embedded in PCL scaffolds for promoting innervation of bioengineered teeth. The results from histological studies showed that the implantation of designed scaffolds in adult ICR mice did not alter the development of teeth. In addition, the transmission electron microscopy (TEM) and indirect immunofluorescence studies showed that 88% of the teeth were innervated upon treating with designed hybrid scaffolds [179].

6. Commercialization Challenges of Electrospinning

Although the benefits of electrospinning have been largely demonstrated in various fields of science, there is still a great need to implement the production in an efficient way. Several challenges relating to the electrospinning process are yet to be addressed. These include: (a) large-scale manufacturing; (b) accuracy and reproducibility during all the fabrication steps; and, (c) safety and environmental aspects of electrospinning [45]. The major challenges involved in mass production of electrospun fibers include low output per spinneret, clogging of the spinneret tip, inter-jet interference, recovery of vaporized solvents involved in the process, and fiber alignment over a large area of substantial thickness. To produce electrospun nanofibers without any morphology defects, the solution concentration is kept to a minimum, with solvent making up more than 70% of the solution mass. Therefore, only a fraction of the solution passing through the spinneret actually contributes to the mass of the nanofiber produced [180]. Also, there is a limit on the feed-rate per nozzle and higher rates might result in dripping of the solution from the nozzle, especially if the nozzle is placed in the middle. This is due to the insufficient electric field experienced by the nozzles, which results in inadequate drawing of the solution.

Clogging of the spinneret due to the solution gelation is highly disruptive and causes production losses. This problem is more apparent with solutions of higher concentration, as they are more viscous [181] and with polymers of high degree of crystallinity [182]. In addition, a solvent with low boiling point also causes clogging of the spinneret tip [183]. While the productivity of the microfiber spinning process can be increased by placing many spinnerets per spinning head, this is not feasible in the case of electrospinning. In electrospinning, the ejected solution spreads out to form an expanding cone and it interferes with the neighboring jets if the spinnerets are packed too close to each other [68]. Uniformity in the fiber layer thickness deposited onto substrate material is also comprised by the inter-jet interference [180].

Another important concern is regarding the solvent used in the electrospinning process. This particular issue is highly important not only for safety reasons during fabrication, but also for the final products, as solvent residues might be trapped inside the electrospun nanofibers. Accurate control over solvent residues becomes crucial in the case of large-volume, solvent-based electrospinning for biomedical and pharmaceutical applications [45]. However, the use of solvent-free spinning should eliminate the risk of solvent residues and recovery of solvents [184]. Due to the lack of reliable and affordable electrospinning technologies, the use of many different active polymeric materials for the fabrication of nanofibers is still limited [45]. In tissue engineering, the other main challenges that impede the progress of electrospinning applications are increasing scaffold thickness and pore size. Moreover, it is highly difficult to produce identical scaffolds, especially between research groups, which narrows the use of electrospun fiber mats for tissue engineering applications. Also, with tailored electrospun fibers, it is challenging to ensure uniformity of the fibers with specific morphologies and properties [185].

The recent development of needleless electrospinning offers the possibility for fabricating electrospun nanofibers on a large scale and addresses the issue of clogging at the spinnerets [186]. Needleless electrospinning systems using rotating disks [187], rollers [188], balls [189], and bubbles [190] that produce huge amounts of nanofibers have been reported by a few researchers. This method involves the formation of numerous small droplets on the drum surface or disk/coil. Moreover, this method does not require the maintenance of Taylor cones throughout the process making it highly advantageous over conventional needle-based method. Nonetheless, this process consumes a lot of energy in order to maintain the high voltage required and thus increases the chance of spark generation in the system. Therefore, solvents with low flash points, such as chloroform, tetrahydrofuran (THF), and toluene cannot be used for needless electrospinning [182]. Another area where considerable progress has been made in recent years is the development of smart electrospun nanofibers. These nanofibers respond to various kinds of stimuli, including pH, ionic strength, temperature, light, electricity, and magnetic field, and undergo physical and/or chemical changes. Studies involving smart electrospun nanofibers, their advantages and shortcomings are detailed in recent review by Weng and Xie [191].

7. Conclusions

The electrospinning process has generated a lot of interest in various medical applications due to its ease of use, adaptability and flexibility in controlling the fiber diameter from the micrometer down to the nanometer range. Though this method has been in use for a few decades now, the techniques and the equipment used in the electrospinning process are ever-evolving. Electrospinning began with a single nozzle configuration and evolved into multi-nozzle configurations through coaxial and emulsion spinning configurations. Further studies are being carried out to modify the nozzle configuration and collector design in order to significantly improve fiber properties and simplify the manufacturing process. This review summarizes several key aspects of electrospinning in the use of electrospun fibers in drug delivery with a special emphasis on electrospun nanofibers impregnated with nanoparticles. Studies involving biomedical applications of electrospun nanofibers are also discussed. By careful selection of polymers, it is now possible to deliver various antibacterial agents and anticancer drugs in a required manner using electrospun nanofibers. In order to make further progress, particularly in the field of drug delivery, it is necessary to identify ways that allow large-scale fabrication of nanofibers with desired morphological and mechanical properties in a reproducible manner. Despite the relentless efforts being made by academic and industrial scientists, much of the research conducted with electrospun fibers is in vitro. Further progress in the field of electrospun nanofibers will require continued assessment in vivo. Scientists working in this field have to identify ways to use nanofibers for immunotherapy, gene therapy and regenerative medicine in order to meet the current, as well as any future, demands in drug delivery.

References

1. Nayak, R.; Padhye, R.; Kyratzis, I.L.; Truong, Y.; Arnold, L. Recent advances in nanofibre fabrication techniques. *Text. Res. J.* **2011**. [CrossRef]
2. Greiner, A.; Wendorff, J.H. Electrospinning: A fascinating method for the preparation of ultrathin fibers. *Angew. Chem. Int. Ed.* **2007**, *46*, 5670–5703. [CrossRef] [PubMed]
3. Reneker, D.H.; Yarin, A.L. Electrospinning jets and polymer nanofibers. *Polymer* **2008**, *49*, 2387–2425. [CrossRef]
4. Kiyohiko, H. Process for Manufacturing Artificial Silk and Other Filaments by Applying Electric Current. U.S. Patents No. US1699615A, 22 January 1929.
5. Huang, Z.-M.; Zhang, Y.-Z.; Kotaki, M.; Ramakrishna, S. A review on polymer nanofibers by electrospinning and their applications in nanocomposites. *Compos. Sci. Technol.* **2003**, *63*, 2223–2253. [CrossRef]
6. Sill, T.J.; von Recum, H.A. Electrospinning: Applications in drug delivery and tissue engineering. *Biomaterials* **2008**, *29*, 1989–2006. [CrossRef] [PubMed]
7. Taylor, G. Electrically driven jets. *Proc. R. Soc. Lond. A Math. Phys. Eng. Sci.* **1969**, *313*, 453–475. [CrossRef]
8. Yarin, A.; Koombhongse, S.; Reneker, D.H. Bending instability in electrospinning of nanofibers. *J. Appl. Phys.* **2001**, *89*, 3018–3026. [CrossRef]
9. Doshi, J.; Reneker, D.H. Electrospinning process and applications of electrospun fibers. *J. Electrost.* **1995**, *35*, 154–160. [CrossRef]
10. Yang, Q.; Li, Z.; Hong, Y.; Zhao, Y.; Qiu, S.; Wang, C.; Wei, Y. Influence of solvents on the formation of ultrathin uniform poly(vinyl pyrrolidone) nanofibers with electrospinning. *J. Polym. Sci. Part B Polym. Phys.* **2004**, *42*, 3721–3726. [CrossRef]
11. Shin, Y.; Hohman, M.; Brenner, M.; Rutledge, G. Electrospinning: A whipping fluid jet generates submicron polymer fibers. *Appl. Phys. Lett.* **2001**, *78*, 1149–1151. [CrossRef]
12. Jaeger, R.; Bergshoef, M.M.; Batlle, C.M.I.; Schönherr, H.; Julius Vancso, G. Electrospinning of ultra-thin polymer fibers. *Macromol. Symp.* **1998**, *127*, 141–150. [CrossRef]
13. Carson, R.; Hendricks, C.; Hogan, J.; Schneider, J. Factors influencing electrically sprayed liquids. *AIAA J.* **1964**, *2*, 1460–1461. [CrossRef]
14. Buchko, C.J.; Chen, L.C.; Shen, Y.; Martin, D.C. Processing and microstructural characterization of porous biocompatible protein polymer thin films. *Polymer* **1999**, *40*, 7397–7407. [CrossRef]
15. Deitzel, J.; Kleinmeyer, J.; Harris, D.; Tan, N.B. The effect of processing variables on the morphology of electrospun nanofibers and textiles. *Polymer* **2001**, *42*, 261–272. [CrossRef]
16. Reneker, D.H.; Chun, I. Nanometre diameter fibres of polymer, produced by electrospinning. *Nanotechnology* **1996**, *7*, 216. [CrossRef]
17. Zhang, C.; Yuan, X.; Wu, L.; Han, Y.; Sheng, J. Study on morphology of electrospun poly(vinyl alcohol) mats. *Eur. Polym. J.* **2005**, *41*, 423–432. [CrossRef]
18. Li, Z.; Wang, C. Effects of working parameters on electrospinning. In *One-Dimensional Nanostructures*; Springer: Berlin, Germany, 2013; pp. 15–28.
19. Megelski, S.; Stephens, J.S.; Chase, D.B.; Rabolt, J.F. Micro-and nanostructured surface morphology on electrospun polymer fibers. *Macromolecules* **2002**, *35*, 8456–8466. [CrossRef]
20. Kilic, A.; Oruc, F.; Demir, A. Effects of polarity on electrospinning process. *Text. Res. J.* **2008**, *78*, 532–539. [CrossRef]
21. Varesano, A.; Carletto, R.A.; Mazzuchetti, G. Experimental investigations on the multi-jet electrospinning process. *J. Mater. Process. Technol.* **2009**, *209*, 5178–5185. [CrossRef]

22. Zargham, S.; Bazgir, S.; Tavakoli, A.; Rashidi, A.S.; Damerchely, R. The effect of flow rate on morphology and deposition area of electrospun nylon 6 nanofiber. *J. Eng. Fibers Fabr.* **2012**, *7*, 42–49.
23. Bhardwaj, N.; Kundu, S.C. Electrospinning: A fascinating fiber fabrication technique. *Biotechnol. Adv.* **2010**, *28*, 325–347. [CrossRef] [PubMed]
24. Nurwaha, D.; Han, W.; Wang, X. Investigation of a new needleless electrospinning method for the production of nanofibers. *J. Eng. Fibers Fabr.* **2013**, *8*, 42–49.
25. Sukigara, S.; Gandhi, M.; Ayutsede, J.; Micklus, M.; Ko, F. Regeneration of Bombyx mori silk by electrospinning—Part 1: Processing parameters and geometric properties. *Polymer* **2003**, *44*, 5721–5727. [CrossRef]
26. Fong, H.; Chun, I.; Reneker, D. Beaded nanofibers formed during electrospinning. *Polymer* **1999**, *40*, 4585–4592. [CrossRef]
27. Baumgarten, P.K. Electrostatic spinning of acrylic microfibers. *J. Colloid Interface Sci.* **1971**, *36*, 71–79. [CrossRef]
28. Meechaisue, C.; Dubin, R.; Supaphol, P.; Hoven, V.P.; Kohn, J. Electrospun mat of tyrosine-derived polycarbonate fibers for potential use as tissue scaffolding material. *J. Biomater. Sci. Polym. Ed.* **2006**, *17*, 1039–1056. [CrossRef] [PubMed]
29. Koski, A.; Yim, K.; Shivkumar, S. Effect of molecular weight on fibrous PVA produced by electrospinning. *Mater. Lett.* **2004**, *58*, 493–497. [CrossRef]
30. Zhao, Y.; Yang, Q.; Lu, X.-F.; Wang, C.; Wei, Y. Study on correlation of morphology of electrospun products of polyacrylamide with ultrahigh molecular weight. *J. Polym. Sci. Part B Polym. Phys.* **2005**, *43*, 2190–2195. [CrossRef]
31. Lyons, J.; Li, C.; Ko, F. Melt-electrospinning part I: Processing parameters and geometric properties. *Polymer* **2004**, *45*, 7597–7603. [CrossRef]
32. Larrondo, L.; St John Manley, R. Electrostatic fiber spinning from polymer melts. I. Experimental observations on fiber formation and properties. *J. Polym. Sci. Polym. Phys. Ed.* **1981**, *19*, 909–920. [CrossRef]
33. Ding, B.; Kim, H.Y.; Lee, S.C.; Shao, C.L.; Lee, D.R.; Park, S.J.; Kwag, G.B.; Choi, K.J. Preparation and characterization of a nanoscale poly(vinyl alcohol) fiber aggregate produced by an electrospinning method. *J. Polym. Sci. Part B Polym. Phys.* **2002**, *40*, 1261–1268. [CrossRef]
34. Inai, R.; Kotaki, M.; Ramakrishna, S. Structure and properties of electrospun PLLA single nanofibres. *Nanotechnology* **2005**, *16*, 208. [CrossRef] [PubMed]
35. Kim, K.-H.; Jeong, L.; Park, H.-N.; Shin, S.-Y.; Park, W.-H.; Lee, S.-C.; Kim, T.-I.; Park, Y.-J.; Seol, Y.-J.; Lee, Y.-M. Biological efficacy of silk fibroin nanofiber membranes for guided bone regeneration. *J. Biotechnol.* **2005**, *120*, 327–339. [CrossRef] [PubMed]
36. Lee, J.S.; Choi, K.H.; Ghim, H.D.; Kim, S.S.; Chun, D.H.; Kim, H.Y.; Lyoo, W.S. Role of molecular weight of atactic poly(vinyl alcohol)(PVA) in the structure and properties of PVA nanofabric prepared by electrospinning. *J. Appl. Polym. Sci.* **2004**, *93*, 1638–1646. [CrossRef]
37. Pillay, V.; Dott, C.; Choonara, Y.E.; Tyagi, C.; Tomar, L.; Kumar, P.; du Toit, L.C.; Ndesendo, V.M. A review of the effect of processing variables on the fabrication of electrospun nanofibers for drug delivery applications. *J. Nanomater.* **2013**, *2013*. [CrossRef]
38. Zong, X.; Kim, K.; Fang, D.; Ran, S.; Hsiao, B.S.; Chu, B. Structure and process relationship of electrospun bioabsorbable nanofiber membranes. *Polymer* **2002**, *43*, 4403–4412. [CrossRef]
39. Hayati, I.; Bailey, A.; Tadros, T.F. Investigations into the mechanisms of electrohydrodynamic spraying of liquids: I. Effect of electric field and the environment on pendant drops and factors affecting the formation of stable jets and atomization. *J. Colloid Interface Sci.* **1987**, *117*, 205–221. [CrossRef]
40. Huang, C.; Chen, S.; Lai, C.; Reneker, D.H.; Qiu, H.; Ye, Y.; Hou, H. Electrospun polymer nanofibres with small diameters. *Nanotechnology* **2006**, *17*, 1558. [CrossRef] [PubMed]
41. Gupta, B.; Revagade, N.; Hilborn, J. Poly(lactic acid) fiber: An overview. *Prog. Polym. Sci.* **2007**, *32*, 455–482. [CrossRef]
42. Cicero, J.A.; Dorgan, J.R.; Garrett, J.; Runt, J.; Lin, J. Effects of molecular architecture on two-step, melt-spun poly (lactic acid) fibers. *J. Appl. Polym. Sci.* **2002**, *86*, 2839–2846. [CrossRef]
43. Kim, M.S.; Kim, J.C.; Kim, Y.H. Effects of take-up speed on the structure and properties of melt-spun poly(L-lactic acid) fibers. *Polym. Adv. Technol.* **2008**, *19*, 748–755. [CrossRef]

44. Postema, A.; Luiten, A.; Pennings, A. High-strength poly(L-lactide) fibers by a dry-spinning/hot-drawing process. I. Influence of the ambient temperature on the dry-spinning process. *J. Appl. Polym. Sci.* **1990**, *39*, 1265–1274. [CrossRef]
45. Persano, L.; Camposeo, A.; Tekmen, C.; Pisignano, D. Industrial upscaling of electrospinning and applications of polymer nanofibers: A review. *Macromol. Mater. Eng.* **2013**, *298*, 504–520. [CrossRef]
46. Tan, E.; Ng, S.; Lim, C. Tensile testing of a single ultrafine polymeric fiber. *Biomaterials* **2005**, *26*, 1453–1456. [CrossRef] [PubMed]
47. Liu, J.; Shen, Z.; Lee, S.-H.; Marquez, M.; McHugh, M.A. Electrospinning in compressed carbon dioxide: Hollow or open-cell fiber formation with a single nozzle configuration. *J. Supercrit. Fluids* **2010**, *53*, 142–150. [CrossRef]
48. Stitzel, J.; Liu, J.; Lee, S.J.; Komura, M.; Berry, J.; Soker, S.; Lim, G.; Van Dyke, M.; Czerw, R.; Yoo, J.J. Controlled fabrication of a biological vascular substitute. *Biomaterials* **2006**, *27*, 1088–1094. [CrossRef] [PubMed]
49. Zhou, Y.; Freitag, M.; Hone, J.; Staii, C.; Johnson, A., Jr.; Pinto, N.J.; MacDiarmid, A. Fabrication and electrical characterization of polyaniline-based nanofibers with diameter below 30 nm. *Appl. Phys. Lett.* **2003**, *83*, 3800–3802. [CrossRef]
50. Agarwal, S.; Burgard, M.; Greiner, A.; Wendorff, J. *Electrospinning: A Practical Guide to Nanofibers*; Walter de Gruyter GmbH & Co KG: Berlin, Germany, 2016.
51. Gupta, P.; Wilkes, G.L. Some investigations on the fiber formation by utilizing a side-by-side bicomponent electrospinning approach. *Polymer* **2003**, *44*, 6353–6359. [CrossRef]
52. Townsend-Nicholson, A.; Jayasinghe, S.N. Cell electrospinning: A unique biotechnique for encapsulating living organisms for generating active biological microthreads/scaffolds. *Biomacromolecules* **2006**, *7*, 3364–3369. [CrossRef] [PubMed]
53. Ravichandran, R.; Venugopal, J.R.; Sundarrajan, S.; Mukherjee, S.; Sridhar, R.; Ramakrishna, S. Expression of cardiac proteins in neonatal cardiomyocytes on PGS/fibrinogen core/shell substrate for Cardiac tissue engineering. *Int. J. Cardiol.* **2013**, *167*, 1461–1468. [CrossRef] [PubMed]
54. Wang, X.; Yuan, Y.; Huang, X.; Yue, T. Controlled release of protein from core–shell nanofibers prepared by emulsion electrospinning based on green chemical. *J. Appl. Polym. Sci.* **2015**, *132*. [CrossRef]
55. Su, Y.; Su, Q.; Liu, W.; Lim, M.; Venugopal, J.R.; Mo, X.; Ramakrishna, S.; Al-Deyab, S.S.; El-Newehy, M. Controlled release of bone morphogenetic protein 2 and dexamethasone loaded in core–shell PLLACL–collagen fibers for use in bone tissue engineering. *Acta Biomater.* **2012**, *8*, 763–771. [CrossRef] [PubMed]
56. Rubert, M.; Dehli, J.; Li, Y.-F.; Taskin, M.B.; Xu, R.; Besenbacher, F.; Chen, M. Electrospun PCL/PEO coaxial fibers for basic fibroblast growth factor delivery. *J. Mater. Chem. B* **2014**, *2*, 8538–8546. [CrossRef]
57. Liao, I.; Chew, S.; Leong, K. Aligned core–shell nanofibers delivering bioactive proteins. *Nanomedicine* **2006**, *1*, 465–471. [CrossRef] [PubMed]
58. Tian, L.; Prabhakaran, M.P.; Ding, X.; Kai, D.; Ramakrishna, S. Emulsion electrospun vascular endothelial growth factor encapsulated poly(L-lactic acid-*co*-ε-caprolactone) nanofibers for sustained release in cardiac tissue engineering. *J. Mater. Sci.* **2012**, *47*, 3272–3281. [CrossRef]
59. Choi, J.S.; Choi, S.H.; Yoo, H.S. Coaxial electrospun nanofibers for treatment of diabetic ulcers with binary release of multiple growth factors. *J. Mater. Chem.* **2011**, *21*, 5258–5267. [CrossRef]
60. Liao, I.-C.; Chen, S.; Liu, J.B.; Leong, K.W. Sustained viral gene delivery through core-shell fibers. *J. Control. Release* **2009**, *139*, 48–55. [CrossRef] [PubMed]
61. Wang, C.; Yan, K.-W.; Lin, Y.-D.; Hsieh, P.C. Biodegradable core/shell fibers by coaxial electrospinning: Processing, fiber characterization, and its application in sustained drug release. *Macromolecules* **2010**, *43*, 6389–6397. [CrossRef]
62. Saraf, A.; Baggett, L.S.; Raphael, R.M.; Kasper, F.K.; Mikos, A.G. Regulated non-viral gene delivery from coaxial electrospun fiber mesh scaffolds. *J. Control. Release* **2010**, *143*, 95–103. [CrossRef] [PubMed]
63. Liao, I.-C.; Leong, K.W. Efficacy of engineered FVIII-producing skeletal muscle enhanced by growth factor-releasing co-axial electrospun fibers. *Biomaterials* **2011**, *32*, 1669–1677. [CrossRef] [PubMed]
64. Huang, W.; Zou, T.; Li, S.; Jing, J.; Xia, X.; Liu, X. Drug-loaded zein nanofibers prepared using a modified coaxial electrospinning process. *AAPS PharmSciTech* **2013**, *14*, 675–681. [CrossRef] [PubMed]
65. Zhu, T.; Chen, S.; Li, W.; Lou, J.; Wang, J. Flurbiprofen axetil loaded coaxial electrospun poly (vinyl

pyrrolidone)–nanopoly(lactic-*co*-glycolic acid) core–shell composite nanofibers: Preparation, characterization, and anti-adhesion activity. *J. Appl. Polym. Sci.* **2015**, *132*. [CrossRef]

66. Ignatova, M.; Rashkov, I.; Manolova, N. Drug-loaded electrospun materials in wound-dressing applications and in local cancer treatment. *Expert Opin. Drug Deliv.* **2013**, *10*, 469–483. [CrossRef] [PubMed]
67. Ding, B.; Kimura, E.; Sato, T.; Fujita, S.; Shiratori, S. Fabrication of blend biodegradable nanofibrous nonwoven mats via multi-jet electrospinning. *Polymer* **2004**, *45*, 1895–1902. [CrossRef]
68. Theron, S.; Yarin, A.; Zussman, E.; Kroll, E. Multiple jets in electrospinning: Experiment and modeling. *Polymer* **2005**, *46*, 2889–2899. [CrossRef]
69. Teo, W.; Ramakrishna, S. Electrospun fibre bundle made of aligned nanofibres over two fixed points. *Nanotechnology* **2005**, *16*, 1878. [CrossRef]
70. Kim, G.; Cho, Y.-S.; Kim, W.D. Stability analysis for multi-jets electrospinning process modified with a cylindrical electrode. *Eur. Polym. J.* **2006**, *42*, 2031–2038. [CrossRef]
71. Hong, Y.; Fujimoto, K.; Hashizume, R.; Guan, J.; Stankus, J.J.; Tobita, K.; Wagner, W.R. Generating elastic, biodegradable polyurethane/poly(lactide-*co*-glycolide) fibrous sheets with controlled antibiotic release via two-stream electrospinning. *Biomacromolecules* **2008**, *9*, 1200–1207. [CrossRef] [PubMed]
72. Wang, X.; Um, I.C.; Fang, D.; Okamoto, A.; Hsiao, B.S.; Chu, B. Formation of water-resistant hyaluronic acid nanofibers by blowing-assisted electro-spinning and non-toxic post treatments. *Polymer* **2005**, *46*, 4853–4867. [CrossRef]
73. Sundaray, B.; Subramanian, V.; Natarajan, T.; Xiang, R.-Z.; Chang, C.-C.; Fann, W.-S. Electrospinning of continuous aligned polymer fibers. *Appl. Phys. Lett.* **2004**, *84*, 1222–1224. [CrossRef]
74. Li, D.; Wang, Y.; Xia, Y. Electrospinning nanofibers as uniaxially aligned arrays and layer-by-layer stacked films. *Adv. Mater.* **2004**, *16*, 361–366. [CrossRef]
75. Ki, C.S.; Kim, J.W.; Hyun, J.H.; Lee, K.H.; Hattori, M.; Rah, D.K.; Park, Y.H. Electrospun three-dimensional silk fibroin nanofibrous scaffold. *J. Appl. Polym. Sci.* **2007**, *106*, 3922–3928. [CrossRef]
76. Smit, E.; Bűttner, U.; Sanderson, R.D. Continuous yarns from electrospun fibers. *Polymer* **2005**, *46*, 2419–2423. [CrossRef]
77. Xu, C.; Inai, R.; Kotaki, M.; Ramakrishna, S. Aligned biodegradable nanofibrous structure: A potential scaffold for blood vessel engineering. *Biomaterials* **2004**, *25*, 877–886. [CrossRef]
78. Bazilevsky, A.V.; Yarin, A.L.; Megaridis, C.M. Co-electrospinning of core-shell fibers using a single-nozzle technique. *Langmuir* **2007**, *23*, 2311–2314. [CrossRef] [PubMed]
79. Bhattarai, N.; Edmondson, D.; Veiseh, O.; Matsen, F.A.; Zhang, M. Electrospun chitosan-based nanofibers and their cellular compatibility. *Biomaterials* **2005**, *26*, 6176–6184. [CrossRef] [PubMed]
80. Theron, A.; Zussman, E.; Yarin, A. Electrostatic field-assisted alignment of electrospun nanofibres. *Nanotechnology* **2001**, *12*, 384. [CrossRef]
81. Zeng, J.; Yang, L.; Liang, Q.; Zhang, X.; Guan, H.; Xu, X.; Chen, X.; Jing, X. Influence of the drug compatibility with polymer solution on the release kinetics of electrospun fiber formulation. *J. Control. Release* **2005**, *105*, 43–51. [CrossRef] [PubMed]
82. Meng, Z.; Xu, X.; Zheng, W.; Zhou, H.; Li, L.; Zheng, Y.; Lou, X. Preparation and characterization of electrospun PLGA/gelatin nanofibers as a potential drug delivery system. *Colloids Surf. B Biointerfaces* **2011**, *84*, 97–102. [CrossRef] [PubMed]
83. Kim, K.; Luu, Y.K.; Chang, C.; Fang, D.; Hsiao, B.S.; Chu, B.; Hadjiargyrou, M. Incorporation and controlled release of a hydrophilic antibiotic using poly(lactide-*co*-glycolide)-based electrospun nanofibrous scaffolds. *J. Control. Release* **2004**, *98*, 47–56. [CrossRef] [PubMed]
84. Jannesari, M.; Varshosaz, J.; Morshed, M.; Zamani, M. Composite poly (vinyl alcohol)/poly (vinyl acetate) electrospun nanofibrous mats as a novel wound dressing matrix for controlled release of drugs. *Int. J. Nanomed.* **2011**, *6*, 993–1003.
85. Nair, R.; Arunkumar, K.; Vishnu Priya, K.; Sevukarajan, M. Recent advances in solid lipid nanoparticle based drug delivery systems. *J. Biomed. Sci. Res.* **2011**, *3*, 368–384.
86. Mickova, A.; Buzgo, M.; Benada, O.; Rampichova, M.; Fisar, Z.; Filova, E.; Tesarova, M.; Lukas, D.; Amler, E. Core/shell nanofibers with embedded liposomes as a drug delivery system. *Biomacromolecules* **2012**, *13*, 952–962. [CrossRef] [PubMed]

87. Volpato, F.Z.; Almodóvar, J.; Erickson, K.; Popat, K.C.; Migliaresi, C.; Kipper, M.J. Preservation of FGF-2 bioactivity using heparin-based nanoparticles, and their delivery from electrospun chitosan fibers. *Acta Biomater.* **2012**, *8*, 1551–1559. [CrossRef] [PubMed]
88. Kim, H.S.; Yoo, H.S. MMPs-responsive release of DNA from electrospun nanofibrous matrix for local gene therapy: In vitro and in vivo evaluation. *J. Control. Release* **2010**, *145*, 264–271. [CrossRef] [PubMed]
89. Mottaghitalab, F.; Farokhi, M.; Mottaghitalab, V.; Ziabari, M.; Divsalar, A.; Shokrgozar, M.A. Enhancement of neural cell lines proliferation using nano-structured chitosan/poly(vinyl alcohol) scaffolds conjugated with nerve growth factor. *Carbohydr. Polym.* **2011**, *86*, 526–535. [CrossRef]
90. Choi, J.S.; Leong, K.W.; Yoo, H.S. In vivo wound healing of diabetic ulcers using electrospun nanofibers immobilized with human epidermal growth factor (EGF). *Biomaterials* **2008**, *29*, 587–596. [CrossRef] [PubMed]
91. Im, J.S.; Yun, J.; Lim, Y.-M.; Kim, H.-I.; Lee, Y.-S. Fluorination of electrospun hydrogel fibers for a controlled release drug delivery system. *Acta Biomater.* **2010**, *6*, 102–109. [CrossRef] [PubMed]
92. Yun, J.; Im, J.S.; Lee, Y.-S.; Kim, H.-I. Electro-responsive transdermal drug delivery behavior of PVA/PAA/MWCNT nanofibers. *Eur. Polym. J.* **2011**, *47*, 1893–1902. [CrossRef]
93. Kim, H.; Yoo, H. Matrix metalloproteinase-inspired suicidal treatments of diabetic ulcers with siRNA-decorated nanofibrous meshes. *Gene Ther.* **2013**, *20*, 378–385. [CrossRef] [PubMed]
94. Luu, Y.; Kim, K.; Hsiao, B.; Chu, B.; Hadjiargyrou, M. Development of a nanostructured DNA delivery scaffold via electrospinning of PLGA and PLA–PEG block copolymers. *J. Control. Release* **2003**, *89*, 341–353. [CrossRef]
95. Zamani, M.; Prabhakaran, M.P.; Ramakrishna, S. Advances in drug delivery via electrospun and electrosprayed nanomaterials. *Int. J. Nanomed.* **2013**, *8*, 2997–3017.
96. Xu, X.; Yang, L.; Xu, X.; Wang, X.; Chen, X.; Liang, Q.; Zeng, J.; Jing, X. Ultrafine medicated fibers electrospun from W/O emulsions. *J. Control. Release* **2005**, *108*, 33–42. [CrossRef] [PubMed]
97. Yang, Y.; Li, X.; Qi, M.; Zhou, S.; Weng, J. Release pattern and structural integrity of lysozyme encapsulated in core–sheath structured poly(DL-lactide) ultrafine fibers prepared by emulsion electrospinning. *Eur. J. Pharm. Biopharm.* **2008**, *69*, 106–116. [CrossRef] [PubMed]
98. He, S.; Xia, T.; Wang, H.; Wei, L.; Luo, X.; Li, X. Multiple release of polyplexes of plasmids VEGF and bFGF from electrospun fibrous scaffolds towards regeneration of mature blood vessels. *Acta Biomater.* **2012**, *8*, 2659–2669. [CrossRef] [PubMed]
99. Yang, Y.; Li, X.; Cheng, L.; He, S.; Zou, J.; Chen, F.; Zhang, Z. Core–sheath structured fibers with pDNA polyplex loadings for the optimal release profile and transfection efficiency as potential tissue engineering scaffolds. *Acta Biomater.* **2011**, *7*, 2533–2543. [CrossRef] [PubMed]
100. Wang, Y.; Qiao, W.; Yin, T. A novel controlled release drug delivery system for multiple drugs based on electrospun nanofibers containing nanoparticles. *J. Pharm. Sci.* **2010**, *99*, 4805–4811. [CrossRef] [PubMed]
101. Xu, J.; Jiao, Y.; Shao, X.; Zhou, C. Controlled dual release of hydrophobic and hydrophilic drugs from electrospun poly(L-lactic acid) fiber mats loaded with chitosan microspheres. *Mater. Lett.* **2011**, *65*, 2800–2803. [CrossRef]
102. Okuda, T.; Tominaga, K.; Kidoaki, S. Time-programmed dual release formulation by multilayered drug-loaded nanofiber meshes. *J. Control. Release* **2010**, *143*, 258–264. [CrossRef] [PubMed]
103. Chunder, A.; Sarkar, S.; Yu, Y.; Zhai, L. Fabrication of ultrathin polyelectrolyte fibers and their controlled release properties. *Colloids Surf. B Biointerfaces* **2007**, *58*, 172–179. [CrossRef] [PubMed]
104. Im, J.S.; Lee, S.K.; Bai, B.C.; Lee, Y.-S. Prediction and characterization of drug release in a multi-drug release system. *J. Ind. Eng. Chem.* **2012**, *18*, 325–330. [CrossRef]
105. Prausnitz, M.R.; Langer, R. Transdermal drug delivery. *Nat. Biotechnol.* **2008**, *26*, 1261–1268. [CrossRef] [PubMed]
106. Suwantong, O.; Ruktanonchai, U.; Supaphol, P. Electrospun cellulose acetate fiber mats containing asiaticoside or Centella asiatica crude extract and the release characteristics of asiaticoside. *Polymer* **2008**, *49*, 4239–4247. [CrossRef]
107. Taepaiboon, P.; Rungsardthong, U.; Supaphol, P. Drug-loaded electrospun mats of poly (vinyl alcohol) fibres and their release characteristics of four model drugs. *Nanotechnology* **2006**, *17*, 2317. [CrossRef]
108. Suwantong, O.; Opanasopit, P.; Ruktanonchai, U.; Supaphol, P. Electrospun cellulose acetate fiber mats containing curcumin and release characteristic of the herbal substance. *Polymer* **2007**, *48*, 7546–7557. [CrossRef]

109. Im, J.S.; Bai, B.C.; Lee, Y.-S. The effect of carbon nanotubes on drug delivery in an electro-sensitive transdermal drug delivery system. *Biomaterials* **2010**, *31*, 1414–1419. [CrossRef] [PubMed]
110. Taepaiboon, P.; Rungsardthong, U.; Supaphol, P. Vitamin-loaded electrospun cellulose acetate nanofiber mats as transdermal and dermal therapeutic agents of vitamin A acid and vitamin E. *Eur. J. Pharm. Biopharm.* **2007**, *67*, 387–397. [CrossRef] [PubMed]
111. Ngawhirunpat, T.; Opanasopit, P.; Rojanarata, T.; Akkaramongkolporn, P.; Ruktanonchai, U.; Supaphol, P. Development of meloxicam-loaded electrospun polyvinyl alcohol mats as a transdermal therapeutic agent. *Pharm. Dev. Technol.* **2009**, *14*, 73–82. [CrossRef] [PubMed]
112. Reda, R.I.; Wen, M.M.; El-Kamel, A.H. Ketoprofen-loaded eudragit electrospun nanofibers for the treatment of oral mucositis. *Int. J. Nanomed.* **2017**, *12*, 2335. [CrossRef] [PubMed]
113. Kenawy, E.-R.; Bowlin, G.L.; Mansfield, K.; Layman, J.; Simpson, D.G.; Sanders, E.H.; Wnek, G.E. Release of tetracycline hydrochloride from electrospun poly(ethylene-*co*-vinylacetate), poly (lactic acid), and a blend. *J. Control. Release* **2002**, *81*, 57–64. [CrossRef]
114. Alhusein, N.; Blagbrough, I.S.; De Bank, P.A. Electrospun matrices for localised controlled drug delivery: Release of tetracycline hydrochloride from layers of polycaprolactone and poly(ethylene-*co*-vinyl acetate). *Drug Deliv. Transl. Res.* **2012**, *2*, 477–488. [CrossRef] [PubMed]
115. Alhusein, N.; De Bank, P.A.; Blagbrough, I.S.; Bolhuis, A. Killing bacteria within biofilms by sustained release of tetracycline from triple-layered electrospun micro/nanofibre matrices of polycaprolactone and poly (ethylene-*co*-vinyl acetate). *Drug Deliv. Transl. Res.* **2013**, *3*, 531–541. [CrossRef] [PubMed]
116. Wang, X.; Yue, T.; Lee, T.-C. Development of Pleurocidin-poly(vinyl alcohol) electrospun antimicrobial nanofibers to retain antimicrobial activity in food system application. *Food Control* **2015**, *54*, 150–157. [CrossRef]
117. Zhang, Y.; Lim, C.T.; Ramakrishna, S.; Huang, Z.-M. Recent development of polymer nanofibers for biomedical and biotechnological applications. *J. Mater. Sci. Mater. Med.* **2005**, *16*, 933–946. [CrossRef] [PubMed]
118. Boateng, J.S.; Matthews, K.H.; Stevens, H.N.; Eccleston, G.M. Wound healing dressings and drug delivery systems: A review. *J. Pharm. Sci.* **2008**, *97*, 2892–2923. [CrossRef] [PubMed]
119. Said, S.S.; Aloufy, A.K.; El-Halfawy, O.M.; Boraei, N.A.; El-Khordagui, L.K. Antimicrobial PLGA ultrafine fibers: Interaction with wound bacteria. *Eur. J. Pharm. Biopharm.* **2011**, *79*, 108–118. [CrossRef] [PubMed]
120. Thakur, R.; Florek, C.; Kohn, J.; Michniak, B. Electrospun nanofibrous polymeric scaffold with targeted drug release profiles for potential application as wound dressing. *Int. J. Pharm.* **2008**, *364*, 87–93. [CrossRef] [PubMed]
121. Wang, A.; Xu, C.; Zhang, C.; Gan, Y.; Wang, B. Experimental investigation of the properties of electrospun nanofibers for potential medical application. *J. Nanomater.* **2015**, *2015*, 5. [CrossRef]
122. GhavamiNejad, A.; Rajan Unnithan, A.; Ramachandra Kurup Sasikala, A.; Samarikhalaj, M.; Thomas, R.G.; Jeong, Y.Y.; Nasseri, S.; Murugesan, P.; Wu, D.; Hee Park, C. Mussel-inspired electrospun nanofibers functionalized with size-controlled silver nanoparticles for wound dressing application. *ACS Appl. Mater. Interfaces* **2015**, *7*, 12176–12183. [CrossRef] [PubMed]
123. Chutipakdeevong, J.; Ruktanonchai, U.; Supaphol, P. Hybrid biomimetic electrospun fibrous mats derived from poly(ε-caprolactone) and silk fibroin protein for wound dressing application. *J. Appl. Polym. Sci.* **2015**, *132*, 41653. [CrossRef]
124. Xu, X.; Chen, X.; Ma, P.; Wang, X.; Jing, X. The release behavior of doxorubicin hydrochloride from medicated fibers prepared by emulsion-electrospinning. *Eur. J. Pharm. Biopharm.* **2008**, *70*, 165–170. [CrossRef] [PubMed]
125. Xu, X.; Chen, X.; Wang, Z.; Jing, X. Ultrafine PEG–PLA fibers loaded with both paclitaxel and doxorubicin hydrochloride and their in vitro cytotoxicity. *Eur. J. Pharm. Biopharm.* **2009**, *72*, 18–25. [CrossRef] [PubMed]
126. Xie, J.; Tan, R.S.; Wang, C.H. Biodegradable microparticles and fiber fabrics for sustained delivery of cisplatin to treat C6 glioma in vitro. *J. Biomed. Mater. Res. Part A* **2008**, *85*, 897–908. [CrossRef] [PubMed]
127. Liu, S.; Zhou, G.; Liu, D.; Xie, Z.; Huang, Y.; Wang, X.; Wu, W.; Jing, X. Inhibition of orthotopic secondary hepatic carcinoma in mice by doxorubicin-loaded electrospun polylactide nanofibers. *J. Mater. Chem. B* **2013**, *1*, 101–109. [CrossRef]
128. Luo, X.; Xie, C.; Wang, H.; Liu, C.; Yan, S.; Li, X. Antitumor activities of emulsion electrospun fibers with core

loading of hydroxycamptothecin via intratumoral implantation. *Int. J. Pharm.* **2012**, *425*, 19–28. [CrossRef] [PubMed]
129. Gupta, S. Biocompatible microemulsion systems for drug encapsulation and delivery. *Curr Sci* **2011**, *101*, 174–188.
130. Chen, P.; Wu, Q.-S.; Ding, Y.-P.; Chu, M.; Huang, Z.-M.; Hu, W. A controlled release system of titanocene dichloride by electrospun fiber and its antitumor activity in vitro. *Eur. J. Pharm. Biopharm.* **2010**, *76*, 413–420. [CrossRef] [PubMed]
131. Shao, S.; Li, L.; Yang, G.; Li, J.; Luo, C.; Gong, T.; Zhou, S. Controlled green tea polyphenols release from electrospun PCL/MWCNTs composite nanofibers. *Int. J. Pharm.* **2011**, *421*, 310–320. [CrossRef] [PubMed]
132. Zahedi, P.; Karami, Z.; Rezaeian, I.; Jafari, S.H.; Mahdaviani, P.; Abdolghaffari, A.H.; Abdollahi, M. Preparation and performance evaluation of tetracycline hydrochloride loaded wound dressing mats based on electrospun nanofibrous poly(lactic acid)/poly(ε-caprolactone) blends. *J. Appl. Polym. Sci.* **2012**, *124*, 4174–4183. [CrossRef]
133. He, C.L.; Huang, Z.M.; Han, X.J.; Liu, L.; Zhang, H.S.; Chen, L.S. Coaxial electrospun poly(L-lactic acid) ultrafine fibers for sustained drug delivery. *J. Macromol. Sci. Part B* **2006**, *45*, 515–524. [CrossRef]
134. He, C.L.; Huang, Z.M.; Han, X.J. Fabrication of drug-loaded electrospun aligned fibrous threads for suture applications. *J. Biomed. Mater. Res. Part A* **2009**, *89*, 80–95. [CrossRef] [PubMed]
135. Gilchrist, S.E.; Lange, D.; Letchford, K.; Bach, H.; Fazli, L.; Burt, H.M. Fusidic acid and rifampicin *co*-loaded PLGA nanofibers for the prevention of orthopedic implant associated infections. *J. Control. Release* **2013**, *170*, 64–73. [CrossRef] [PubMed]
136. Zamani, M.; Morshed, M.; Varshosaz, J.; Jannesari, M. Controlled release of metronidazole benzoate from poly ε-caprolactone electrospun nanofibers for periodontal diseases. *Eur. J. Pharm. Biopharm.* **2010**, *75*, 179–185. [CrossRef] [PubMed]
137. Toncheva, A.; Paneva, D.; Maximova, V.; Manolova, N.; Rashkov, I. Antibacterial fluoroquinolone antibiotic-containing fibrous materials from poly (L-lactide-*co*-D, L-lactide) prepared by electrospinning. *Eur. J. Pharm. Sci.* **2012**, *47*, 642–651. [CrossRef] [PubMed]
138. Spasova, M.; Manolova, N.; Paneva, D.; Rashkov, I. Preparation of chitosan-containing nanofibres by electrospinning of chitosan/poly(ethylene oxide) blend solutions. *e-Polymers* **2004**, *4*, 624–635. [CrossRef]
139. Verreck, G.; Chun, I.; Rosenblatt, J.; Peeters, J.; Van Dijck, A.; Mensch, J.; Noppe, M.; Brewster, M.E. Incorporation of drugs in an amorphous state into electrospun nanofibers composed of a water-insoluble, nonbiodegradable polymer. *J. Control. Release* **2003**, *92*, 349–360. [CrossRef]
140. Huang, L.-Y.; Branford-White, C.; Shen, X.-X.; Yu, D.-G.; Zhu, L.-M. Time-engineeringed biphasic drug release by electrospun nanofiber meshes. *Int. J. Pharm.* **2012**, *436*, 88–96. [CrossRef] [PubMed]
141. Jiang, Y.-N.; Mo, H.-Y.; Yu, D.-G. Electrospun drug-loaded core–sheath PVP/zein nanofibers for biphasic drug release. *Int. J. Pharm.* **2012**, *438*, 232–239. [CrossRef] [PubMed]
142. Jiang, H.; Fang, D.; Hsiao, B.; Chu, B.; Chen, W. Preparation and characterization of ibuprofen-loaded poly(lactide-*co*-glycolide)/poly(ethylene glycol)-*g*-chitosan electrospun membranes. *J. Biomater. Sci. Polym. Ed.* **2004**, *15*, 279–296. [CrossRef] [PubMed]
143. Lu, T.; Jing, X.; Song, X.; Wang, X. Doxorubicin-loaded ultrafine PEG-PLA fiber mats against hepatocarcinoma. *J. Appl. Polym. Sci.* **2012**, *123*, 209–217. [CrossRef]
144. Ranganath, S.H.; Wang, C.-H. Biodegradable microfiber implants delivering paclitaxel for post-surgical chemotherapy against malignant glioma. *Biomaterials* **2008**, *29*, 2996–3003. [CrossRef] [PubMed]
145. Xie, J.; Wang, C.-H. Electrospun micro-and nanofibers for sustained delivery of paclitaxel to treat C6 glioma in vitro. *Pharm. Res.* **2006**, *23*, 1817–1826. [CrossRef] [PubMed]
146. Liu, D.; Liu, S.; Jing, X.; Li, X.; Li, W.; Huang, Y. Necrosis of cervical carcinoma by dichloroacetate released from electrospun polylactide mats. *Biomaterials* **2012**, *33*, 4362–4369. [CrossRef] [PubMed]
147. Xu, X.; Zhuang, X.; Chen, X.; Wang, X.; Yang, L.; Jing, X. Preparation of core-sheath composite nanofibers by emulsion electrospinning. *Macromol. Rapid Commun.* **2006**, *27*, 1637–1642. [CrossRef]
148. Chew, S.Y.; Wen, J.; Yim, E.K.; Leong, K.W. Sustained release of proteins from electrospun biodegradable fibers. *Biomacromolecules* **2005**, *6*, 2017–2024. [CrossRef] [PubMed]
149. Rujitanaroj, P.-o.; Wang, Y.-C.; Wang, J.; Chew, S.Y. Nanofiber-mediated controlled release of siRNA complexes for long term gene-silencing applications. *Biomaterials* **2011**, *32*, 5915–5923. [CrossRef] [PubMed]

150. Cao, H.; Jiang, X.; Chai, C.; Chew, S.Y. RNA interference by nanofiber-based siRNA delivery system. *J. Control. Release* **2010**, *144*, 203–212. [CrossRef] [PubMed]
151. Schneider, A.; Wang, X.; Kaplan, D.; Garlick, J.; Egles, C. Biofunctionalized electrospun silk mats as a topical bioactive dressing for accelerated wound healing. *Acta Biomater.* **2009**, *5*, 2570–2578. [CrossRef] [PubMed]
152. Zhang, X.; Shi, Z.; Fu, W.; Liu, Z.; Fang, Z.; Lu, W.; Wang, Y.; Chen, F. In vitro biocompatibility study of electrospun copolymer ethylene carbonate-ε-caprolactone and vascular endothelial growth factor blended nanofibrous scaffolds. *Appl. Surf. Sci.* **2012**, *258*, 2301–2306. [CrossRef]
153. Cho, Y.I.; Choi, J.S.; Jeong, S.Y.; Yoo, H.S. Nerve growth factor (NGF)-conjugated electrospun nanostructures with topographical cues for neuronal differentiation of mesenchymal stem cells. *Acta Biomater.* **2010**, *6*, 4725–4733. [CrossRef] [PubMed]
154. Han, N.; Johnson, J.; Lannutti, J.J.; Winter, J.O. Hydrogel–electrospun fiber composite materials for hydrophilic protein release. *J. Control. Release* **2012**, *158*, 165–170. [CrossRef] [PubMed]
155. Chen, G.; Lv, Y. Immobilization and application of electrospun nanofiber scaffold-based growth factor in bone tissue engineering. *Curr. Pharm. Des.* **2015**, *21*, 1967–1978. [CrossRef] [PubMed]
156. Ren, S.; Dong, L.; Zhang, X.; Lei, T.; Ehrenhauser, F.; Song, K.; Li, M.; Sun, X.; Wu, Q. Electrospun Nanofibers Made of Silver Nanoparticles, Cellulose Nanocrystals, and Polyacrylonitrile as Substrates for Surface-Enhanced Raman Scattering. *Materials* **2017**, *10*, 68. [CrossRef] [PubMed]
157. Segala, K.; Nista, S.V.G.; Cordi, L.; Bizarria, M.T.M.; Ávila Júnior, J.D.; Kleinubing, S.A.; Cruz, D.C.; Brocchi, M.; Lona, L.M.F.; Caballero, N.E.D. Silver nanoparticles incorporated into nanostructured biopolymer membranes produced by electrospinning: A study of antimicrobial activity. *Braz. J. Pharm. Sci.* **2015**, *51*, 911–921. [CrossRef]
158. Li, J.; Chen, X.; Ai, N.; Hao, J.; Chen, Q.; Strauf, S.; Shi, Y. Silver nanoparticle doped TiO_2 nanofiber dye sensitized solar cells. *Chem. Phys. Lett.* **2011**, *514*, 141–145. [CrossRef]
159. Cui, H.; Yuan, L.; Li, W.; Lin, L. Antioxidant property of SiO_2-eugenol liposome loaded nanofibrous membranes on beef. *Food Packag. Shelf Life* **2017**, *11*, 49–57. [CrossRef]
160. Yarin, A.L.; Pourdeyhimi, B.; Ramakrishna, S. *Fundamentals and Applications of Micro-and Nanofibers*; Cambridge University Press: Cambridge, UK, 2014.
161. Zou, H.; Lv, P.F.; Wang, X.; Wu, D.; Yu, D.G. Electrospun poly(2-aminothiazole)/cellulose acetate fiber membrane for removing Hg (II) from water. *J. Appl. Polym. Sci.* **2017**, *134*. [CrossRef]
162. Zhou, J.; Zhang, J.; Rehman, A.U.; Kan, K.; Li, L.; Shi, K. Synthesis, characterization, and ammonia gas sensing properties of Co_3O_4@ CuO nanochains. *J. Mater Sci.* **2016**, *52*, 1–14. [CrossRef]
163. Homaeigohar, S.; Elbahri, M. Nanocomposite electrospun nanofiber membranes for environmental remediation. *Materials* **2014**, *7*, 1017–1045. [CrossRef] [PubMed]
164. Lee, S.J.; Heo, D.N.; Moon, J.-H.; Ko, W.-K.; Lee, J.B.; Bae, M.S.; Park, S.W.; Kim, J.E.; Lee, D.H.; Kim, E.-C. Electrospun chitosan nanofibers with controlled levels of silver nanoparticles. Preparation, characterization and antibacterial activity. *Carbohydr. Polym.* **2014**, *111*, 530–537. [CrossRef] [PubMed]
165. Shi, Q.; Vitchuli, N.; Nowak, J.; Caldwell, J.M.; Breidt, F.; Bourham, M.; Zhang, X.; McCord, M. Durable antibacterial Ag/polyacrylonitrile (Ag/PAN) hybrid nanofibers prepared by atmospheric plasma treatment and electrospinning. *Eur. Polym. J.* **2011**, *47*, 1402–1409. [CrossRef]
166. Castro-Mayorga, J.; Randazzo, W.; Fabra, M.; Lagaron, J.; Aznar, R.; Sánchez, G. Antiviral properties of silver nanoparticles against norovirus surrogates and their efficacy in coated polyhydroxyalkanoates systems. *LWT Food Sci. Technol.* **2017**, *79*, 503–510. [CrossRef]
167. Nie, H.; Wang, C.-H. Fabrication and characterization of PLGA/HAp composite scaffolds for delivery of BMP-2 plasmid DNA. *J. Control. Release* **2007**, *120*, 111–121. [CrossRef] [PubMed]
168. Tanaka, K.; Shiga, T.; Katayama, T. Fabrication of Hydroxyapatite/PLA Composite Nanofiber by Electrospinning. *WIT Trans. Built Environ.* **2016**, *166*, 371–379.
169. Chen, M.; Gao, S.; Dong, M.; Song, J.; Yang, C.; Howard, K.A.; Kjems, J.; Besenbacher, F. Chitosan/siRNA nanoparticles encapsulated in PLGA nanofibers for siRNA delivery. *ACS Nano* **2012**, *6*, 4835–4844. [CrossRef] [PubMed]
170. Chew, S.Y.; Mi, R.; Hoke, A.; Leong, K.W. Aligned Protein–Polymer Composite Fibers Enhance Nerve Regeneration: A Potential Tissue-Engineering Platform. *Adv. Funct. Mater.* **2007**, *17*, 1288–1296. [CrossRef] [PubMed]

171. Kowalczyk, T.; Nowicka, A.; Elbaum, D.; Kowalewski, T.A. Electrospinning of bovine serum albumin. Optimization and the use for production of biosensors. *Biomacromolecules* **2008**, *9*, 2087–2090. [CrossRef] [PubMed]
172. Li, X.; Su, Y.; Liu, S.; Tan, L.; Mo, X.; Ramakrishna, S. Encapsulation of proteins in poly (L-lactide-*co*-caprolactone) fibers by emulsion electrospinning. *Colloids Surf. B Biointerfaces* **2010**, *75*, 418–424. [CrossRef] [PubMed]
173. Huang, L.; Apkarian, R.P.; Chaikof, E.L. High-resolution analysis of engineered type I collagen nanofibers by electron microscopy. *Scanning* **2001**, *23*, 372–375. [CrossRef] [PubMed]
174. Huang, L.; Nagapudi, K.; Apkarian, R.P.; Chaikof, E.L. Engineered collagen–PEO nanofibers and fabrics. *J. Biomater. Sci. Polym. Ed.* **2001**, *12*, 979–993. [CrossRef] [PubMed]
175. Zhang, E.; Zhu, C.; Yang, J.; Sun, H.; Zhang, X.; Li, S.; Wang, Y.; Sun, L.; Yao, F. Electrospun PDLLA/PLGA composite membranes for potential application in guided tissue regeneration. *Mater. Sci. Eng. C* **2016**, *58*, 278–285. [CrossRef] [PubMed]
176. Sudakaran, S.V.; Venugopal, J.R.; Vijayakumar, G.P.; Abisegapriyan, S.; Grace, A.N.; Ramakrishna, S. Sequel of MgO nanoparticles in PLACL nanofibers for anti-cancer therapy in synergy with curcumin/β-cyclodextrin. *Mater. Sci. Eng. C* **2017**, *71*, 620–628. [CrossRef] [PubMed]
177. Khalil, I.S.; Abdel-Kader, R.M.; Gomaa, I.E.; Serag, N.; Klingner, A.; Elwi, M. Targeting of Cancer Cells using Controlled Nanoparticles and Robotics Sperms. *Int. J. Adv. Robot. Syst.* **2016**, *13*, 123. [CrossRef]
178. Sezer, U.A.; Ozturk, K.; Aru, B.; Demirel, G.Y.; Sezer, S.; Bozkurt, M.R. Zero valent zinc nanoparticles promote neuroglial cell proliferation: A biodegradable and conductive filler candidate for nerve regeneration. *J. Mater. Sci. Mater. Med.* **2017**, *28*, 19. [CrossRef] [PubMed]
179. Kuchler-Bopp, S.; Larrea, A.; Petry, L.; Idoux-Gillet, Y.; Sebastian, V.; Ferrandon, A.; Schwinté, P.; Arruebo, M.; Benkirane-Jessel, N. Promoting Bioengineered Tooth Innervation Using Nanostructured and Hybrid Scaffolds. *Acta Biomater.* **2017**, *50*, 493–501. [CrossRef] [PubMed]
180. Teo, W.-E. Addressing the Needs of Nanofiber Mass Production (Limitation of Nozzle System). Available online: http://electrospintech.com/mpchallenge.html#.WK2nq28rLIX (accessed on 27 October 2018).
181. Li, L.; Frey, M.W.; Green, T.B. Modification of air filter media with nylon-6 nanofibers. *J. Eng. Fibers Fabr.* **2006**, *1*, 1–22.
182. Moon, S.; Gil, M.; Lee, K.J. Syringeless Electrospinning toward Versatile Fabrication of Nanofiber Web. *Sci. Rep.* **2017**, *7*, 41424. [CrossRef] [PubMed]
183. Liu, W.; Huang, C.; Jin, X. Electrospinning of grooved polystyrene fibers: Effect of solvent systems. *Nanoscale Res. Lett.* **2015**, *10*, 237. [CrossRef] [PubMed]
184. Zhang, B.; Yan, X.; He, H.-W.; Yu, M.; Ning, X.; Long, Y.-Z. Solvent-free electrospinning: Opportunities and challenges. *Polym. Chem.* **2017**, *8*, 333–352. [CrossRef]
185. Fakirov, S. *Nano-Size Polymers: Preparation, Properties, Applications*; Springer: Berlin, Germany, 2016.
186. Niu, H.; Lin, T. Fiber generators in needleless electrospinning. *J. Nanomater.* **2012**, 12. [CrossRef]
187. Niu, H.; Lin, T.; Wang, X. Needleless electrospinning. I. A comparison of cylinder and disk nozzles. *J. Appl. Polym. Sci.* **2009**, *114*, 3524–3530. [CrossRef]
188. Cengiz, F.; Dao, T.A.; Jirsak, O. Influence of solution properties on the roller electrospinning of poly(vinyl alcohol). *Polym. Eng. Sci.* **2010**, *50*, 936–943. [CrossRef]
189. Niu, H.; Wang, X.; Lin, T. Needleless electrospinning: Influences of fibre generator geometry. *J. Text. Inst.* **2012**, *103*, 787–794. [CrossRef]
190. Liu, Y.; He, J. Bubble electrospinning for mass production of nanofibers. *Int. J. Nonlinear Sci. Numer. Simul.* **2007**, *8*, 393. [CrossRef]
191. Weng, L.; Xie, J. Smart electrospun nanofibers for controlled drug release: Recent advances and new perspectives. *Curr. Pharm. Des.* **2015**, *21*, 1944–1959. [CrossRef] [PubMed]

10

Hydrophobic Amino Acid Tryptophan Shows Promise as a Potential Absorption Enhancer for Oral Delivery of Biopharmaceuticals

Noriyasu Kamei, Hideyuki Tamiwa, Mari Miyata, Yuta Haruna, Koyo Matsumura, Hideyuki Ogino, Serena Hirano, Kazuhiro Higashiyama and Mariko Takeda-Morishita *

Laboratory of Drug Delivery Systems, Faculty of Pharmaceutical Sciences, Kobe Gakuin University, 1-1-3 Minatojima, Chuo-ku, Kobe, Hyogo 650-8586, Japan; noriyasu@pharm.kobegakuin.ac.jp (N.K.); hideyuki.ko192@gmail.com (H.T.); poffc263@s.kobegakuin.ac.jp (M.M.); pphgl074@s.kobegakuin.ac.jp (Y.H.); pohje089@s.kobegakuin.ac.jp (K.M.); pooww214@s.kobegakuin.ac.jp (H.O.); pofip292@s.kobegakuin.ac.jp (S.H.); podtk272@s.kobegakuin.ac.jp (K.H.)

* Correspondence: mmtakeda@pharm.kobegakuin.ac.jp

Abstract: Cell-penetrating peptides (CPPs) have great potential to efficiently deliver drug cargos across cell membranes without cytotoxicity. Cationic arginine and hydrophobic tryptophan have been reported to be key component amino acids for cellular internalization of CPPs. We recently found that L-arginine could increase the oral delivery of insulin in its single amino acid form. Therefore, in the present study, we evaluated the ability of another key amino acid, tryptophan, to enhance the intestinal absorption of biopharmaceuticals. We demonstrated that co-administration with L-tryptophan significantly facilitated the oral and intestinal absorption of the peptide drug insulin administered to rats. Furthermore, L-tryptophan exhibited the ability to greatly enhance the intestinal absorption of other peptide drugs such as glucagon-like peptide-1 (GLP-1), its analog Exendin-4 and macromolecular hydrophilic dextrans with molecular weights ranging from 4000 to 70,000 g/mol. However, no intermolecular interaction between insulin and L-tryptophan was observed and no toxic alterations to epithelial cellular integrity—such as changes to cell membranes, cell viability, or paracellular tight junctions—were found. This suggests that yet to be discovered inherent biological mechanisms are involved in the stimulation of insulin absorption by co-administration with L-tryptophan. These results are the first to demonstrate the significant potential of using the single amino acid L-tryptophan as an effective and versatile bioavailability enhancer for the oral delivery of biopharmaceuticals.

Keywords: tryptophan; oral delivery; insulin; GLP-1; intestinal absorption; amino acid; cell-penetrating peptide

---

1. Introduction

During the past few decades, cell-penetrating peptides (CPPs) have been established as potential tools for delivering bioactive macromolecules and lipidic or polymeric particulate carriers into cells via mainly covalent conjugation [1,2]. Conversely, our recent studies demonstrate that CPPs can dramatically accelerate the intestinal and nasal absorption of therapeutic peptides and proteins including insulin and the GLP-1 receptor agonist, Exendin-4, by the means of noncovalent co-administration [3–5]. In particular, we found that artificial cationic peptides such as octaarginine (R8) and the amphipathic sequence derived from antennapedia homeoprotein—penetratin—are CPPs that have shown the greatest potential to act as bioavailability enhancers for facilitating mucosal absorption of poorly absorbable peptides and proteins [3,6]. Several reports suggested that CPPs may enter into cells by multiple internalization mechanisms including endocytosis, mainly macropinocytosis and energy-independent direct translocation into the cytoplasm compartment [7–10].

Alternatively, in an earlier study examining the effects of arginine peptides with different chain lengths (4–16 residues), Futaki and coworkers found that the cationic amino acid arginine is a key common amino acid in arginine-rich CPPs, including the human immunodeficiency virus (HIV)-1 Tat peptide and identified an optimal arginine chain length that maximized cellular internalization efficiency [11]. We also examined the relationship between chain length of arginine peptides and their ability to enhance the intestinal absorption of insulin and confirmed that the effect of R8 was stronger than that of shorter or longer peptides [12]. Apart from the discussion regarding the effects of peptides with different numbers of amino acids, we recently found that the L-form of the amino acid arginine (L-arginine) could strongly enhance the intestinal absorption of insulin in its single amino acid form, although its effectiveness was relatively less than peptide forms of arginine [13]. Other studies suggest that when hydrophobic moieties such as stearyl groups or hydrophobic amino acids such as tryptophan are found within the peptide structure they synergistically enhance the potential of the original arginine-rich peptides [14–17]. R8 modified with a stearyl group and penetratin containing tryptophan residues are typical examples of CPPs with both cationic and amphipathic properties [18–20]. In fact, we demonstrated the stronger effect of penetratin over R8 on the intestinal and nasal absorption of various peptide and protein drugs [3,6,21,22]. These findings have shown the importance of the hydrophobic amino acid tryptophan for boosting the action of arginine-rich peptides in the facilitation of the intestinal absorption of insulin. It was expected that single amino acid tryptophan would affect the modulation of intestinal absorption of insulin similar to L-arginine. However, little is known about the ability of tryptophan to enhance the absorption of insulin.

Therefore, in the present study, we examined the effects of single amino acid tryptophan on the intestinal absorption of insulin and compared its effectiveness to other useful and conventional absorption enhancers including CPP (penetratin), tight junction-modulator (sodium caprate, C10) [23–25] and lipid membrane-disrupting bile acid (sodium taurodeoxycholate) [26,27]. Among the diversity of biopharmaceuticals currently available, the majority include peptides and proteins that must be administered as injectable forms [28]. Therefore, we further evaluated the applicability of tryptophan to enhance intestinal absorption of other biopharmaceuticals including peptide drugs (GLP-1 and Exendin-4) and different sizes of model hydrophilic macromolecules (dextrans, FD-4, FD-20 and FD-70; with molecular weights of 4000, 20,000 and 70,000 g/mol, respectively). Regarding the safe use of tryptophan as a potential absorption enhancer, we evaluated the irreversibility of action and possible cytotoxic effects on the intestinal mucosa. Furthermore, to better understand the mechanism of action, the structural isomeric difference and its specificity among hydrophobic amino acids on the ability of tryptophan and the possibility of intermolecular interaction between insulin and tryptophan in absorption enhancement were examined. As the possible transepithelial pathway utilized by tryptophan, the involvement of paracellular transport via tight junction opening effect of tryptophan itself or its major metabolite serotonin was examined. In addition, the ability of tryptophan to protect the peptide drugs from intestinal enzymatic degradation was tested.

2. Materials and Methods

2.1. Materials

Recombinant human insulin (27.5 IU/mg) and amino acids (L-tryptophan, D-tryptophan, L-phenylalanine, L-isoleucine and L-proline) were purchased from Wako Pure Chemical Industries, Ltd. (Osaka, Japan). Exendin-4 was synthesized by Sigma Genosys, Life Science Division of Sigma-Aldrich Japan Co. (Hokkaido, Japan). L-Penetratin (RQIKIWFQNRRMKWKK; capital letters indicate the L-form of amino acids) and GLP-1 were synthesized by Toray Research Center, Inc. (Tokyo, Japan). D-R8 (rrrrrrrr; lowercase letters indicate the D-form of amino acids) was synthesized by Scrum Inc. (Tokyo, Japan). Fluorescein isothiocyanate-labeled dextran with average molecular weights 4400,

20,000 and 70,000 g/mol (FD-4, FD-20 and FD-70, respectively), sodium taurodeoxycholate and Triton X-100 were purchased from Sigma-Aldrich Co. (Darmstadt, Germany). C10 was purchased from Tokyo Chemical Industry, Co. Ltd. (Tokyo, Japan). Methylcellurose (MC, METOLOSE) was purchased from Shin-Etsu Chemical Co., Ltd. (Tokyo, Japan). Human colon adenocarcinoma-derived Caco-2 cell line was purchased form the American Type Culture Collection (Rockville, MD, USA) at passage 18. Dulbecco's modified Eagle's medium (DMEM) with 4.5 g/L glucose, nonessential amino acids (NEAA), antibiotic mixture (10,000 U/mL penicillin, 10,000 μg/mL streptomycin and 29.2 mg/mL L-glutamine in 10 mM citric acid-buffered saline), 0.05% trypsin-ethylenediaminetetraacetic acid (EDTA) and Hanks' balanced salt solution (HBSS) were purchased from Gibco Laboratories (Lenexa, KS, USA). Fetal bovine serum (FBS) was purchased from Biowest (Nuaillé, France). Carboxymethyl dextran (CM5)-coated sensor chips were purchased from GE Healthcare (Little Chalfont, Buckinghamshire, UK). All other chemicals were of analytical grade and are commercially available.

2.2. Preparation of Mixed Solutions of Peptide Drugs and Amino Acids or CPPs

To prepare the insulin solution, specific amounts of recombinant human insulin were dissolved in 100 μL of 0.1 M HCl. The insulin solution was diluted with 0.8 mL of phosphate buffered saline (PBS, pH 7.4) (137 mM NaCl, 2.7 mM KCl, 8.1 mM Na_2HPO_4 and 1.47 KH_2PO_4 without calcium and magnesium) containing 0.001% MC, which prevents the adsorption of insulin and penetratin to the tube surface and was then normalized with 100 μL of 0.1 M NaOH. The final insulin concentration of the stock solution was 40 IU/mL. Stock solutions of other peptide drugs (GLP-1 and Exendin-4) and macromolecular compounds (FD-4, FD-20 and FD-70) were created by dissolving in PBS (pH 7.4) containing 0.001% MC (1.0 mg/mL and 8.0 mg/mL, respectively). Two times concentrations of amino acids (L-arginine, L- or D-tryptophan, L-phenylalanine, L-isoleucine and L-proline) were prepared using PBS (pH 7.4) containing 0.001% MC. To aid in the dissolution of high concentrations of hydrophobic amino acids such as L- or D-tryptophan and L-phenylalanine, the solutions were immersed in a water bath at 60 °C resulting in a clear solution. To create the solution used for the intestinal absorption study, two times concentrations of peptide drugs or macromolecular compounds and amino acid stock solutions were mixed together in equal volumes.

In the comparison study, specific amounts of L-penetratin, D-R8, C10, or sodium taurodeoxycholate were dissolved in PBS (pH 6.0 or 7.4) containing 0.001% MC at appropriate concentrations. For the in vitro study with Caco-2 cells, HBSS (LDH assay and transepithelial electrical resistance [TEER] measurement) or completed DMEM (WST-8 assay) were used instead of PBS to produce the test solution.

2.3. Animal Study

Animal experiments were performed at Kobe Gakuin University and complied with the regulations of the Committee on Ethics in the Care and Use of Laboratory Animals (approved as A16-15 and A17-4). Male Sprague Dawley rats weighing 180–220 g and male ddY mice weighing 30–40 g were purchased from Japan SLC, Inc. (Shizuoka, Japan), housed in temperature controlled rooms (23 ± 1 °C) with a relative humidity of 55 ± 5% and had free access to water and food during acclimatization. Animals were fasted for 18 h (rats) and 24 h (mice) before the experiments; however, they were allowed to drink water ad libitum.

2.4. In Situ Closed Ileum Loop Administration Study

Following anesthetization by intraperitoneal (i.p.) injection of sodium pentobarbital (50 mg/kg, Somnopentyl®, Kyoritsu Seiyaku Corp., Tokyo, Japan), which has been conventionally used in our insulin delivery study as confirmed to have a minimal effect on the blood glucose levels, rats were restrained in a supine position on a thermostatically controlled board at 37 °C. Additional i.p. injections of sodium pentobarbital (12.5 mg/kg) were administered every 1 h to maintain anesthesia. The ileum was exposed following a small midline incision made carefully in the abdomen. Its proximal to ileocecal junction segments (length = 10 cm) were cannulated at both ends using polypropylene tubing and ligated securely to prevent fluid loss. To wash out the intestinal contents, PBS warmed to 37 °C was circulated through the cannula at 5.0 mL/min for 4 min using an infusion pump. The cannulation tubing was removed, the segments were closed tightly and returned carefully to their original location inside the peritoneal cavity. Rats were kept on the board at 37 °C for an additional 30 min to calm biological reactions such as elevated blood glucose levels resulting from the stress imposed by surgery. After 30 min rest period, 0.5 mL of test insulin or other drug solution with or without amino acids and/or L-penetratin was administered directly into a 6 cm ileal loop created from the 10 cm pretreated segment. The insulin dose was administered at 50 IU/kg body weight (20 IU/mL) for all animal experiments. To examine dose dependency, the final concentrations of tryptophan were adjusted to 4, 8, 16 and 32 mM. In the comparison study with three hydrophobic amino acids or metabolite of L-tryptophan, the final concentrations of L-isoleucine, L-proline, L-phenylalanine and serotonin were 32 mM. In the study examining the synergistic effect of L-arginine and L-tryptophan, the final concentration of L-arginine was fixed at 40 mM. The doses of GLP-1 and Exendin-4 were both 1.25 mg/kg (0.5 mg/mL) and the doses of FDs were all 10 mg/kg (4 mg/mL). In the study examining the effect of pretreatment with L-tryptophan, D-R8, L-penetratin and other positive controls, ileal loop was exposed to these solutions during 30 min rest period after surgery and before the administration of insulin solution. For a part of above experiments involving pretreatment with L-tryptophan, C10 and sodium taurodeoxycholate for 30 min, an additional rest period of 30 min was added before the administration of insulin.

During the experiment, 0.25 mL blood aliquots were taken from the jugular vein at 0, 5, 10, 15, 30, 60, 120 and 180 min after dosing. The tuberculin syringes (1 mL, Terumo Corp., Tokyo, Japan) were heparinized by the standard procedure of coating the syringe wall with aspirated heparin and then expelling all the heparin. Plasma was separated by centrifugation at 13,400× g for 1 min and stored at −80 °C until analysis. The plasma concentrations of insulin, GLP-1 and Exendin-4 were determined using a human insulin ELISA kit (Mercodia AB, Uppsala, Sweden), GLP-1 ELISA kit (Wako Pure Chemical Industries, Ltd.) and Exendin-4 EIA kit (Phoenix Pharmaceuticals, Inc., Burlingame, CA, USA), respectively. The plasma concentrations of FDs were measured with a microplate fluorimeter (Synergy HT, BioTek Instruments Inc., Winooski, VT, USA) at excitation and emission wavelengths of 485 and 528 nm, respectively. The total area under the drug concentration time curve (AUC) from 0–3 h was estimated using the sum of successive trapezoids fitted between each set of data points in the time profiles of the plasma drug concentration.

2.5. *Pharmacokinetic Analysis*

The bioavailability of intestinal administered insulin was calculated relative to the subcutaneous (s.c.) route. Briefly, an insulin solution was prepared by dissolving an appropriate amount of insulin in PBS for s.c. injection (1 IU/kg). The peak plasma concentration (C_{max}) and time to reach C_{max} (T_{max}) were determined directly from the plasma insulin concentration–time curves. The total area under the insulin concentration–time curve (AUC) for 0–3 h was estimated from the sum of successive trapezoids between each data point. The relative bioavailability (BA) of insulin was calculated relative to the s.c. injection as follows:

$$BA\ (\%) = ([AUC]/dose)/([AUC]_{s.c.}/dose_{s.c.}) \times 100$$

2.6. *In Vivo Oral Administration Study*

After 24 h fasting, mice were dosed with insulin (50 IU/kg) with or without L-tryptophan (32 mM) (100 μL) by using oral gavage tube (i.d. 0.9 × length 50 mm) (Natsume Seisakusho Co., Ltd., Tokyo, Japan). Blood glucose levels were measured (One Touch Ultra View, Johnson & Johnson K.K., Tokyo, Japan) by collection of blood (one drop) from a small cut in the tail vein at t = 0 (prior to dosing), 15, 30, 60, 120, 180, 240, 300 and 360 min after administration. Blood glucose levels are depicted as percentage of the initial value in same mouse. Mice were trained with oral dosing and tail cutting at 24 h and

60 min prior to actual drug administration to avoid the unexpected elevation of blood glucose levels during experiments.

2.7. *Insulin Degradation in Intestinal Enzymatic Fluid*

Intestinal fluid was collected from male Sprague-Dawley rats by inserting a Sonde needle into the upper portion of the small intestine and the intestine was then cannulated on the lower side (length = 20 cm) to remove the intestinal fluid. The contents of the small intestine were washed out with 30 mL of PBS. Because intestinal fluid contains a high lipid content, the efflux solution was treated with equal volume of methylene chloride to remove any lipids that might interfere with the analysis of insulin by HPLC. This removal of lipid contents was repeated five times. L- or D-tryptophan (8–32 mM as final concentration) was mixed with insulin (10 IU/mL final concentration) and incubated in the intestinal fluid at 37 °C. At 5, 15, 30, 45 and 60 min, 50 μL was collected and added to 50 μL of ice-cold mobile phase solution to terminate the reaction. L- or D-penetratin (0.25 mM as final concentration) and STI (1.25 mg/mL final concentration) were used as a CPP and positive conventional inhibitor, respectively. Insulin concentration was measured by HPLC (LaChrom Elite System, Hitachi High-Technologies Corporation, Tokyo, Japan) using the following conditions: mobile phase, acetonitrile, trifluoroacetic acid (0.1%) and sodium chloride (31:69:0.58, *v*/*v*/*w*); 20 μL injection volume; 1.0 mL/min flow rate; 220 nm wave length; analytical column (4.6 × 150 mm; 5 μm) with guard column (4.6 × 150 mm; 5 μm) (ChemcoPak Nucleosil 5C18, Chemco Plus Scientific Co., Ltd., Osaka, Japan).

2.8. *Cell Culture*

Caco-2 cells were cultured in 75 cm^2 culture dishes (Nippon Becton Dickinson, Tokyo, Japan) with 10 mL of culture medium. The culture medium consisted of DMEM containing 10% FBS, 0.1 mM NEAA, 2 mM glutamine, 100 U/mL penicillin and 100 μg/mL streptomycin (completed DMEM). The seeding density for cultivation was 8.0×10^5 cells/dish. The cells were maintained in an incubator at 37 °C, 95% relative humidity and 5% CO_2. The culture medium was replaced with fresh medium every second day for approximately 7 days until the cells reached 80% confluence, at which time they were subcultured. For the subculture procedure, the cells were detached from the culture dishes by trypsinization with 0.05% trypsin–EDTA, counted with a hemocytometer and transferred at the desired seeding density to new culture dishes or experimental wells. We used cells between passages 25 and 35.

2.9. *In Vitro and In Situ the Lactate Dehydrogenase (LDH) Leakage*

To assess the cytotoxic effects of L-tryptophan, the integrity of the cell membrane after treatment with the CPPs was examined by measuring the lactate dehydrogenase (LDH) released from the cytoplasm under both in vitro and in situ conditions.

In the in vitro assay, the Caco-2 cells were grown in 24-well plates with a 1.88 cm^2 culture area (Nippon Becton Dickinson) at the density of 1.0×10^5 cells/cm^2 and then grown in completed DMEM for 3 or 4 days. Before the addition of L-tryptophan, cell membranes were allowed to equilibrate in 0.5 mL of assay buffer for 30 min. HBSS containing 0.001% MC (pH 7.4) was added to the wells as the transport buffer. After a 30 min pre-incubation with transport buffer, the assay was initiated by replacing 50 μL of transport buffer with 50 μL of L-tryptophan stock solution (ten times concentration) or transport buffer. Various concentrations (300–2400 μM) of L-tryptophan were incubated in Caco-2-seeded wells for 120 min at 37 °C. The incubation buffer was collected and LDH released from the cytoplasm into the incubation buffer was determined using a CytoTox 96 Non-Radioactive Cytotoxicity Assay kit (Promega Corp., Madison, WI, USA). Cytotoxicity was expressed as the percentage calculated by dividing the absorbance of the vehicle (HBSS) or the L-tryptophan-treated sample by that of a sample treated with 0.8% Triton X-100, according to the instructions of assay kit.

In the in situ assay, various concentrations of L-tryptophan solution (16, 32 or 50 mM) with 50 IU/kg insulin were administered into rat ileal segments in the same manner as the closed loop administration study described above. For the trial with the highest concentration of L-tryptophan (50 mM), L-arginine (40 mM) was added as a solubilizing agent. For this test, 5% sodium taurodeoxycholate was used as a positive control. At 60 min after administration, the ileal loop was washed with 5.0 mL of PBS and then intestinal fluid was collected. After adjusting the collected intestinal fluid to a total volume of 6.0 mL with PBS, the activity of LDH (Unit) leaked into the intestinal fluid was determined using an LDH kit (Promega Corp.).

2.10. Cell Viability Assay

To examine the cellular viability of Caco-2 cells exposed to L-tryptophan, a WST-8 assay was performed with Cell Counting Kit-8 (CCK-8, Dojindo Laboratories, Kumamoto, Japan). The Caco-2 cells were grown in 96-well plates with a 0.33 cm^2 culture area (Nippon Becton Dickinson) to a density of 3.0×10^4 cells/cm^2 and then grown in 100 μL of completed DMEM for 3 or 4 days. In this assay, the completed DMEM was used in place of the incubation buffer to prevent the possible loss of cell viability during total 5 h incubation in HBSS. First, 10 μL of L-tryptophan stock solution (eleven times concentration) or transport buffer was added to 100 μL of completed DMEM and the cells were incubated with various concentrations of L-tryptophan (600–2400 μM) for 2 h. Then, 10 μL of CCK-8 reagent was added to the wells and the cells were incubated for an additional 3 h to allow for the reductive reaction of WST-8. The resulting absorbances of the incubated solution in the wells were read with a microplate reader (Synergy HT, BioTek Instruments Inc.) at a wavelength of 450 nm. In this assay, 0.8% of Triton X-100 was used as a positive control, same as the LDH assay.

2.11. Transcellular Transport Assay

For TEER measurement, Caco-2 cells were grown in 12-well transwell plates with a 1.13 cm^2 culture area (collagen-coated polytetrafluoroethylene (PTFE) membrane with 0.4 μm pore size, Corning Inc., Corning, NY, USA). The cells were cultured to a density of 1.0×10^5 cells/cm^2. The cells were grown in completed DMEM for 21 days until they achieved a constant TEER reading of >500 Ω cm^2, which indicated that tight junctions had formed in the monolayer. The culture medium was changed every second day and the electrical resistance was monitored by the method described below. Each well consisted of apical (top) and basal (bottom) chambers, which were separated by a collagen-coated polytetrafluoroethylene membrane with a pore size of 0.4 μm and a filter area of 1.12 cm^2.

In preparation for the assays, the cell membranes were allowed to equilibrate for 30 min in transport buffer; HBSS (pH 7.4) with 0.001% MC was added to the apical (0.5 mL) and basal (1.5 mL) chambers of the transwell. After a 30 min pre-incubation for equilibration, an initial TEER measurement was taken of the monolayer in each well and then 100 μL of transport buffer was removed from the apical chamber and replaced with 50 μL of insulin and 50 μL of L-tryptophan or serotonin stock solutions (ten times concentration) or transport buffer. L-tryptophan (600, 1200 or 16,000 μM) or serotonin (2.4 or 16 mM) was incubated with insulin (15 μM) in the apical chamber of the Caco-2-seeded transwell for 2 h. During the incubation, the Caco-2 monolayer was kept at physiological temperature (37 °C).

2.12. TEER Measurement

The TEER of the Caco-2 monolayer was measured to confirm cell growth and differentiation on the insert filter of the transwell using a Millicell ERS-2 (Millipore Corp., Bedford, MA, USA). Before seeding the Caco-2 cells, the electrical resistance of the insert filter in the medium was measured and subtracted from the total electrical resistance determined for the monolayer to calculate the intrinsic TEER of the monolayer. The TEER of the monolayer was measured at the end of the 2 h incubation to detect any negative effects of the applied L-tryptophan on the intercellular tight junctions. The TEER is expressed as a percentage calculated by dividing the TEER value (Ω cm^2) at 2 h by the initial value.

2.13. Surface Plasmon Resonance (SPR)-Based Binding Assay

The intermolecular interactions between insulin and L-tryptophan or L-penetratin were analyzed by SPR (Biacore X-100, GE Healthcare). To measure the binding of L-tryptophan or L-penetratin to insulin, insulin was immobilized at the carboxymethyl dextran surface of a CM5 sensor chip by using an amine coupling method. For the immobilization procedure, insulin was diluted to a concentration of 50 μg/mL using acetate buffer at pH 4.5 and immobilized on the chip surface in separate flow cells at 5 μL/min for 7 min. Reference surfaces were prepared by amine coupling activation followed by immediate deactivation. For binding measurements, different concentrations of L-tryptophan or L-penetratin (2–200 μM) were injected for 90 s followed by an additional 90 s dissociation phase. At the end of each cycle, the surface was regenerated by a 30 s injection of 1 M NaCl. Measurements were carried out in HBSS (pH 7.4) supplied with 0.001% MC at 20 μL/min at 25 °C. Each sensorgram was determined by subtracting nonspecific binding on the surface of the reference flow cell from total binding on the immobilized-insulin surface.

2.14. Statistical Analysis

Each value is expressed as the mean and standard error of the mean (SEM) of multiple determinations. The significance of the differences in the mean values of multiple groups was evaluated using analysis of variance with Dunnett's test. IBM SPSS Statistics (version 24; IBM Corp., Armonk, NY, USA) was used for statistical analysis. Differences were considered significant when the p value was less than 0.05.

3. Results

3.1. Stimulatory Effect of L-Tryptophan on the Intestinal Absorption of Insulin

It was reported that tryptophan residues at position 6 and 14 in the penetratin amino acid sequence aid in lipid interaction in cell membranes and are therefore an important moiety involved in the cellular internalization of penetratin [18]. To test the ability of hydrophobic amino acid tryptophan as an absorption enhancer for insulin, we first conducted an in situ absorption study in which insulin was administered with various concentrations of the L-form of tryptophan (8–32 mM) into rat ileal closed loops. As shown in Figure 1A, the plasma insulin concentration increased after administration of insulin with L-tryptophan in a concentration dependent manner and with a late onset of action 30–60 min after administration. This result suggests that L-tryptophan has the potential to strongly enhance the intestinal absorption of insulin as single amino acid form. On the other hand, we confirmed the effect of the amphipathic CPP penetratin on the intestinal absorption of insulin. The effect of L-penetraitn shown in Figure 1A was consistent with our previous publication using L-penetratin [3,6], in which insulin co-administered with L-penetratin was absorbed immediately at 15 min post administration. The difference of action onset between L-tryptophan and L-penetratin suggested that L-tryptophan as single amino acid played a role in increasing absorption of insulin in a different way from tryptophan residues as a component of the peptide structure of L-penetratin. We further compared the effect of other hydrophobic amino acids such as phenylalanine, proline and isoleucine on the absorption of insulin. The results in Figure 1B show that there was no stimulatory effect on insulin absorption by these three hydrophobic amino acids suggesting that the bioenhancing effect is unique to tryptophan among the hydrophobic amino acids. The pharmacokinetic parameters are summarized in Table 1.

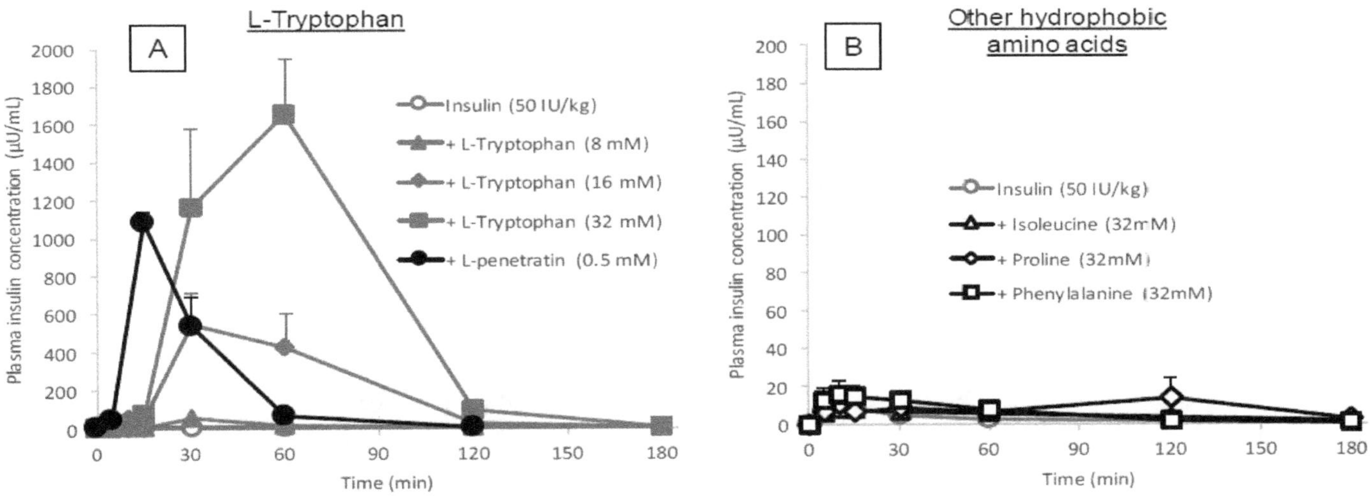

Figure 1. Time profiles of plasma insulin concentration after in situ administration of insulin (50 IU/kg) with or without L-tryptophan, L-penetratin or other hydrophobic amino acid additives into rat ileal loop. Panel (**A**), L-tryptophan (8–32 mM) or L-penetratin (0.5 mM); panel (**B**), hydrophobic amino acids (L-isoleucine, L-proline and L-phenylalanine, 32 mM). Each data point represents the mean ± SEM of N = 3–8, except for the group with L-tryptophan (8 mM, N = 2).

Table 1. Pharmacokinetic parameters following in situ administration of insulin with various amino acid additives, L-penetratin, or after pretreatment of amino acids or control reagents.

		Experiment	C_{max} (μU/mL)	T_{max} (min)	AUC (μU·h/mL)	BA (%)
Insulin (50 IU/kg)		8	10.6 ± 2.4	9.4 ± 1.1	8.5 ± 2.5	0.1 ± 0.0
+L-Tryptophan	(8 mM)	2	52.9	30	35.8	0.4
	(16 mM)	4	563.0 ± 162.4	45.0 ± 8.7	558.4 ± 195.2 **	5.8 ± 2.0 **
	(32 mM)	4	2008.2 ± 196.9	52.5 ± 7.5	1785.7 ± 153.5 **	18.7 ± 1.6 **
+D-Tryptophan	(16 mM)	3	84.7 ± 35.8	60.0 ± 0.0	75.4 ± 30.2	0.8 ± 0.3
	(32 mM)	3	723.5 ± 153.0	60.0 ± 0.0	606.3 ± 132.8 **	6.3 ± 1.4 **
+L-penetratin (0.5 mM)		4	1079.0 ± 54.4	15.0 ± 0.0	481.8 ± 85.0 **	5.0 ± 0.9 **
+Serotonin (32 mM)		3	258.3 ± 124.7	60.0 ± 0.0	304.8 ± 174.1	3.2 ± 1.8
Pretreatment study						
+PBS		4	1.7 ± 0.3	7.5 ± 2.5	2.0 ± 0.2	0.0 ± 0.0
+L-Tryptophan (32 mM)		4	1040.5 ± 455.9	18.8 ± 3.8	582.1 ± 229.2	6.1 ± 2.4
+D-R8 (0.5 mM)		3	22.7 ± 5.2	8.3 ± 3.3	22.5 ± 6.7	0.2 ± 0.1
+L-penetratin (0.5 mM)		3	356.3 ± 241.3	5.0 ± 0.0	141.0 ± 73.8	1.5 ± 0.8
+C10 (100 mM)		3	1574.8 ± 772.9	20.0 ± 5.0	1235.9 ± 686.2	12.9 ± 7.2
+Sodium taurodeoxycholate (5%)		3	4038.0 ± 1685.4	8.3 ± 3.3	2386.2 ± 1114.6 *	25.0 ± 11.7 *
Pretreatment with 30 min rest						
+L-Tryptophan (32 mM)		3	41.2 ± 11.2	11.7 ± 3.3	25.8 ± 5.4	0.3 ± 0.1
+C10 (100 mM)		3	165.1 ± 22.7	11.7 ± 3.3	128.3 ± 35.6	1.3 ± 0.4
+ Sodium taurodeoxycholate (5%)		3	393.7 ± 225.2	8.3 ± 3.3	203.3 ± 121.3	2.1 ± 1.3
Insulin s.c. (1 IU/kg)		3	133.8 ± 3.4	25.0 ± 5.0	191.2 ± 5.2	100

C_{max}, the maximum concentration; T_{max}, the time to reach the C_{max}; AUC, the area under the curve; BA, relative bioavailability compared to subcutaneous injection. Each data point represents the mean ± SEM of N =3–8, except for the group with L-tryptophan (8 mM, N = 2). * $p < 0.05$, ** $p < 0.01$, significantly different with corresponding control insulin (50 IU/kg).

3.2. Identification of the Ability of L-Tryptophan as the Oral Absorption Enhancer for Insulin

The above-mentioned results suggested that L-tryptophan has the ability to effectively increase the intestinal absorption of insulin. Therefore, the potential of L-tryptophan as oral absorption enhancer was further tested after in vivo oral administration of insulin to mice. As shown in Figure 2, the hypoglycemic reaction elevated after oral administration of insulin (50 IU/kg) with L-tryptophan (32 mM) suggested that L-tryptophan could enhance the oral absorption of insulin. The elevation in the blood glucose levels just after oral administration in all groups might be because of the stress by oral gavage, even though mice were trained before administration.

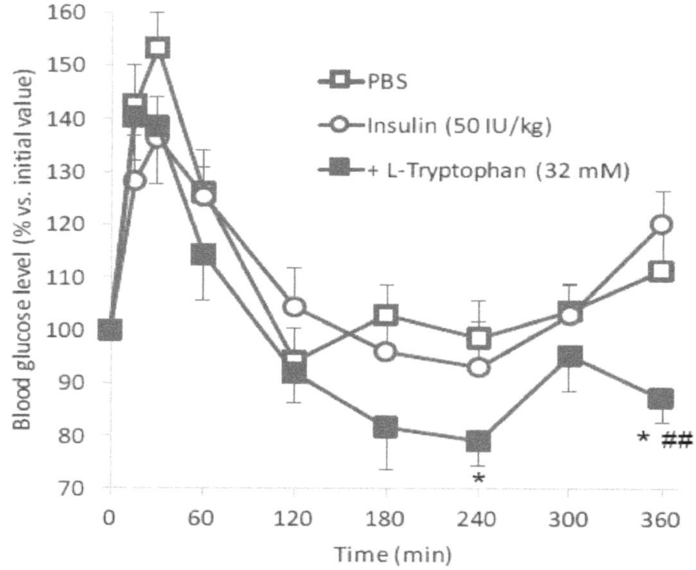

Figure 2. Blood glucose levels in mice following oral administration of insulin (50 IU/kg) with or without L-tryptophan (32 mM). Each data point represents the mean ± SEM of N = 6–8. * $p < 0.05$, ## $p < 0.01$, significantly different with PBS and insulin (50 IU/kg), respectively.

3.3. Applicability of L-Tryptophan to Enhance the Intestinal Absorption of Various Biopharmaceuticals

Although the mechanism involved in the absorption-stimulatory effect of L-tryptophan is still unclear, our results strongly suggest that L-tryptophan has potential as an effective absorption enhancer for the oral delivery of insulin. We additionally researched the ability of L-tryptophan to aid in the delivery of other biopharmaceuticals.

To examine the ability of L-tryptophan to assist in the transport of a range of differently sized potential drug cargo, we evaluated the effect of L-tryptophan co-administered with fluorescently labeled hydrophilic dextrans of various molecular weights (4400, 20,000 and 70,000 g/mol). As shown in Figure 3A–C, the intestinal absorption of all dextrans (FD-4, FD-20 and FD-70) was effectively enhanced by co-administration with L-tryptophan (32 mM), although the effectiveness of enhancement tended to decrease with increase in the molecular weight of the cargo compounds. Furthermore, the effect of L-tryptophan on the intestinal absorption of other peptide drugs, GLP-1 and Exendin-4, was examined. As shown in Figure 4A,B, these peptide drugs were efficiently absorbed in the presence of L-tryptophan (32 mM). Thus, L-tryptophan has the potential to enhance the intestinal absorption of a wide variety of biopharmaceuticals in a safe manner. The AUC values of dextrans and peptide drugs are summarized in Table 2.

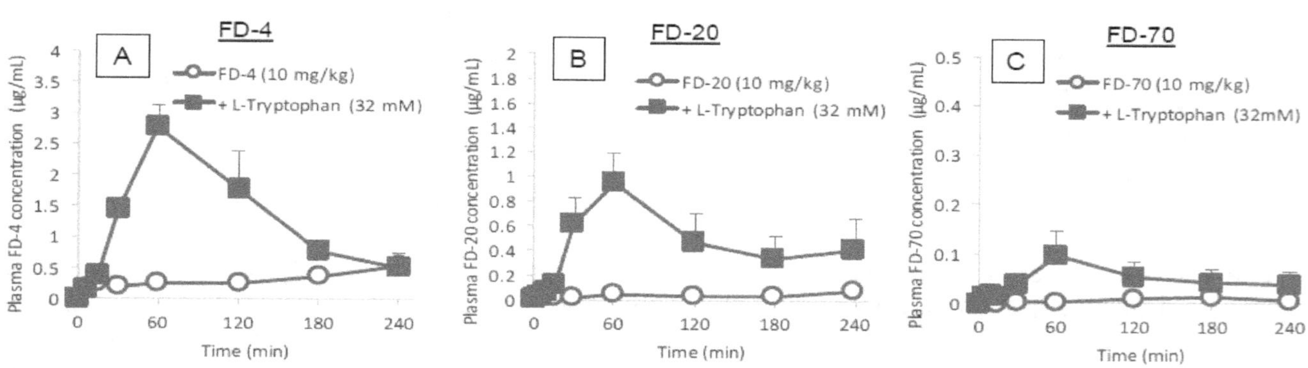

Figure 3. Time profiles of plasma concentrations of model hydrophilic macromolecules (FD-4, FD-20 and FD-70) after their in situ administration with or without L-tryptophan (32 mM) into rat ileal loop. Panels (**A**–**C**) show the absorption of FD-4, FD-20 and FD-70, respectively. Each data point represents the mean ± SEM of N = 3–8.

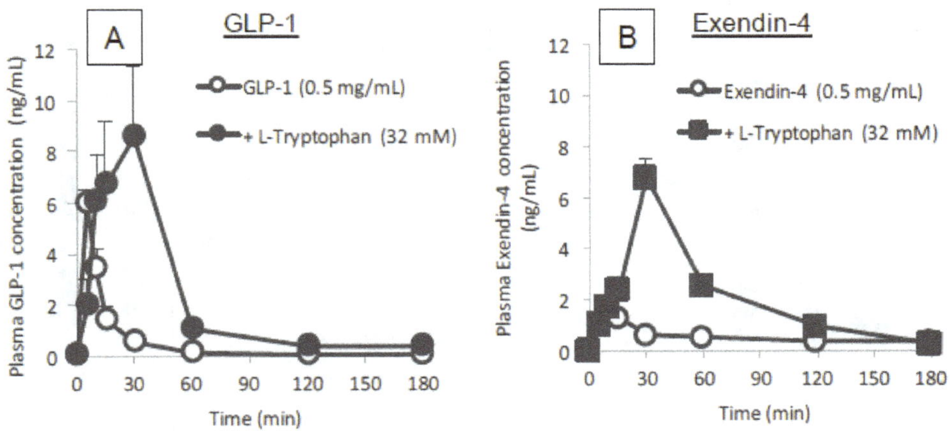

Figure 4. Time profiles of plasma concentrations of peptide drugs (GLP-1 and Exendin-4) after their in situ administration with or without L-tryptophan (32 mM) into rat ileal loop. Panels (**A**) and (**B**) show the absorption of GLP-1 and Exendin-4, respectively. Each data point represents the mean ± SEM of $N = 4$.

Table 2. AUCs following in situ administration of dextrans (FD-4, FD-20 and FD-70) with L-tryptophan into rat ileal loop.

	AUC (ng·h/mL)	
	−L-Tryptophan	**+L-Tryptophan (32 mM)**
FD-4 (10 mg/kg)	1194.2 ± 463.2	5512.7 ± 1034.9**
FD-20 (10 mg/kg)	146.0 ± 44.8	1973.2 ± 801.8*
FD-70 (10 mg/kg)	25.4 ± 24.6	205.6 ± 115.0
GLP-1 (0.5 mg/mL)	1.35 ± 0.27	6.35 ± 2.06*
Exendin-4 (0.5 mg/mL)	1.54 ± 0.62	6.17 ± 0.67**

AUC, the area under the curve. Each data point represents the mean ± SEM of $N = 3$–8. * $p < 0.05$, ** $p < 0.01$, significantly different with corresponding control without L-tryptophan.

3.4. Mucosal Cytotoxic Examinations for Intestinal Administration of L-Tryptophan

3.4.1. Effect of L-Tryptophan on the Membrane Integrity and Cell Viability in the Intestinal Epithelium

The intestinal absorption of insulin accelerated by co-administration with L-tryptophan might be attributed to the modulation of biological structures and functions in the intestinal mucosa. To establish the safety of L-tryptophan as a potential absorption enhancer for biopharmaceuticals, changes in the integrity of epithelial cell membranes, cellular viability and the tightness of the paracellular junctions after administration of L-tryptophan were examined.

Figure 5A,B shows the leakage of an intracellular protein, LDH, from intestinal epithelial cells after in situ administration into rat ileal loop (A) and in vitro exposure onto the epithelial model Caco-2 cells (B). In Figure 5A, the leakage of LDH was negligible after in situ administration of insulin with L-tryptophan at all tested concentrations (16 and 32 mM) and these measurements were significantly low when compared to the positive control (the administration of 5% sodium taurodeoxycholate). Similarly, in the in vitro assay (Figure 5B), no release of LDH into the media was observed after the exposure of Caco-2 cells to L-tryptophan at all concentrations (300–2400 µM). Figure 5C shows the viability of Caco-2 cells after applying L-tryptophan to culture media. The results indicate no decrease in cell viability after addition of L-tryptophan at all concentrations (600–2400 µM). The toxicity examinations suggest that L-tryptophan has no adverse effect on the intestinal mucosa and may therefore become a potentially safe absorption enhancer.

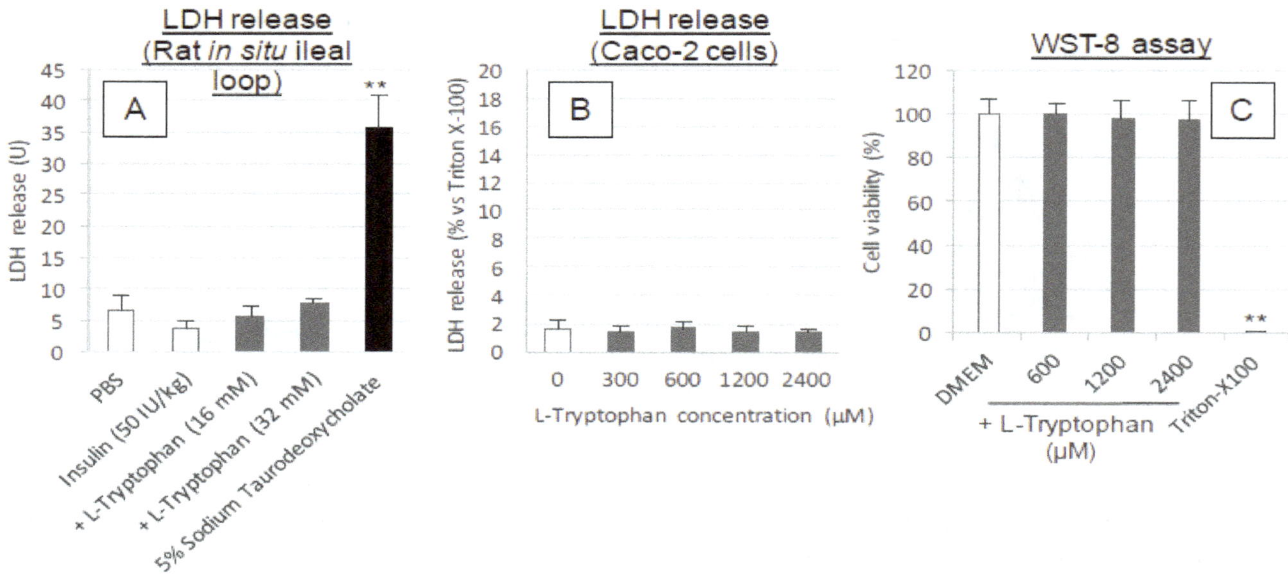

Figure 5. Cytotoxicity examinations after the exposure of intestinal epithelium to L-tryptophan. Panel (**A**), the LDH release in the intestinal fluid collected at 60 min after ileal administration of PBS, insulin (50 IU/kg) with or without L-tryptophan (16–50 mM) and sodium taurodeoxycholate (5%). Panel (**B**), LDH released from the cytoplasm into the incubation medium (HBSS) after incubation with various concentrations of L-tryptophan (200–2400 μM). The value is expressed as a percentage calculated by dividing the absorbance of the L-tryptophan treated medium sample by that of the sample treated with Triton X-100 (0.8%). Panel C, cell viability after incubation with various concentrations of L-tryptophan (600–2400 μM). Each data point represents the mean ± SEM of $N = 3$, 3 and 6–11 for panels (**A–C**), respectively. * $p < 0.05$, ** $p < 0.01$, significantly different with corresponding control PBS- (panel (**A**)), or DMEM- (panel (**C**)) treatment group.

3.4.2. Effect of Intestinal Pretreatment with L-Tryptophan on the Intestinal Absorption of Insulin

The results from the previous section suggest that L-tryptophan can enhance the intestinal absorption of insulin via functional and structural modification of the intestinal mucosa, while not exhibiting cytotoxicity (Figure 5). When further considering the safe use of absorption enhancers, it is important that these agents exhibit either no effect or only a temporal effect on the functions of the mucosal membrane since this membrane is an integral component of the defense system protecting against exogenous pathogens. To assess the reversibility of L-tryptophan activity, an insulin solution was administered to rat ileal loop after pretreatment with L-tryptophan (32 mM), CPPs (D-R8 and L-penetratin), or conventional enhancers (C10 and sodium taurodeoxycholate) for 30 min and then washing the pretreated ileal segment with fresh PBS.

As shown in Figure 6A, an increase in plasma insulin concentration was observed after the administration of insulin to the ileal loop pretreated with L-tryptophan and L-penetratin, however, the extent of insulin absorption was lower than the effect of co-administration with these enhancers (Figure 1A). In addition, the onset of insulin absorption could be shifted to an early time point, (5 min after administration of insulin), by pretreating withL-tryptophan. In contrast, pretreatment with C10 and sodium taurodeoxycholate had a stronger stimulatory response on intestinal absorption of insulin than L-tryptophan and L-penetratin (Figure 6B). When insulin was administered into the ileal loop after 30 min of pretreatment with L-tryptophan followed by washing and further rest for 30 min, the increase in the plasma insulin concentration was almost completely eliminated (Figure 6C), suggesting that the action of L-tryptophan was temporal and reversible. The pharmacokinetic parameters are summarized in Table 1.

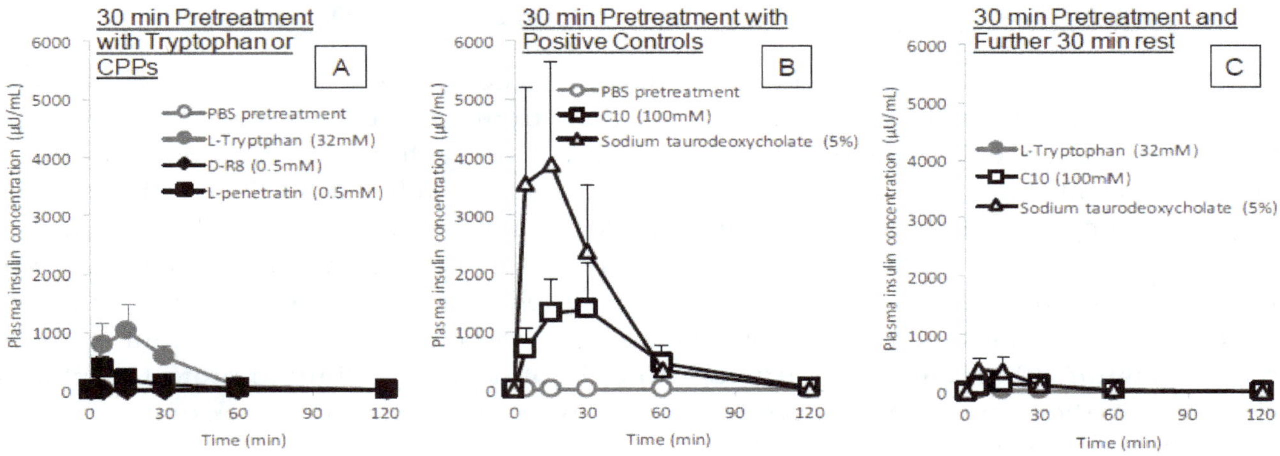

Figure 6. Time profiles of plasma insulin concentration after in situ administration of insulin (50 IU/kg) into rat ileal loop pretreated with L-tryptophan (32 mM), D-R8 (0.5 mM), L-penetratin (0.5 mM), C10 (100 mM), or sodium taurodeoxycholate (5%). In the results shown in Panels (**A**,**B**), insulin solution was administered immediately after washing the pretreatment solution from the ileal loop. For the results shown in Panel (**C**), insulin solution was administered at 30 min after washing out the pretreatment solution. Each data point represents the mean ± SEM of $N = 3$–4.

3.5. Mechanistic Analysis for the Intestinal Absorption of Insulin Facilitated by L-Tryptophan

3.5.1. Possibility of the Intermolecular Interaction between Insulin and L-Tryptophan

The above-mentioned results suggest that single amino acid L-tryptophan is unique in its ability to enhance the intestinal absorption of insulin. The binding affinity of L-tryptophan with insulin and/or possible activity of L-tryptophan in the modulation of biological functions and structures may explain its specificity for absorption enhancement. In this section, we analyzed the intermolecular interaction between insulin and L-tryptophan using a SPR-based assay.

Figure 7 shows the binding sensorgrams obtained from the assay. Various concentrations of L-tryptophan (2–200 μM) or L-penetratin (2–200 μM) were injected into the flow cells containing immobilized insulin. The resulting sensorgrams do not show an increase after the injection of L-tryptophan at any concentration (Figure 7A). For comparison, L-penetratin was bound to the insulin-immobilized flow cells depending on the applied insulin concentration (Figure 7B) in a manner consistent with our previous publications [29]. These results suggest that L-tryptophan can enhance the absorption of insulin without intermolecular interaction and that the modulation of mucosal epithelial structure might be important for the enhancement of intestinal insulin absorption mediated by L-tryptophan.

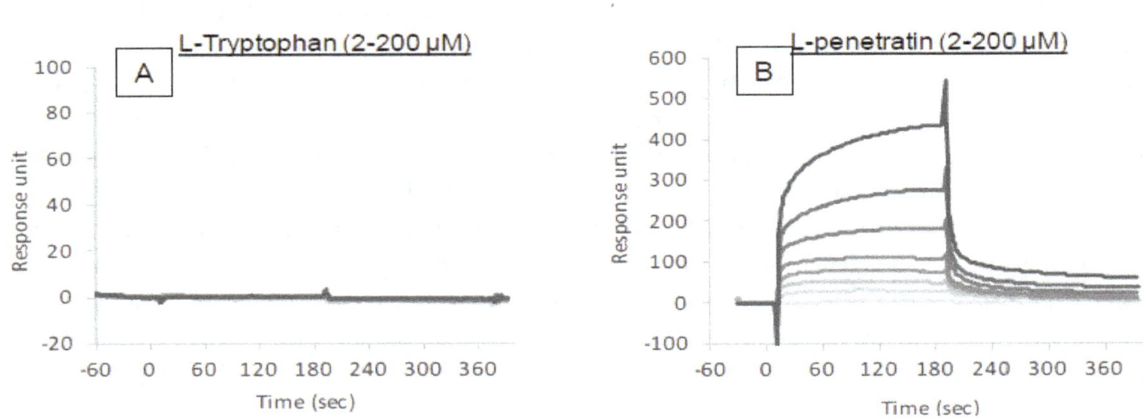

Figure 7. Binding sensorgrams obtained by SPR analysis. Various concentrations of L-tryptophan (**A**) or L-penetratin (**B**) solutions (pH 7.4) were injected into insulin-immobilized flow cells.

3.5.2. Possible Ability of Tryptophan to Protect Insulin from Enzymatic Degradation

The formation of the complex via intermolecular interaction between insulin and L-tryptophan or L-penetratin might be related to the protection of insulin from the intestinal enzymatic degradation. Therefore, we further evaluated the protective effect of L-tryptophan and L-penetratin on the degradation of insulin in the intestinal enzymatic fluid. As shown in Figure 8B, the positive control STI (1.25 mg/mL) completely abolished the activity of proteases in the intestinal fluid and the co-incubation with L-penetratin partially protected insulin from the enzymatic degradation. This was consistent with the result in our previous work [6]. This suggested that the stabilization of insulin in the presence of L-penetratin could be probably explained by steric hindrance via their intermolecular interaction (Figure 7B). In contrast, L-tryptophan did not have the ability to protect insulin from intestinal enzymatic degradation (Figure 8A). This may be attributed to the lack of intermolecular interaction between insulin and L-tryptophan (Figure 7A).

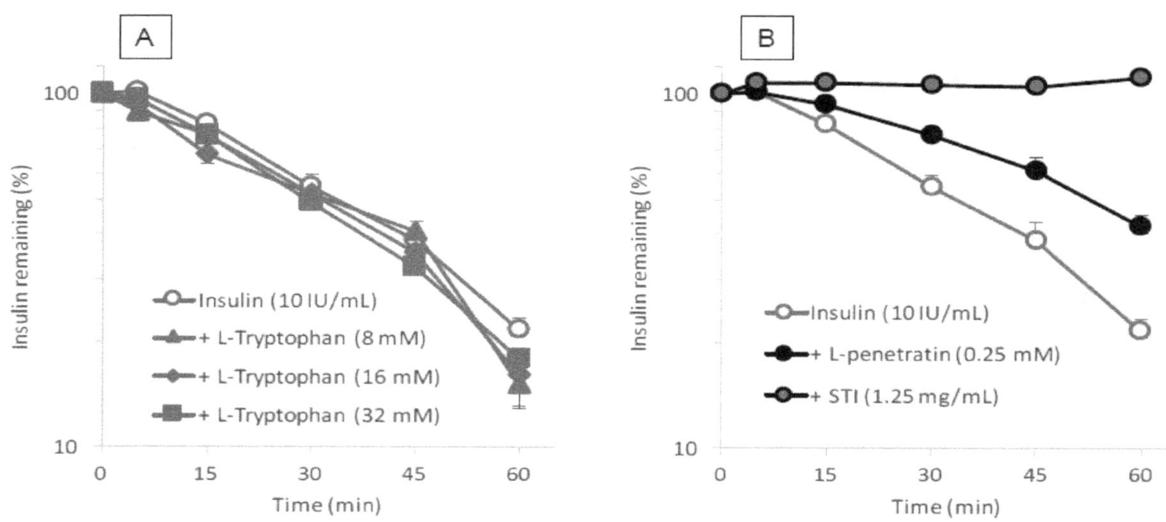

Figure 8. Degradation profiles of insulin in the presence of tryptophan or positive controls (penetratin and STI) in rat intestinal enzymatic fluid. Panel (**A**), various concentrations of L-tryptophan (8–32 mM); panel (**B**), L-penetratin (0.25 mM) or STI (positive control, 1.25 mg/mL). Each data point represents the mean ± SEM of $N = 3$.

3.5.3. Possibility of Paracellular Transport via Tight Junction Opening Effect Induced by L-Tryptophan and Its Metabolite

The temporal effect of pretreatment with L-tryptophan on the intestinal absorption of insulin (Figure 6A,C) suggested that L-tryptophan could possibly modify the structure of the lipid membrane or tight junctions in the intestinal epithelium, resulting in enhanced transcellular or paracellular transport of insulin. Therefore, the epithelial transport of insulin in the in vitro Caco-2 cell monolayer model was then examined in the absence or presence of L-tryptophan. Figure 9A shows the TEER values which reflect the integrity of paracellular tight junctions after the application of L-tryptophan into Caco-2 cells grown in transwells. No change in the TEER values was observed after addition of L-tryptophan at all concentrations examined (600–16,000 μM), although a significant reduction in TEER was observed after addition of typical enhancer C10. The maintained TEER confirmed that the cellular lipid membrane was retained after addition of L-tryptophan, consistent with the LDH release assays (Figure 5A,B). Consistent with the result in TEER measurement, Figure 9B showed no change in the in vitro epithelial permeation of insulin after co-incubation with various concentrations of L-tryptophan.

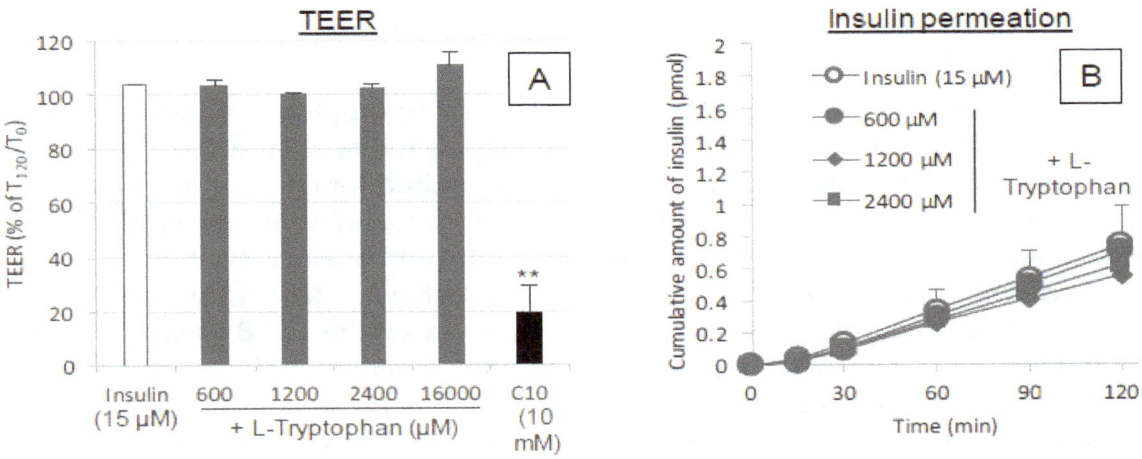

Figure 9. Cytotoxicity examinations after the exposure of intestinal epithelium to L-tryptophan. Panel (**A**), changes in the TEER of Caco-2 cell monolayers after the incubation with insulin (15 μM) and various concentrations of L-tryptophan (600–16,000 μM). The values are expressed as a percentage calculated by dividing the TEER measurement (Ω cm^2) at 120 min by the initial value. Panel (**B**), time courses of permeation of insulin through Caco-2 monolayer in the presence or absence of L-Tryptophan (600–2400 μM). Each data point represents the mean ± SEM of $N = 3$. * $p < 0.05$, ** $p < 0.01$, significantly different with corresponding insulin control group.

3.5.4. Isomeric Dependent Effect of Tryptophan Co-Administration on the Intestinal Absorption of Insulin

The lack of L-tryptophan effect in the in vitro transport assay (Figure 9B) contradicted the in situ and in vivo effect of L-tryptophan on the absorption of insulin (Figures 1A and 2), suggesting that inherent active transport systems might potentially be associated with the action of L-tryptophan but that these transport systems might be diminished or deficient in Caco-2 cells. In our recent work, we found that only the L-form of arginine in its amino acid form can facilitate the intestinal absorption of insulin [13]. As it is possible that the effect of tryptophan may also vary between L- and D-forms, we conducted an in situ absorption study of insulin with D-tryptophan (16 and 32 mM) and compared its effectiveness to that of L-tryptophan (Figure 1A). The results in Figure 10 show that the effect of D-tryptophan appears much weaker than that of L-tryptophan but the onset of action by D-tryptophan (60 min after administration) was similar to that of L-tryptophan.

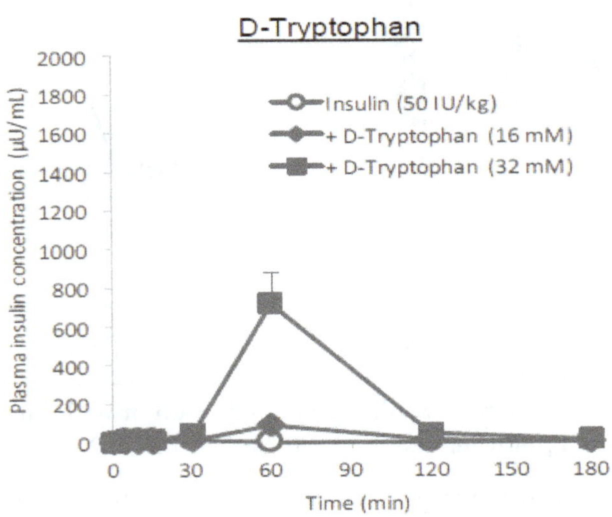

Figure 10. Time profiles of plasma insulin concentration after in situ administration of insulin (50 IU/kg) with or without D-tryptophan (16 or 32 mM) into rat ileal loop. Each data point represents the mean ± SEM of $N = 3$.

3.5.5. Possible Involvement of Serotonin as Active Metabolite of L-Tryptophan to Enhance the Intestinal Absorption of Insulin

On the other hand, it is possible that the metabolite of L-tryptophan, serotonin, has the potential to enhance the epithelial permeability of insulin and other macromolecular drugs [30] and the delayed action of L-tryptophan might be attributed to the time required for conversion from tryptophan to serotonin after administration to the intestine. Therefore, we then tested the effect of serotonin on the permeation and absorption of insulin under the in vitro and in situ conditions. The result of the permeation study with Caco-2 cell monolayer (Figure 11A,B) showed that serotonin had no stimulatory effect on the permeation of insulin, in fact, serotonin increased the TEER as shown in Figure 11C, suggesting that paracellular space was tightened by addition of serotonin. Consistent with the increase in TEER, the permeability of insulin through the Caco-2 cell monolayer decreased by co-incubation with serotonin (Figure 11B). On the other hand, serotonin (32 mM) could enhance the intestinal absorption of insulin after administration to a rat ileal loop but it was less effective than L-tryptophan (Figure 11D). The pharmacokinetic parameters are summarized in Table 1. The relationship between results in the in vitro and in vivo conditions is unknown.

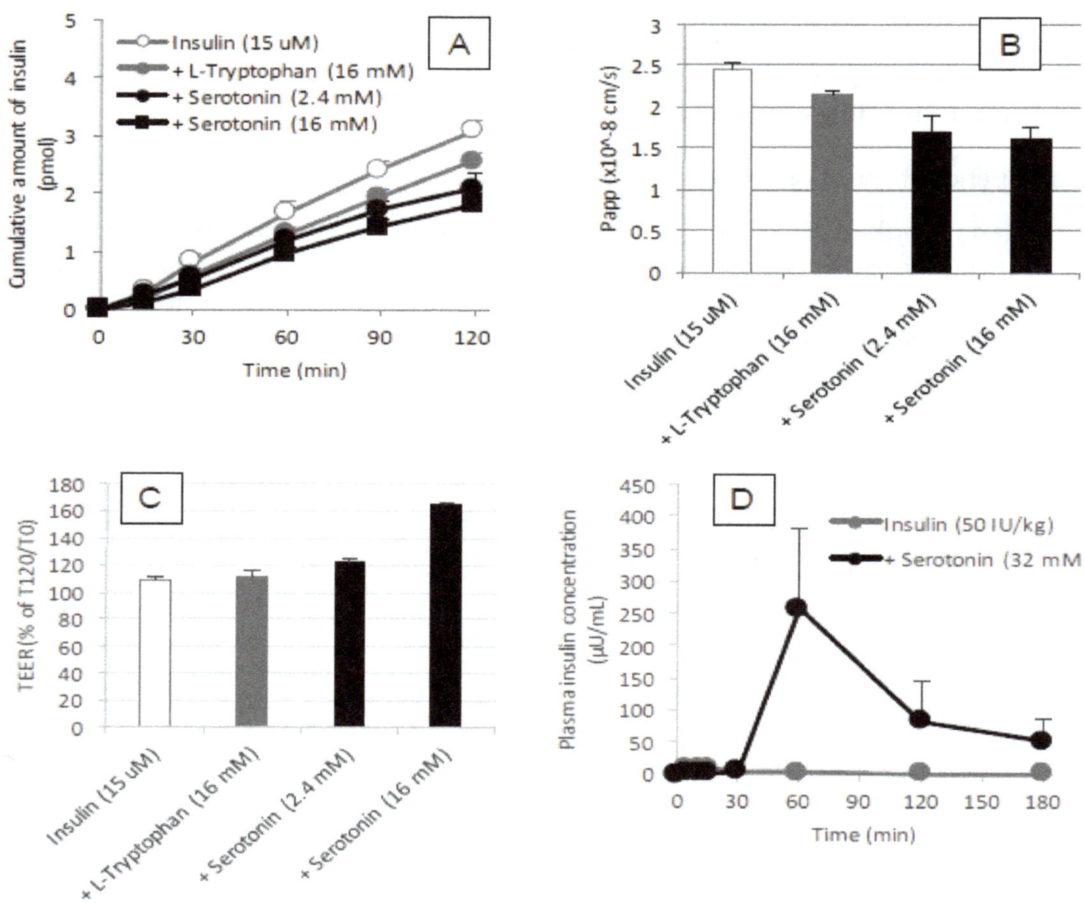

Figure 11. Permeation of insulin through the Caco-2 cell monolayer panels (**A**,**B**) and TEER values panel (**C**) during coincubation with L-tryptophan (16 mM) or serotonin (2.4 or 16 mM) and the absorption of insulin after its in situ administration of insulin (50 IU/kg) with or without serotonin (32 mM) into rat ileal loop panel (**D**). Each data point represents the mean ± SEM of $N = 3$.

3.5.6. Combined Effect of Co-Administration of L-Tryptophan with L-Penetratin on the Intestinal Absorption of Macromolecules

The difference in the action onset between L-tryptophan (slow) and L-penetratin (rapid) shown in Figure 1A suggested that these two enhancers used different pathways to enhance the intestinal absorption of insulin and other macromolecular drugs. No intermolecular interaction between insulin and L-tryptophan (Figure 7A,B) confirmed that L-tryptophan uses a different mechanism than L-penetratin. Therefore, we then examined the additive or synergistic potential of the combination of L-tryptophan and L-penetratin to increase the intestinal absorption of macromolecular dextran (FD-4) in the in situ ileal loop administration study.

As shown in Figure 12, the individual effect of L-tryptophan (16 mM) and L-penetratin (0.5 mM) on the absorption of FD-4 was confirmed as being delayed and rapid onset, respectively, consistent with the above-mentioned results with insulin (Figure 1). Contrary to our expectation, the effect of the combined co-administration with L-tryptophan (16 mM) and L-penetratin (0.5 mM) on the absorption of FD-4 was almost equal to that co-administered with only L-penetratin (0.5 mM). As L-penetratin had the capacity to interact with FD-4 similar to insulin, L-tryptophan might be deprived of a chance to facilitate the absorption of FD-4. Possibly, a large part of FD-4 administered to the intestine could be systemically and quickly absorbed by complexing with L-penetratin, while FD-4 which could be delivered by L-tryptophan was scarce due to the slow mechanism of action. The results suggested that the action mechanism of L-tryptophan to facilitate the intestinal absorption of macromolecular drugs was different from that of L-penetratin.

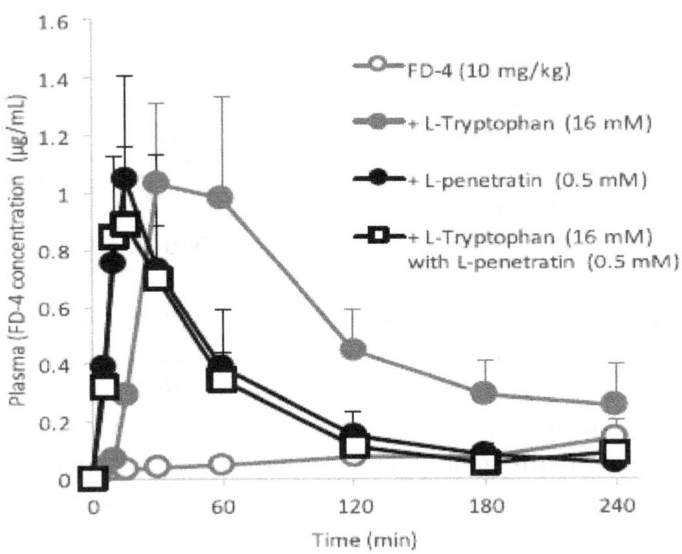

Figure 12. Time profiles of plasma concentrations of FD-4 after its in situ administration with or without L-tryptophan (16 mM) and/or L-penetratin (0.5 mM) into rat ileal loop. Each data point represents the mean ± SEM of $N = 3–4$.

4. Discussion

We recently discovered that single amino acid arginine, particularly the L-form of arginine, an important component in cationic CPPs, has the potential to facilitate the intestinal absorption of insulin without being part of a peptide structure such as arginine-rich CPPs [13]. Another amino acid, the hydrophobic amino acid tryptophan, is known to play an important role in the cellular association and internalization of the amphipathic CPP, penetratin [16,18]. In fact, our previous study demonstrated that the amphipathic CPP enhanced the intestinal absorption of insulin to a greater degree than cationic CPPs such as R8 and Tat peptide [3]. Therefore, we hypothesized that addition of tryptophan to insulin might potentially improve the intestinal absorption of insulin.

The data showed that the intestinal absorption of insulin was significantly enhanced by co-administration with L-tryptophan (16 or 32 mM, Figure 1A and Table 1), comparable to the effect of L-penetratin (0.5 mM). Interestingly, the onset patterns of insulin absorption after co-administration were quite different between L-arginine (T_{max} 12.8 ± 0.9 min at 40 mM) and L-tryptophan (T_{max} 52.5 ± 7.5 min at 32 mM), as shown in Figure 1A, Table 1 and our previous publication [13], suggesting that different mechanisms might be associated with the absorption enhancement by cationic arginine versus hydrophobic tryptophan. On the other hand, we showed in our previous publications that the simple cationic CPP (R8) generated a relatively slow enhancing effect, whereas the typical amphipathic CPP (penetratin), containing two tryptophan residues, rapidly enhanced the absorption of insulin [3,21], contradicting the effect of amino acids, L-arginine and L-tryptophan, observed in the present and current studies [13]. This suggests that L-tryptophan and L-arginine could enhance intestinal absorption via mechanisms distinctly different from that involving CPPs.

The binding analysis showed no intermolecular interaction between insulin and L-tryptophan (Figure 7), implying that L-tryptophan has no capacity to bring the noncovalently mixed drugs as a delivery carrier. L-arginine also showed no binding with insulin (data not shown). This observation is quite different from the mechanism of penetratin and R8 in which intermolecular interaction is essential to their ability as absorption enhancers. There was no protective effect of L-tryptophan on the enzymatic degradation of insulin (Figure 8A), confirming no possible interaction between insulin and L-tryptophan. With respect to the opening of tight junctions as a possible mechanism, the examination in our recent report suggested that no opening of tight junctions was observed after adding the effective concentrations of L-arginine (9.6 mM equivalent to 4.2 mg/kg in the animal study) to the transwell with Caco-2 cell monolayers [13]. In regard to tryptophan, while there is an earlier report suggesting that mucosal exposure of L-tryptophan (1 mM or more) increases the paracellular permeability of macromolecules in an energy- and sodium-dependent manner [31], more recent study suggests that indole-containing molecules like tryptophan strengthen the epithelial barrier function via the increased expression of tight junction-related proteins such as claudins and occludins [32,33]. No change in the TEER values of Caco-2 cell monolayers was observed after addition of various concentrations of L-tryptophan (600–16,000 μM) (Figure 9A). Therefore, it is expected that the mechanism resulting in the enhancement of the mucosal absorption by both amino acids does not occur via opening of tight junctions.

Interestingly, it was suggested that the enteric nervous system was associated with the intestinal transport of low molecular weight compounds and hydrophilic macromolecules [34,35]. While the adrenergic stimulation has been known to decrease the intestinal absorption of dextran with molecular weights of 20,000 and 40,000 g/mol [35], vascular perfusion with the cholinergic agonist bethanechol can contribute to the increase in intestinal drug transport [34]. Furthermore, serotonin, a major metabolite of tryptophan, is known to promote the secretion of acetylcholine via the stimulation of the serotonin 5-HT$_4$ receptor, possibly contributing to the increased intestinal absorption of macromolecules [30]. No enhancement of the epithelial permeation of insulin in the presence of L-tryptophan (Figure 9B) may strengthen the hypothesis that L-tryptophan needs to be metabolized for enhancing the epithelial permeation of drugs. However, our in vivo data (Figure 11D) in the present study was inconsistent with such a hypothesis, as the effect of serotonin (32 mM) on the intestinal absorption of insulin was weaker than that of L-tryptophan (32 mM) and the action onset of serotonin was delayed compared to L-tryptophan. Furthermore, our in vitro data partially negated the possible cholinergic contribution, as serotonin appeared to tighten the paracellular space and decrease the epithelial transport of insulin through a Caco-2 cell monolayer (Figure 11A–C). In the present study regarding the ability of tryptophan to enhance intestinal absorption, the L-form is more effective than the D-form (Figure 10), similar to arginine. Considering the differences between how L- and D-amino acids affect insulin absorption, endogenous systems such as the enteric nervous system, the transporter-mediated influx, or receptor-mediated influx mechanisms might be involved either directly or indirectly. Although some effects of D-tryptophan remained at the higher dose (32 mM), it was considerably small compared to that of L-tryptophan (Figure 10 and Table 1), suggesting that stereospecificity might be partially involved in their absorption enhancing mechanisms.

The in situ administration study conducted after pretreatment with L-tryptophan indicated its reversibility in the enhancement of the intestinal absorption of insulin. As shown in Figure 6C, the absorption stimulatory effect of L-tryptophan greatly diminishes at 30 min after pretreatment with L-tryptophan followed by washing, like the effect of conventional positive controls such as C10 and sodium taurodeoxycholate. These results along with the cytotoxic analysis (Figure 5A–C and Figure 9A) suggest L-tryptophan has no irreversible effect on the mucosal structure, which means that L-tryptophan does not induce permanent functional change to the intestinal membrane. Future studies are needed to clarify the mechanism.

Based on the results of the in situ intestinal insulin absorption study, we examined the potential of L-tryptophan as an oral absorption enhancer for insulin in vivo. Figure 2 clearly showed the hypoglycemic effects after oral administration of insulin (50 IU/kg) with L-tryptophan (32 mM). In this study, insulin and L-tryptophan were administered just as a solution, therefore, the development of an appropriate formulation could be expected to increase the biological effect of insulin. Figures 3 and 4 clearly demonstrates the wide applicability of L-tryptophan as an absorption enhancer for macromolecules having peptide- to protein-sized molecular weights. In contrast, L-arginine had no effect on the intestinal absorption of such peptide drugs (data not shown). The effectiveness of absorption enhancement by L-tryptophan was comparable to that by L-penetratin, although L-tryptophan required relatively higher concentrations (16 mM or more) than L-penetratin (0.5 mM). Since L-tryptophan is currently used as an oral supplement and it appears to facilitate the intestinal absorption of a wide variety of biopharmaceuticals, its potential as an intestinal absorption enhancer is meritorious and quite unique.

As mentioned above, tryptophan is first metabolized into serotonin which stimulates the cholinergic nervous system, balancing neural activity. Therefore, although L-tryptophan is one of the essential amino acids, its excess use has to be carefully considered for safe pharmacotherapy. In addition, another metabolite from tryptophan, melatonin, is used as a sleep-inducing agent and therefore may affect circadian rhythm. The required dose of L-tryptophan for inducing sleepiness is roughly to 1500–3000 mg$\cdot$day$^{-1}\cdot$human^{-1}, which is comparable to the maximum dose used to enhance the intestinal absorption of biopharmaceuticals (32 mM equivalent to 16.3 mg/kg) in this study. However, the dose of L-tryptophan used as an absorption enhancer could be further optimized by precisely evaluating the relation between its co-administered concentration and the efficiency of the resultant absorption enhancement. Considering the effective plasma concentration of insulin (<100 μU/mL), it is expected that the dose of L-tryptophan can be reduced to 10 mM, the equivalent to 5.1 mg/kg (300 mg/human). Further examination will be essential to establish the potential of L-tryptophan as a safe and effective absorption enhancer for the oral delivery of biopharmaceuticals.

5. Conclusions

In the process of studying the role of the hydrophobic amino acid tryptophan, which was widely known as a key amino acid in the function of CPPs, we discovered that tryptophan singly improves the intestinal absorption of various biopharmaceuticals having peptide to protein molecular sizes. When examining the absorption of insulin in particular, the bioavailability enhancement effect of L-tryptophan was far stronger than that of L-arginine [13], another key cationic amino acid component of CPPs and comparable to the potent CPP, L-penetratin. However, the mechanism of action remains unclear. In the present study, the cell integrity of the intestinal epithelium (demonstrated by assessing cell viability, cell membrane integrity and the tightness of paracellular junctions) was not changed in the presence of L-tryptophan. Furthermore, no intermolecular interaction between insulin and L-tryptophan was observed and insulin was not protected from enzymatic degradation when in the presence of L-tryptophan. Tryptophan is the precursor of a wide array of bioactive compounds, such as serotonin, melatonin and so forth. [36]. Considering the stronger action of L-tryptophan as an absorption enhancer relative to the D-form, inherent biological functions might be involved in its action mechanisms. To utilize L-tryptophan as a safe absorption enhancer, further studies are required to identify the complete mechanism of action.

Author Contributions: M.T.-M. conceived the study and acquired research grants. N.K. and M.T.-M. designed the study. H.T. and M.M. conducted in situ loop absorption experiments. H.T., M.M. and K.H. conducted in vivo oral absorption experiments. H.T conducted in situ intestinal toxicity examinations (LDH assay). H.O. and S.H.

conducted in vitro cytotoxicity examinations (LDH and WST-8 assays) and transcellular transport assays. M.M. conducted SPR-binding assays. Y.H. and K.M. conducted enzymatic degradation assays. N.K. prepared the manuscript. All authors analyzed and discussed the results and reviewed the manuscript.

Acknowledgments: The authors are grateful to Matthew Miller (Laboratory of Biomaterials, Drug Delivery, and Bionanotechnology, McKetta Department of Chemical Engineering, Cockrell School of Engineering, The University of Texas at Austin) for his assistance in improving English in the manuscript.

References

1. Komin, A.; Russell, L.M.; Hristova, K.A.; Searson, P.C. Peptide-based strategies for enhanced cell uptake, transcellular transport, and circulation: Mechanisms and challenges. *Adv. Drug Deliv. Rev.* **2017**, *110–111*, 52–64. [CrossRef] [PubMed]
2. Salzano, G.; Torchilin, V.P. Intracellular delivery of nanoparticles with cell penetrating peptides. *Methods Mol. Biol.* **2015**, *1324*, 357–368. [PubMed]
3. Kamei, N.; Morishita, M.; Eda, Y.; Ida, N.; Nishio, R.; Takayama, K. Usefulness of cell-penetrating peptides to improve intestinal insulin absorption. *J. Control. Release* **2008**, *132*, 21–25. [CrossRef] [PubMed]
4. Kamei, N.; Morishita, M.; Takayama, K. Importance of intermolecular interaction on the improvement of intestinal therapeutic peptide/protein absorption using cell-penetrating peptides. *J. Control. Release* **2009**, *136*, 179–186. [CrossRef] [PubMed]
5. Khafagy, E.-S.; Morishita, M.; Kamei, N.; Eda, Y.; Ikeno, Y.; Takayama, K. Efficiency of cell-penetrating peptides on the nasal and intestinal absorption of therapeutic peptides and proteins. *Int. J. Pharm.* **2009**, *381*, 49–55. [CrossRef] [PubMed]
6. Khafagy, E.S.; Iwamae, R.; Kamei, N.; Takeda-Morishita, M. Region-dependent role of cell-penetrating peptides in insulin absorption across the rat small intestinal membrane. *AAPS J.* **2015**, *17*, 1427–1437. [CrossRef] [PubMed]
7. Brock, R. The uptake of arginine-rich cell-penetrating peptides: Putting the puzzle together. *Bioconjug. Chem.* **2014**, *25*, 863–868. [CrossRef] [PubMed]
8. Copolovici, D.M.; Langel, K.; Eriste, E.; Langel, U. Cell-penetrating peptides: Design, synthesis, and applications. *ACS Nano* **2014**, *8*, 1972–1994. [CrossRef] [PubMed]
9. Bechara, C.; Sagan, S. Cell-penetrating peptides: 20 years later, where do we stand? *FEBS Lett.* **2013**, *587*, 1693–1702. [CrossRef] [PubMed]
10. Kamei, N.; Onuki, Y.; Takayama, K.; Takeda-Morishita, M. Mechanistic study of the uptake/permeation of cell-penetrating peptides across a caco-2 monolayer and their stimulatory effect on epithelial insulin transport. *J. Pharm. Sci.* **2013**, *102*, 3998–4008. [CrossRef] [PubMed]
11. Futaki, S.; Suzuki, T.; Ohashi, W.; Yagami, T.; Tanaka, S.; Ueda, K.; Sugiura, Y. Arginine-rich peptides. An abundant source of membrane-permeable peptides having potential as carriers for intracellular protein delivery. *J. Biol. Chem.* **2001**, *276*, 5836–5840. [CrossRef] [PubMed]
12. Morishita, M.; Kamei, N.; Ehara, J.; Isowa, K.; Takayama, K. A novel approach using functional peptides for efficient intestinal absorption of insulin. *J. Control. Release* **2007**, *118*, 177–184. [CrossRef] [PubMed]
13. Kamei, N.; Khafagy, E.S.; Hirose, J.; Takeda-Morishita, M. Potential of single cationic amino acid molecule "arginine" for stimulating oral absorption of insulin. *Int. J. Pharm.* **2017**, *521*, 176–183. [CrossRef] [PubMed]
14. Bechara, C.; Pallerla, M.; Zaltsman, Y.; Burlina, F.; Alves, I.D.; Lequin, O.; Sagan, S. Tryptophan within basic peptide sequences triggers glycosaminoglycan-dependent endocytosis. *FASEB J.* **2013**, *27*, 738–749. [CrossRef] [PubMed]
15. Jobin, M.L.; Bonnafous, P.; Temsamani, H.; Dole, F.; Grelard, A.; Dufourc, E.J.; Alves, I.D. The enhanced membrane interaction and perturbation of a cell penetrating peptide in the presence of anionic lipids: Toward an understanding of its selectivity for cancer cells. *Biochim. Biophys. Acta* **2013**, *1828*, 1457–1470. [CrossRef] [PubMed]
16. Jobin, M.L.; Blanchet, M.; Henry, S.; Chaignepain, S.; Manigand, C.; Castano, S.; Lecomte, S.; Burlina, F.; Sagan, S.; Alves, I.D. The role of tryptophans on the cellular uptake and membrane interaction of arginine-rich cell penetrating peptides. *Biochim. Biophys. Acta* **2015**, *1848*, 593–602. [CrossRef] [PubMed]
17. Crombez, L.; Aldrian-Herrada, G.; Konate, K.; Nguyen, Q.N.; McMaster, G.K.; Brasseur, R.; Heitz, F.; Divita, G. A new potent secondary amphipathic cell-penetrating peptide for sirna delivery into mammalian cells. *Mol. Ther.* **2009**, *17*, 95–103. [CrossRef] [PubMed]

18. Christiaens, B.; Grooten, J.; Reusens, M.; Joliot, A.; Goethals, M.; Vandekerckhove, J.; Prochiantz, A.; Rosseneu, M. Membrane interaction and cellular internalization of penetratin peptides. *Eur. J. Biochem.* **2004**, *271*, 1187–1197. [CrossRef] [PubMed]
19. Futaki, S.; Ohashi, W.; Suzuki, T.; Niwa, M.; Tanaka, S.; Ueda, K.; Harashima, H.; Sugiura, Y. Stearylated arginine-rich peptides: A new class of transfection systems. *Bioconjug. Chem.* **2001**, *12*, 1005–1011. [CrossRef] [PubMed]
20. Khalil, I.A.; Futaki, S.; Niwa, M.; Baba, Y.; Kaji, N.; Kamiya, H.; Harashima, H. Mechanism of improved gene transfer by the n-terminal stearylation of octaarginine: Enhanced cellular association by hydrophobic core formation. *Gene Ther.* **2004**, *11*, 636–644. [CrossRef] [PubMed]
21. Kamei, N.; Morishita, M.; Kanayama, Y.; Hasegawa, K.; Nishimura, M.; Hayashinaka, E.; Wada, Y.; Watanabe, Y.; Takayama, K. Molecular imaging analysis of intestinal insulin absorption boosted by cell-penetrating peptides by using positron emission tomography. *J. Control. Release* **2010**, *146*, 16–22. [CrossRef] [PubMed]
22. Khafagy, E.-S.; Morishita, M.; Isowa, K.; Imai, J.; Takayama, K. Effect of cell-penetrating peptides on the nasal absorption of insulin. *J. Control. Release* **2009**, *133*, 103–108. [CrossRef] [PubMed]
23. Maher, S.; Leonard, T.W.; Jacobsen, J.; Brayden, D.J. Safety and efficacy of sodium caprate in promoting oral drug absorption: From in vitro to the clinic. *Adv. Drug Deliv. Rev.* **2009**, *61*, 1427–1449. [CrossRef] [PubMed]
24. Krug, S.M.; Amasheh, M.; Dittmann, I.; Christoffel, I.; Fromm, M.; Amasheh, S. Sodium caprate as an enhancer of macromolecule permeation across tricellular tight junctions of intestinal cells. *Biomaterials* **2013**, *34*, 275–282. [CrossRef] [PubMed]
25. Brayden, D.J.; Maher, S.; Bahar, B.; Walsh, E. Sodium caprate-induced increases in intestinal permeability and epithelial damage are prevented by misoprostol. *Eur. J. Pharm. Biopharm.* **2015**, *94*, 194–206. [CrossRef] [PubMed]
26. Swenson, E.S.; Milisen, W.B.; Curatolo, W. Intestinal permeability enhancement: Efficacy, acute local toxicity, and reversibility. *Pharm. Res.* **1994**, *11*, 1132–1142. [CrossRef] [PubMed]
27. Whitehead, K.; Karr, N.; Mitragotri, S. Safe and effective permeation enhancers for oral drug delivery. *Pharm. Res.* **2008**, *25*, 1782–1788. [CrossRef] [PubMed]
28. Karsdal, M.A.; Riis, B.J.; Mehta, N.; Stern, W.; Arbit, E.; Christiansen, C.; Henriksen, K. Lessons learned from the clinical development of oral peptides. *Br. J. Clin. Pharmacol.* **2015**, *79*, 720–732. [CrossRef] [PubMed]
29. Kamei, N.; Aoyama, Y.; Khafagy, E.-S.; Henmi, M.; Takeda-Morishita, M. Effect of different intestinal conditions on the intermolecular interaction between insulin and cell-penetrating peptide penetratin and on its contribution to stimulation of permeation through intestinal epithelium. *Eur. J. Pharm. Biopharm.* **2015**, *94*, 42–51. [CrossRef] [PubMed]
30. Hiraoka, H.; Kimura, N.; Furukawa, Y.; Ogawara, K.; Kimura, T.; Higaki, K. Up-regulation of p-glycoprotein expression in small intestine under chronic serotonin-depleted conditions in rats. *J. Pharmacol. Exp. Ther.* **2005**, *312*, 248–255. [CrossRef] [PubMed]
31. Madara, J.L.; Carlson, S. Supraphysiologic l-tryptophan elicits cytoskeletal and macromolecular permeability alterations in hamster small intestinal epithelium in vitro. *J. Clin. Investig.* **1991**, *87*, 454–462. [CrossRef] [PubMed]
32. Bansal, T.; Alaniz, R.C.; Wood, T.K.; Jayaraman, A. The bacterial signal indole increases epithelial-cell tight-junction resistance and attenuates indicators of inflammation. *Proc. Natl. Acad. Sci. USA* **2010**, *107*, 228–233. [CrossRef] [PubMed]
33. Shimada, Y.; Kinoshita, M.; Harada, K.; Mizutani, M.; Masahata, K.; Kayama, H.; Takeda, K. Commensal bacteria-dependent indole production enhances epithelial barrier function in the colon. *PLoS ONE* **2013**, *8*, e80604. [CrossRef] [PubMed]
34. Higaki, K.; Sone, M.; Ogawara, K.; Kimura, T. Regulation of drug absorption from small intestine by enteric nervous system i: A poorly absorbable drug via passive diffusion. *Drug Metab. Pharmacokinet.* **2004**, *19*, 198–205. [CrossRef] [PubMed]
35. Kimoto, T.; Takanashi, M.; Mukai, H.; Ogawara, K.; Kimura, T.; Higaki, K. Effect of adrenergic stimulation on drug absorption via passive diffusion in caco-2 cells. *Int. J. Pharm.* **2009**, *368*, 31–36. [CrossRef] [PubMed]
36. Kaluzna-Czaplinska, J.; Gatarek, P.; Chirumbolo, S.; Chartrand, M.S.; Bjorklund, G. How important is tryptophan in human health? *Crit. Rev. Food Sci. Nutr.* **2017**, 1–17. [CrossRef] [PubMed]

11

Chitosan Plus Compound 48/80: Formulation and Preliminary Evaluation as a Hepatitis B Vaccine Adjuvant

Dulce Bento [1,2], Sandra Jesus [1,2], Filipa Lebre [1,2], Teresa Gonçalves [1,3] and Olga Borges [1,2,*]

1 CNC-Center for Neuroscience and Cell Biology, University of Coimbra, 3004-0504 Coimbra, Portugal; dfbento@gmail.com (D.B.); sjesus.mg@gmail.com (S.J.); filipalebre@sapo.pt (F.L.); tgoncalves@fmed.uc.pt (T.G.)

2 Faculty of Pharmacy, University of Coimbra, Pólo das Ciências da Saúde, Azinhaga de Santa Comba, 3000-548 Coimbra, Portugal

3 Faculty of Medicine, University of Coimbra, 3004-504 Coimbra, Portugal

* Correspondence: olga@ci.uc.pt

Abstract: Current vaccine research is mostly based on subunit antigens. Despite the better toxicity profile of these antigens they are often poorly immunogenic, so adjuvant association has been explored as a strategy to obtain a potent vaccine formulation. Recently, mast cell activators were recognized as a new class of vaccine adjuvants capable of potentiating mucosal and systemic immune responses. In this study, a co-adjuvanted delivery system was developed and characterized, combining the mast cell activator C48/80 with chitosan nanoparticles (Chi-C48/80 NPs), and the results were compared with plain chitosan nanoparticles. The adsorption of model antigens onto the NP surface as well as the biocompatibility of the system was not affected by the incorporation of C48/80 in the formulation. The stability of the nanoparticles was demonstrated by studying the variation of size and zeta potential at different times, and the ability to be internalized by antigen presenting cells was confirmed by confocal microscopy. Vaccination studies with hepatitis B surface antigen loaded Chi-C48/80 NPs validated the adjuvanticity of the delivery system, demonstrating for the first time a successful association between a mast cell activator and chitosan nanoparticles as a vaccine adjuvant for hepatitis B virus, applied to a nasal vaccination strategy.

Keywords: compound 48/80; chitosan; nanoparticles; mast cell activator; vaccine adjuvant; nasal vaccination

---

1. Introduction

Traditional vaccines consisting of live attenuated or inactivated pathogens are highly immunogenic, but, due to safety concerns, development of new vaccines is being focused on the use of recombinant subunit antigens. Recombinant antigens are safer but they are often poorly immunogenic, requiring the use of adjuvants to enhance the resultant immune response. Therefore, different adjuvant approaches have been studied to enhance and/or modulate vaccine response to subunit antigens. Among them is the use of nanotechnology, a strategy that has been extensively explored and holds great promise [1,2]. Formulation of antigens in nanoparticles may offer several attractive features, namely an enhanced uptake by antigen presenting cells (APCs) [3], a depot effect with gradual release of the antigen [1,4], a cross-presentation of antigens [1,5], slower antigen processing than antigens in solution, which can result in a prolonged antigen presentation [6], and the co-delivery of antigens and adjuvants to the same cell population [2]. Besides, particulate antigens are generally more immunogenic than soluble antigens [7] and can be used to modulate the type of immune response [1]. Different nano-sized platforms such as virus-like particles, liposomes, immune stimulating complexes

(ISCOMs), nanoemulsions, and polymeric nanoparticles have been explored as potential vaccine delivery systems [8,9]. Chitosan and its derivatives are among the most studied compounds for development of polymeric vaccines [10,11] because of their attractive characteristics for biomedical applications. Chitosan is a biocompatible, biodegradable, and non-toxic polysaccharide [12], obtained by deacetylation of chitin, consisting of β-(1-4)-linked D-glucosamine and *N*-acetyl-D-glucosamine monomer units. Its cationic nature, mucoadhesivity and immunostimulating properties [10] make it an attractive polymer, particularly for the design of nanoparticulate vaccines for mucosal delivery.

Despite the potential of nanoparticles as vaccine adjuvants, it is possible to obtain a more potent adjuvant formulation by association with immunopotentiators. In fact, the concept of concomitant delivery of antigens and immunostimulatory molecules through delivery systems gained increased attention and has been appointed as a promising approach in vaccine development [2,13,14].

Mast cells (MCs), strategically located at the host surface contact with pathogens, have been recognized in recent years as important players in the development of protective immune responses [15–17], and the use of mast cell activators as a new class of vaccine adjuvants has begun to be explored [18]. Since then, additional studies confirmed the immunopotentiator properties of the mast cell activator compound 48/80 (C48/80) [19–21]. In this study, we explore the feasibility of combining the mast cell activator with chitosan nanoparticles to prepare a new adjuvant formulation for nasal vaccination. The strategy proposed here could be advantageous because, while chitosan could extend the residence time of the antigen on the nasal mucosa, MC activation could promote a local environment favorable to the development of an immune response. In particular, the application of this strategy to the hepatitis B recombinant antigen could allow the development of a nasal vaccine suitable for developing countries, where the possibility of self-administration could improve patient ease of access and compliance. Additionally, nasal vaccines are known to induce the generation of mucosal immune responses in the genital tract [22,23], which is highly attractive considering the sexual transmission of the virus. One of the biggest obstacles for vaccine development is the lack of knowledge on how to formulate complex adjuvant systems combining immunopotentiators and delivery systems [24]. Therefore, the publication of innovative methodologies for the preparation of these co-adjuvanted formulations is of utmost importance. These approaches would allow other researchers to have access to a broader range of adjuvants to test as vaccine candidates. Considering this, the present paper describes the design and characterization of a novel co-adjuvanted formulation consisting of chitosan nanoparticles associated with the mast cell activator C48/80. Stability, biocompatibility, and uptake by macrophages of the obtained nanoparticles were assessed in vitro. Finally, we tested the potential of C48/80 loaded chitosan NPs to modulate the adaptive immune response following nasal immunization using the recombinant hepatitis B surface antigen (HBsAg). To the authors' knowledge, this was the first time C48/80 was used as a co-adjuvant for hepatitis B vaccination.

2. Materials and Methods

2.1. Materials

A low molecular weight chitosan (deacetylation degree 95%) was purchased from Primex BioChemicals AS (Avaldsnes, Norway). Compound 48/80, bovine serum albumin (BSA), MTT (3-[4, 5-dimethylthiazol-2-yl]-2,5-diphenyl tetrazolium bromide), albumin-fluorescein isothiocyanate conjugate (FITC-BSA), trehalose, Dulbecco's modified Eagle medium (DMEM) and Roswell Park Memorial Institute (RPMI) 1640 were obtained from Sigma-Aldrich (Sintra, Portugal). Bicinchoninic acid (BCA) assay and micro BCA kits were obtained from Pierce Chemical Company (Rockford, IL, USA). FITC was purchased to Santa Cruz Biotechnology (Santa Cruz, CA, USA). Fetal bovine serum (FBS), wheat germ agglutinin Alexa Fluor® 350 Conjugate and Lysotracker® Red DND 99 were obtained from Life Technologies Corporation (Paisley, UK). HBsAg was purchased from Aldevron. All other reagents used were of analytical grade.

2.2. Chitosan Purification

Chitosan was purified by a method described elsewhere [25] with slight modifications. Briefly, 1 *g* of chitosan was suspended in 10 mL of a 1 M NaOH solution, and stirred for 3 h at 50 °C. The mixture was then filtered (0.45 μm membrane, MerckMillipore, Darmstadt, Germany), and the resultant pellet washed with 20 mL of deionized water. The recovered chitosan was dissolved in 200 mL of 1% (*v*/*v*) acetic acid solution and stirred for 1 h. The solution was filtered (0.45 μm membrane), and 1 M NaOH was used to adjust the filtrate to pH 8.0, resulting in purified chitosan in the form of precipitates. Purified chitosan was freeze-dried for 48 h with a Labconco freeze-dryer, model 77530 (Labconco, Kansas City, MO, USA) equipment.

2.3. Characterization of the Purified Chitosan by Fourier-Transform Infrared Spectroscopy (FTIR)

The FTIR spectra of purified and non-purified chitosan were recorded using an FTIR spectrometer (Spectrum 400, PerkinElmer, Villepinte, France) with an attenuated total reflection (ATR) top-plate accessory. The instrument operated with a resolution of 2 cm^{-1}, and 30 scans were collected for each sample. Spectra were recorded between 650 and 4000 cm^{-1}.

2.4. Nanoparticle Preparation

C48/80 loaded chitosan nanoparticles (Chi-C48/80 NPs) were prepared by adding dropwise 3 mL of an alkaline solution (5 mM NaOH) of C48/80 and Na_2SO_4 (0.3 mg/mL and 2.03 mg/mL, respectively) to 3 mL of a chitosan solution (1 mg/mL in acetic acid 0.1%) under high-speed vortexing. The nanoparticles were formed after further maturation for 60 min under magnetic stirring. Blank chitosan particles (Chi NPs) were obtained by preparing nanoparticles in exactly the same conditions but without C48/80.

To evaluate the stability after freeze-drying, nanoparticles were lyophilized with 1%, 2.5%, or 5% of trehalose as cryoprotectant. All samples were lyophilized for 48 h with a Labconco freeze-dryer, model 77530 (Labconco, Kansas City, USA), at −50 °C and 100 mbar.

Chitosan–aluminum nanoparticles (Chi-Al NPs) and chitosan–poly epsilon caprolactone (Chi-PCL) NPs used in the immunogenicity study were produced as previously described by our group [26,27]

2.5. Characterization of Nanoparticles

2.5.1. Size and Zeta Potential

Particle size was measured by dynamic light scattering (DLS) using a Delsa™ Nano C (Beckman Coulter). Samples were diluted in milli-Q water and analyzed at a detection angle of 160° and a temperature of 25 °C. Zeta potential was measured by electrophoretic light scattering (ELS), after dispersion of the nanoparticles in a solution of 1 mM NaCl.

2.5.2. Morphology

Particle morphology was evaluated by scanning electron microscopy (SEM) in a field emission scanning electron microscope (FEI Quanta 400 FEG ESEM, ThermoFisher Scientific, Waltham, MA, USA). One drop of nanoparticle suspension was mounted on a microscope stub using a double-stick carbon tape and allowed to dry overnight. Prior to image acquisition, samples were coated with gold.

2.5.3. Quantification of C48/80 Loading Efficacy

In order to evaluate the loading efficacy (LE) of C48/80, nanoparticles were centrifuged for 20 min at 8000 *g*, and C48/80 was quantified in the supernatant using a method validated by our group [28]. Briefly, 25 μL of carbonate buffer pH 9.6 was added to 175 μL of sample in a 96-well plate. Subsequently,

50 μL of a 15% acetaldehyde solution containing 1.5% of sodium nitroprusside was added and the absorbance measured at 570 nm. The loading efficacy was calculated according to Equation (1).

$$\text{C48/80 LE (\%)} = \frac{\text{total C48/80 (μg/mL)} - \text{free C48/80 in supernatant (μg/mL)}}{\text{total C48/80 (μg/mL)}} \times 100 \quad (1)$$

2.5.4. FTIR Analysis

FTIR analysis of lyophilized chitosan, C48/80, Chi NPs, and Chi-C48/80 NPs was performed according to Section 2.3.

2.6. Stability Studies

The short term stability of freshly prepared nanoparticle suspensions stored either at 4 °C or at room temperature (RT) was studied for a period of 15 days. Size, polydispersity index (PI), and zeta potential of three independent batches of Chi-C48/80 NPs and Chi NPs were measured. Samples were withdrawn and characterized at Days 0, 3, 5 and 15.

The stability of lyophilized Chi-C48/80 NPs was also investigated after storage for a period of 4 months at RT. At the end of the test period, samples were resuspended in milli-Q water, NPs were characterized, and the parameters were compared to the values before lyophilization.

2.7. Evaluation of Loading Efficacy and Loading Capacity of Model Antigens

Loading of model antigens on a nanoparticle surface was performed by physical adsorption. Nanoparticles were centrifuged for 30 min at 4500 *g* and resuspended in acetate buffer, pH 5.7, 25 mM. Nanoparticles at a final concentration of 2.5 mg/mL were incubated with BSA, ovalbumin (OVA), or myoglobin in acetate buffer for 60 min at RT. Ratios from 7:1 to 1:1 (NP/protein) were tested for BSA, while OVA and myoglobin were incubated at a fixed weight ratio of 7:1. After incubation, particles were centrifuged at 12,000 *g* for 20 min, and the supernatant was collected. The amount of protein loaded on nanoparticles was determined indirectly by measuring the concentration of non-bound protein in the nanoparticle supernatant using the BCA or Micro-BCA protein assay (Pierce, ThermoFisher Scientific, Waltham, MA, USA) according to the manufacturer's instructions. Loading efficacy and loading capacity (LC) were determined by Equations (2) and (3), respectively.

$$\text{LE (\%)} = \frac{\text{total amount of BSA} - \text{non bound BSA}}{\text{total amount of BSA}} \times 100 \quad (2)$$

$$\text{LC (\%)} = \frac{\text{total amount of BSA} - \text{non bound BSA}}{\text{weight of nanoparticles}} \times 100. \quad (3)$$

2.8. In Vitro Cytotoxicity Studies

Single cell suspensions of spleens from 8-week old female C57BL/6 mice (Charles River) were prepared according to a method previously described [29]. Cells were seeded in a 96-well plate at a density of 1×10^6 cells/well in an RPMI 1640 medium (supplemented with 10% (*v*/*v*) fetal bovine serum, 2 mM glutamine, 1% (*v*/*v*) penicillin/streptomycin, and 20 mM HEPES) and incubated together with different concentrations of nanoparticles. After 24 h of incubation, cellular viability was assessed by MTT assay. Briefly, 20 μL of 5 mg/mL MTT in PBS, pH 7.4, was added to each well and incubated for more 4 h. The plate was centrifuged for 25 min, at 800 *g*, and the supernatants were removed. Finally, the formazan crystals produced by viable cells were solubilized with 200 μL of DMSO per well, and the optical density values were measured at 540 nm with 630 nm as a wavelength reference. The viability of non-treated cells (culture medium only) was defined as 100% and the relative cell viability calculated using Equation (4).

$$\text{Cell viability } (\%) = \frac{\text{OD sample } (540 \text{ nm}) - \text{OD sample } (630 \text{ nm})}{\text{OD control } (540 \text{ nm}) - \text{OD control } (630 \text{ nm})} \times 100. \quad (4)$$

A549 cells (American Type Culture Collection, ATCC) were seeded in a 96-well plate at a density of 10^5 cells/mL, at 37 °C and 5% CO_2, in a nutrient mixture F12-Ham with 10% (*v*/*v*) fetal bovine serum supplemented with 1% (*v*/*v*) penicillin/streptomycin, and incubated with different concentrations of nanoparticles. MTT assay was performed as described previously for spleen cells with minor modifications: incubation with MTT was performed over 1.5 h, and the cell supernatants were directly removed without centrifuging.

2.9. Particle Uptake by Macrophages

FITC-labeled NPs were prepared by the method described in Section 2.4 using FITC-labeled chitosan. The synthesis of FITC-labeled chitosan was based on the reaction between the isothiocyanate group of FITC (Ex/Em—490/525) and the primary amino group of chitosan established by our group [30]. Briefly, chitosan was labeled by mixing 35 mL of dehydrated methanol containing 25 mg of FITC to 25 mL of a 1% (*w*/*v*) chitosan in 0.1 M acetic acid. After 3 h of reaction in the dark at RT, the FITC-labeled chitosan was precipitated with 0.2 M NaOH until pH 10. FITC-labeled chitosan was obtained by centrifugation for 30 min at 4500 *g* and the resultant pellet was washed 3 times with a mixture of methanol/water (70:30, *v*/*v*). The labeled chitosan was resuspended in 15 mL of 0.1 M acetic acid and stirred overnight. A polymer solution was dialyzed in the dark against 2.5 L of deionized water for 3 days before freeze-drying using a freeze-dry system (FreezeZone 6, Labconco, Kansas City, MO, USA).

The ability of nanoparticles to be internalized by antigen presenting cells was assessed on the mouse macrophage cell line RAW 264.7 (ECACC, Salisbury, UK). Cells were maintained in Dulbecco's modified Eagle medium (DMEM, Sigma Aldrich, Sintra, Portugal) supplemented with 1 mM HEPES, 1 mM sodium pyruvate, and 10% of non-inactivated FBS. To evaluate the uptake of nanoparticles, RAW 264.7 cells were seeded on glass coverslips in 12-well plates at a density of 2.5×10^5 cells per well and cultured at 37 °C in 5% CO_2 overnight. On the next day, RAW 264.7 were pre-labeled with 300 nM Lysotracker® Red DND 99 (Ex/Em—577/590 nm) for 30 min at 37 °C, and the culture medium was replaced by a fresh one. The cells were then incubated for 4 h with FITC-Chi NPs and FITC-Chi-C48/80 NPs at 100 µg/mL or FITC-BSA loaded nanoparticles at 50 µg/mL in DMEM.

Following uptake, cells were washed three times with phosphate-buffered saline pH 7.4 (PBS) and fixed with 4% paraformaldehyde in PBS for 15 min at 37 °C. The plasma membrane of pre-fixed cells was then labeled with 5 µg/mL of wheat germ agglutinin Alexa Fluor 350 conjugate (Ex/Em—346/442 nm) in PBS for 10 min at RT. After labeling, cells were washed twice with PBS and the coverslips mounted in microscope slides with DAKO mounting medium and examined under an inverted laser scanning confocal microscope (Zeiss LSM 510 META, Carl Zeiss, Oberkochen, Germany) equipped with imaging software (LSM 5 software, version 3.2, Carl Zeiss, Oberkochen, Germany).

2.10. Immunogenicity Study

2.10.1. Nasal Vaccination

Female C57BL/6 mice of 6–8 weeks of age were purchased from Charles River (Écully, France) and housed in the Center for Neuroscience and Cell Biology (CNC) animal facility (Coimbra, Portugal) and provided food and water ad libitum. All experiments were carried out in accordance with institutional ethical guidelines and with national (Dec. No. 1005/92, 23 October 2018) and international (normative 2010/63 from EU) legislation. Groups of 5 mice were intranasally immunized on Days 0, 7, and 21 with 15 µL of vaccine formulation (7.5 µL per nostril), under slight isoflurane anesthesia. All mice, except for those in the naïve group (Group I), received 10 µg of HBsAg adsorbed onto Chi-C48/80 NPs (Group II), Chi-Al NPs (Group III), or Chi-PCL NPs (Group IV).

Samples were collected and processed as previously described [31]. Briefly, blood was collected by a submandibular lancet method on Days 21 and 42 and allowed to coagulate for 30 min prior to centrifugation at 1000 g for 10 min. Nasal and vaginal washes were collected on Day 42. Vaginal washes were collected by instilling 100 μL of PBS into the vaginal cavity, and the lavage fluid was flushed in and out a few times before collection. Samples were centrifuged at 11,500 g for 10 min, and supernatants were stored. Nasal lavage samples were collected from euthanized mice. The lower jaw of the mice was cut way and the nasal lavage collected by instilling 200 μL of sterile PBS posteriorly into the nasal cavity. Fluid exiting the nostrils was collected and spun at 11,500 g at 4 °C for 20 min. Collected and processed samples were stored until further analysis.

2.10.2. Determination of Serum IgG, IgG1, IgG2c, and Secretory IgA

Quantification of immunoglobulins was performed using a protocol optimized by our group [27,30]. The endpoint titers presented in the results represent the antilog of the last log2 dilution, for which the OD values were at least two-fold higher than that of the naive sample, equally diluted. The log 2 end-point titers were used for statistical analysis.

2.11. Statistical Analysis

Statistical analysis was performed with GraphPad Prism v 5.03 (GraphPad Software Inc., La Jolla, CA, USA). Student's t-test and ANOVA followed by Tukey's post-test were used for two samples or multiple comparisons, respectively. A p-value <0.05 was considered statistically significant (* $p < 0.05$; ** $p < 0.01$; *** $p < 0.001$).

3. Results and Discussion

3.1. Purification of Chitosan

Before use chitosan was submitted to a purification process to ensure the removal of any possible impurities. FTIR analysis was performed before and after the purification process to confirm the preservation of structure and integrity of the commercial polymer. The spectra obtained were in agreement with previously published data [32,33]. FTIR spectrum of chitosan showed a broad band between 3500 and 3200 cm^{-1} (Figure 1) corresponding to the stretching vibration of O–H. The peak of N–H stretching from primary amine groups was overlapped in the same region. The peak at 2869 cm^{-1} indicates C–H stretching vibrations. Peaks at 1650 and 1588 cm^{-1} correspond to C=O stretch and N–H bending, respectively. The peak at 1419 cm^{-1} belongs to the N–C stretching and the bands at 1150 and 1025 cm^{-1} are characteristic of the CO stretching vibration. No differences were observed between the spectra of non-purified and purified chitosan, which indicates that the purification process had no effect on the structure of the polymer.

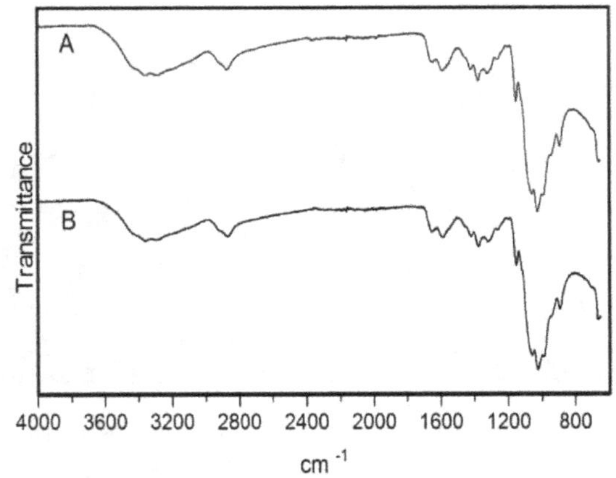

Figure 1. Fourier-transform infrared spectroscopy (FTIR) spectra of chitosan after and before the purification process. (A) Purified chitosan. (B) Non-purified chitosan.

3.2. Development and Physicochemical Characterization of C48/80-Chitosan Nanoparticles

C48/80 loaded chitosan nanoparticles were prepared by ionotropic gelation of cationic chitosan with sulfate anions from Na_2SO_4. C48/80 was added to a crosslink solution and entrapped during NP formation. This method of nanoparticle preparation is extremely simple and involves mixing two aqueous solutions at RT. Despite the simplicity of the method, different conditions were tested in the laboratory before getting the final nanoparticle formulation. Based on previous data collected from our group, different concentrations of the nanoparticles components, as well as different pH and incubation conditions, were tested in order to achieve nanoparticles with the desired characteristics: submicron size, a good polydispersity, and a reasonable encapsulation of the mast cell activator C48/80. The main challenge was to associate a cationic compound, the mast cell activator C48/80, with the also positively charged chitosan. Typically, interactions with chitosan amine group are electrostatic, which favors the interaction of the polymer with anionic compounds. Consequently, the association of cationic compounds with chitosan can be trickier due to partial repulsion, since both are positively charged [34]. At the end, the preparation of chitosan nanoparticles loaded with the mast cell activator C48/80 was possible by mixing the compound with an alkalinized sodium sulfate solution prior to the preparation of the nanoparticles.

Figure 2A summarizes Chi NP and Chi-C48/80 NP characteristics. The unloaded Chi NPs had an average size of 396.2 ± 35.0 nm, while the formulation loaded with the mast cell activator, Chi-C48/80 NPs, had an average size of 500.9 ± 65.15 nm. Images from scanning electron microscopy confirmed the size measured by DLS (Figure 2B1,B2). Both formulations had a narrow size distribution (PI < 0.170) and were positively charged. The incorporation of C48/80 in Chi NPs led to an increase of about 100 nm in the nanoparticle size ($p < 0.001$, Student's t-test), but the nanoparticle surface charge remained unaltered. The increased mean size was a good indicator of the association of C48/80 in the nanoparticles, but the incorporation was definitively confirmed after quantification of the amount of C48/80 in the nanoparticles by a validated method [28]. The results showed that the compound was successfully incorporated into Chi NPs with a loading efficacy of 18.6%. Even if the attempts to correlate particle size and the resultant immune responses lead to conflicting findings [4,35], previous studies showed that 500 nm is in the optimal size range for uptake by APCs [36]. Therefore, not only the Chi-C48/80 NPs and Chi NPs have a suitable size for uptake, but also their positive charge is an advantage since it favors mucoadhesion, through interaction with the negatively charged sites on cell surfaces, and should also facilitate the uptake by antigen-presenting cells.

A

Formulation	Size (nm)	PI[a]	ZP (mV)[b]	% LE (C48/80)[c]
Chi-C48/80 NP	500.9 ± 65.2	0.161 ± 0.051	+ 23.83 ± 3.76	18.6
Chi NP	396.2 ± 35.0	0.156 ± 0.037	+ 21.59 ± 2.81	-

[a]Polydispersity index; [b] Zeta Potential; [c] C48/80 loading efficacy

B

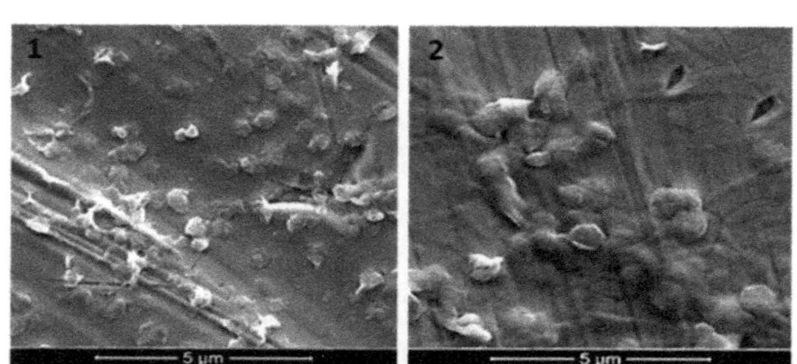

Figure 2. Characterization of C48/80 loaded and unloaded chitosan nanoparticles. (**A**) Size and zeta potential were measured by dynamic light scattering and electrophoretic light scattering, respectively, with a Delsa™ Nano C. C48/80 loading efficacy was measured by a colorimetric method. Mean $\pm$ SD, $n \geq 3$. (**B**) SEM images of (**1**) Chi NP and (**2**) Chi-C48/80 NP. Magnification 15,000×, scale 5 µm.

3.3. FTIR Analysis of Nanoparticles

FTIR is an important tool to analyze the interactions between groups and useful for the study of nanomaterial surface [37]. Therefore, chitosan, Chi NPs, Chi-C48/80 NPs, and C48/80 were analyzed by FTIR to characterize any potential interactions in the nanoparticles. Comparison of chitosan polymer (Figure 3A) with Chi NPs (Figure 3B) showed a shift of peaks from 1650 and 1558 cm^{-1} to 1631 and 1532 cm^{-1}, respectively. This difference can be explained by the interaction between the amino groups of chitosan and sulfate ions, which resulted in the formation of the NPs by ionic crosslink [33]. The broad band between 3500 and 3200 cm^{-1} attributed to O–H and N–H bonds shifted to a lower wavelength in Chi NPs, indicating an enhancement of the hydrogen bonds interactions [38]. The same band appeared to be broader in Chi-C48/80 NPs (Figure 3C) than in Chi NPs, which also indicates enhanced hydrogen bonding in the loaded formulation [32]. No peak exclusively characteristic from C48/80 (Figure 3D) was observed on the FTIR spectrum of Chi-C48/80 NPs. This may be due to the small amount of C48/80 and therefore its chemical groups, present in the nanoparticles, which may be masked by the much higher amount of chitosan.

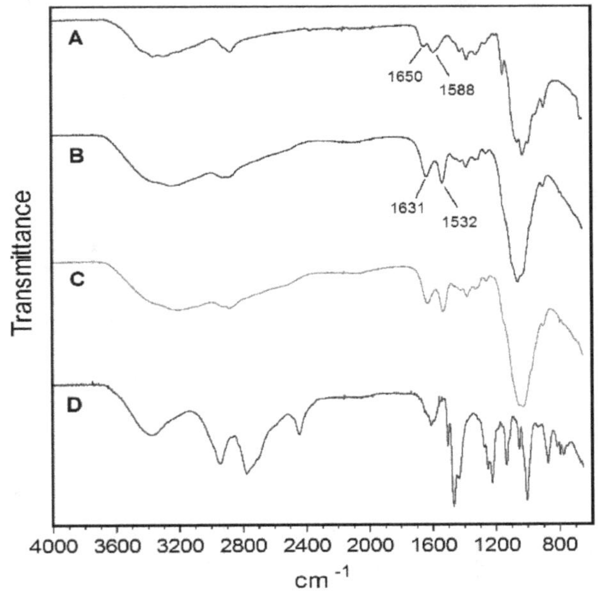

Figure 3. FTIR spectra of (A) Chitosan, (B) Chi NPs, (C) Chi-C48/80 NPs, and (D) C48/80.

3.4. Stability Studies of the Nanoparticles

A particle-based vaccine should be stable in relation to size throughout the process of preparation, storage, and administration. Considering this, the short-term stability of aqueous suspensions of Chi-C48/80 NPs was assessed by measuring the size, PI, and zeta potential during storage at 25 °C or at 4 °C for 15 days. Chi-C48/80 NPs showed a consistent particle size with a uniform size distribution during the test period (Figure 4A,B). Additionally, no changes in zeta potential of nanoparticles were observed (Figure 4C,D).

The results showed that Chi-C48/80 NPs were stable up to 15 days at the tested conditions. However, it should be noted that the target function of these formulation is to act as an adjuvant for nasal vaccination after association with an antigen of interest. It is known that instability during the storage of vaccines can lead to physicochemical changes of the formulation and antigen degradation, often requiring additional steps to improve its long-term stability [4]. One effective way to guarantee this stability and to prevent antigen degradation is to lyophilize the vaccine formulation [39]. It is important that this procedure does not affect the original particle size and size distribution of the formulation since it would also influence the immune responses. Thus, the potential impact of these processes should be investigated at early stages of formulation design [4]. Considering this, we explored the feasibility of lyophilizing the developed formulations by evaluating the impact of this technique on the physicochemical properties of Chi-C48/80 NPs and Chi NPs. The preliminary data obtained revealed that freeze-drying of the developed formulations without any cryoprotectant resulted in great particle aggregation (data not shown). This destabilization of nanoparticle suspensions is very common and most likely is a result of the stress of freezing and dehydration inherent to the technique [40]. Therefore, to avoid that, in this study a fixed concentration of nanoparticles (2 mg/mL) was lyophilized with different concentrations of trehalose (1%, 2.5%, and 5% (w/v)). The physicochemical characteristics of the delivery systems were then measured after reconstitution in water and compared to the initial ones (pre-lyophilization) to see if the concentrations of cryoprotectant used were sufficient to stabilize the formulations (Figure 5).

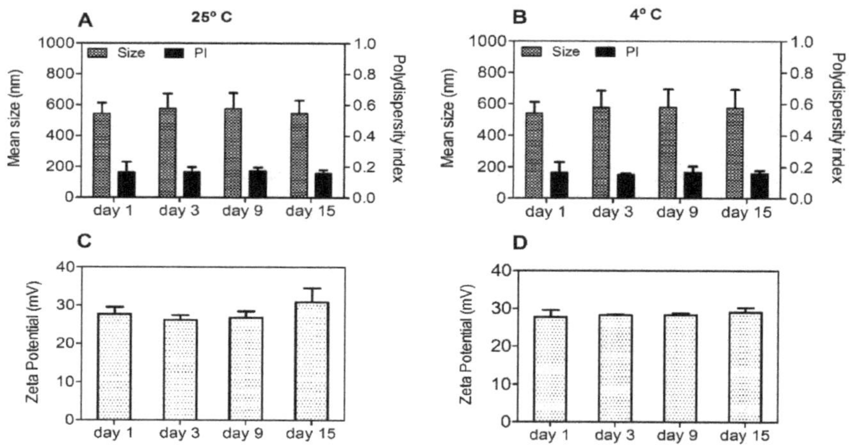

Figure 4. Short-term stability of Chi-C48/80 NPs at 25 °C (**A**,**C**) and 4 °C (**B**,**D**). Size, polydispersity index (PI), and zeta potential of the C48/80 loaded formulation were measured during storage up to 15 days at 25 °C or at 4 °C. Data are expressed as mean ± standard deviation (SD), n = 3.

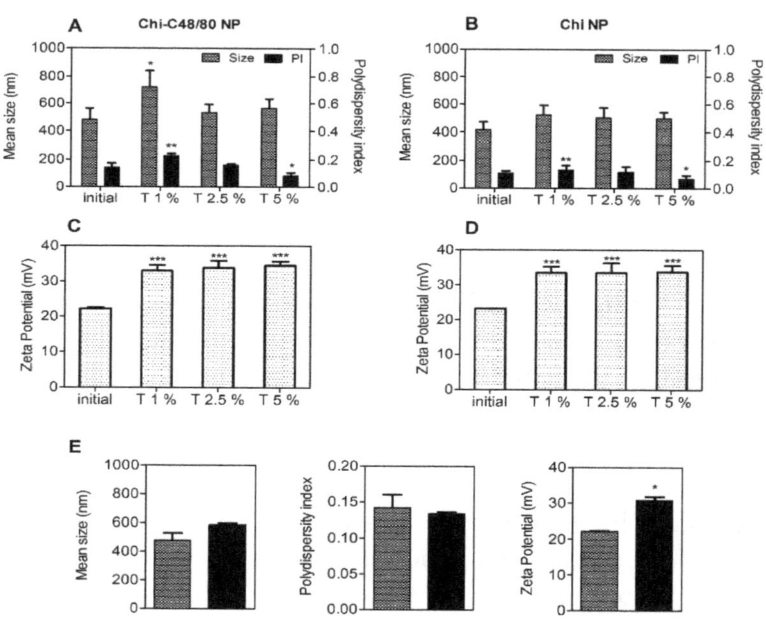

Figure 5. Effect of lyophilization with different concentrations of trehalose on the characteristics of nanoparticles. Size, polydispersion index, and zeta potential of Chi-C48/80 NPs (**A**,**C**) and Chi NPs (**B**,**D**) were measured before and after liophilization with 1%, 2.5%, and 5% of trehalose. (**E**) To evaluate the long-term stability of the lyophilized nanoparticles, Chi-C48/80 NPs plus 2.5% of trehalose were characterized after 4 months at room temperature (RT). Data are expressed as mean ± SD, n = 3.

Trehalose was selected as a cryoprotectant because it has been successfully used to preserve not only the characteristics of chitosan nanoparticles [38] but also the bioactivity of both C48/80 and an antigen [21]. The size of Chi NPs remains the same after lyophilization with all trehalose concentrations tested (Figure 5A,B). On the other hand, differences in size and PI for Chi-C48/80 NPs indicate that an adequate reconstitution was only achieved when using 2.5% or 5% of the cryoprotectant. Zeta potential of nanoparticles increased after the lyophilization with trehalose (Figure 5C,D). This can result from either a change in charge distribution on the NP surface or from the presence of trehalose on the on the NP suspension. The results suggest that 2.5% of trehalose was sufficient to achieve a successful cryopreservation of both delivery systems.

To assess if the lyophilized nanoparticles would be feasible to avoid the cold chain, Chi-C48/80 NPs lyophilized with 2.5% of trehalose were characterized after storage at RT for 4 months. Results showed that nanoparticles preserved the initial size and polydispersity for at least 4 months of storage (Figure 5E).

Overall, the results suggest that the stability of Chi NPs was not impaired by the association with C48/80. However, it is noteworthy that, even if these studies on the stability of the nanoparticles provided us with an indication about the potential of the formulations for long-term storage, they do not exclude the requirement of a more complete stability study, including antigen potency evaluation over time, for guarantee that the immunogenicity of the vaccine candidate is not affected. That would be particularly important during the development of vaccines designed to avoid the cold chain.

3.5. Loading of Model Antigens

In this study, BSA, OVA, and myoglobin were used as model antigens to confirm the adsorption of proteins onto the surface of nanoparticles. The use of three different proteins with different isoelectric points (IPs) allowed us to assess the suitability of the developed delivery systems for loading different antigens of interest. The loading of proteins on nanoparticles was made by physical adsorption, a mild technique that involves simply the incubation of nanoparticles with an aqueous solution of the antigen. This approach not only helps to preserve the structure of antigen but also allows a repetitive antigen display to the APC, which mimics pathogens [1].

Initially different NP/BSA ratios were tested to evaluate the more efficient weight ratio of NP/protein for loading. BSA loading efficacies were very similar for both Chi-C48/80 NPs and Chi NPs (Figure 6A,B). The LE was dependent on the ratio NP/BSA: the higher the ratio, the higher the amount of protein adsorbed on NP surface, ranging from 50.8% to 94.1% and from 52.2% and 95.5%, for Chi-C48/80 NPs and Chi NPs, respectively. The LC of nanoparticles was also calculated; it represents the amount of protein that the nanoparticles are able to carry. Unlike LE, the LC of the nanoparticles decreased with the increase in the NP/BSA ratio. Loading capacity was maximum at the lower ratio tested (1:1) for both Chi NPs and Chi-C48/80 NPs. However, even if the incubation with higher amounts of protein allows the nanoparticles to carry a higher amount of the protein of interest, generally it is preferable to use the NP/protein ratio that allows the highest LE because the antigen is usually the most expensive component of the vaccine. The LE near 95%, achieved for NP/BSA = 7:1, is very favorable in formulation development since almost the entire amount of antigen used would be associated with the nanoparticles. Therefore, this ratio was selected to test the loading of OVA and myoglobin on the NP surface.

LE of OVA and myoglobin on nanoparticles was around 70% and 10%, respectively, for both Chi-C48/80 NPs and Chi NPs (Figure 6C). These values were significantly lower than those observed for BSA. The isoelectric points of BSA, OVA, and myoglobin (4.7, 4.9, and 7.2, respectively) can help one to understand the observed results. BSA and OVA displayed high adsorption efficacies to the surface of the NPs that can be associated with the electrostatic interactions between the positively charged amino groups of chitosan and the negatively charged carboxyl groups of the proteins. On the other hand, at pH 5.7, both nanoparticles and myoglobin are positively charged, which explains the very low LE % observed for this protein. However, despite the similarity in the isoelectric points of BSA and

OVA, the adsorption of these proteins was different within the same delivery system. That is because, even if the IP is helpful for predicting the loading of proteins on the NP surface, the adsorption is a complex process depending on several other factors [41]. Overall, the results suggested that the developed formulations are suitable for loading negatively charged antigens and that the adsorption of protein onto the Chi NP surface was not affected by the presence of C48/80.

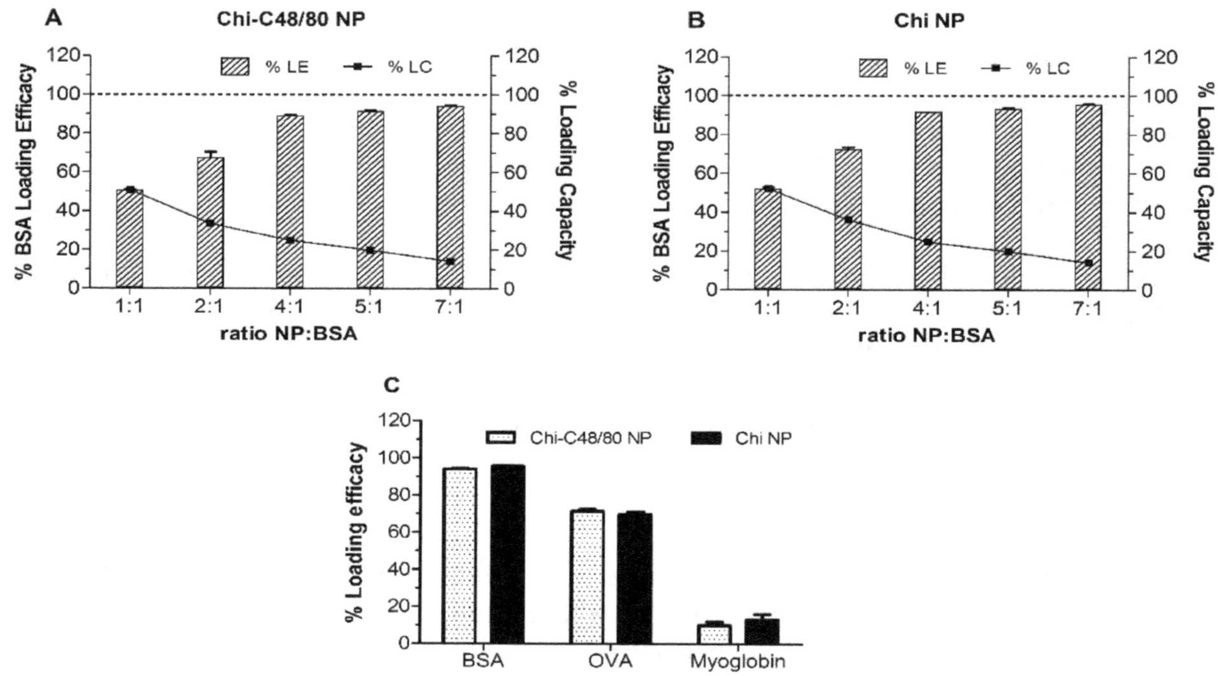

Figure 6. Loading of model antigens. Effect of NP/protein ratio on the protein adsorption to (**A**) Chi-C48/80 NPs and (**B**) Chi NPs. (**C**) Loading efficacy for bovine serum albumin (BSA), ovalbumin (OVA) and myoglobin at the NP/protein ratio of 7:1. Nanoparticles were incubated with different proteins for 60 min in acetate buffer, pH = 5.7 at RT. Loading efficacy (% LE) and loading capacity (% LC) were determined after quantification of unbound protein in the supernatant using the Bicinchoninic acid (BCA) assay. Bars represent mean ± SD, n = 3.

3.6. *Cytotoxicity*

The cytotoxicity of Chi-C48/80 NPs and Chi NPs was evaluated in spleen cells and in the A549 cell line using the MTT assay. Spleen cells were chosen because they are a good representation of the different cells of the immune system and have been already used to test the toxicity of vaccine delivery systems [29,42]. Since the aim of this study was to evaluate the incorporation of a mast cell activator in a delivery system, the A549 cell line, a model of alveolar basal epithelium, was used to evaluate the potential harmful effect of the nanoparticles at the administration site. As expected, the results show that cytotoxicity was concentration-dependent. Higher concentrations of nanoparticles resulted in a decreased cell viability (Figure 7).

In spleen cells, the incorporation of C48/80 in Chi NPs did not affect the toxicity of formulations, with both formulations showing no cytotoxicity for concentrations up to 2000 μg/mL (Figure 7A). With the A549 cell line, cell viability was above 70% for concentrations up to 750 μg/mL, for both formulations (Figure 7B). However, in these cells, the presence of C48/80 in the nanoparticles reduced the cell viability more rapidly than did Chi NPs. Note that 1500 μg/mL is a very high concentration and out of the range normally used in in vitro studies. These results are in agreement with others that have demonstrated that chitosan nanoparticles are nontoxic [29,43,44].

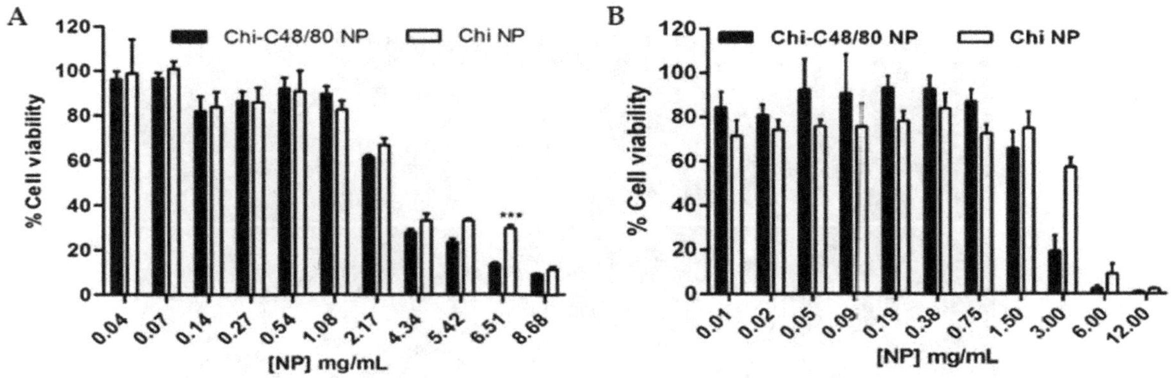

Figure 7. Effect of Chi-C48/80 NPs and Chi NPs on viability of spleen cells (**A**) and epithelial A549 cells (**B**). Different concentrations of nanoparticles were incubated with cells for 24 h. The cell viability was measured by MTT assay. Each result is representative of two independent experiments performed in quadruplicate for spleen cells and three independent experiments performed in quadruplicate for A549 cells (mean ± SD).

3.7. Uptake Studies

The uptake of nanoparticles by antigen presenting cells is favorable to an adaptive immune response [45]. Therefore, we investigated the ability of both developed formulations to be internalized by RAW 264.7 cells, a macrophage cell line widely used to explore the uptake and immune effect of vaccine delivery systems [3,7]. To visualize particle uptake by the macrophage cell line RAW 264.7, cells were incubated with FITC-labeled Chi NPs or Chi-C48/80 NPs. The intracellular location of nanoparticles was analyzed by labeling the cells with Lysotracker Red, which accumulates in the acidic endolysosomes. The results showed that the NPs were efficiently taken up by macrophages (Figure 8A). After 4 h of incubation, the FITC-NPs (green) were mostly detected on the cell cytoplasm. However, some of the compartments enclosing NPs showed acidification, as observed in the merged images between green fluorescent NPs and red fluorescent vesicles, appearing in yellow, indicating maturation of the phagolysosome (Figure 8A). To confirm that not only the nanoparticles but also the associated antigens would be internalized by antigen presenting cells, uptake studies were repeated with nanoparticles loaded with a fluorescently labeled protein. The confocal images showed an extensive internalization of FITC-BSA loaded on both Chi-C48/80 NPs and Chi NPs (Figure 8B). Similarly to what was observed with FITC-labeled NPs, the fluorescence signal of BSA was detected mostly on cell cytoplasm with only a few yellow co-localization signals observed.

These results suggest that NPs and protein-loaded NPs might escape from the endosomes to cytoplasm which can facilitate cross-presentation and potentially mediate the MHC I antigen presentation pathway, associated with an induction of CD8+ T cell response [3]. In fact, it was demonstrated by others that chitosan-based nanoparticles could escape from endosomes [46] and that antigens delivered by Chi NPs mediate antigen presentation through both MHC I and MHC II pathways [7]. This escape mechanism and consequent cross-presentation of antigens is particularly important for the development of vaccines that require cellular immune response.

Overall, the results showed that there were no significant differences regarding the uptake and distribution of Chi-C48/80 NPs and Chi NPs. This means that the association of the mast cell activator with the NPs not only did not impair the characteristics of nanoparticle and antigen uptake by antigen-presenting cells but also proved to be an effective antigen delivery system.

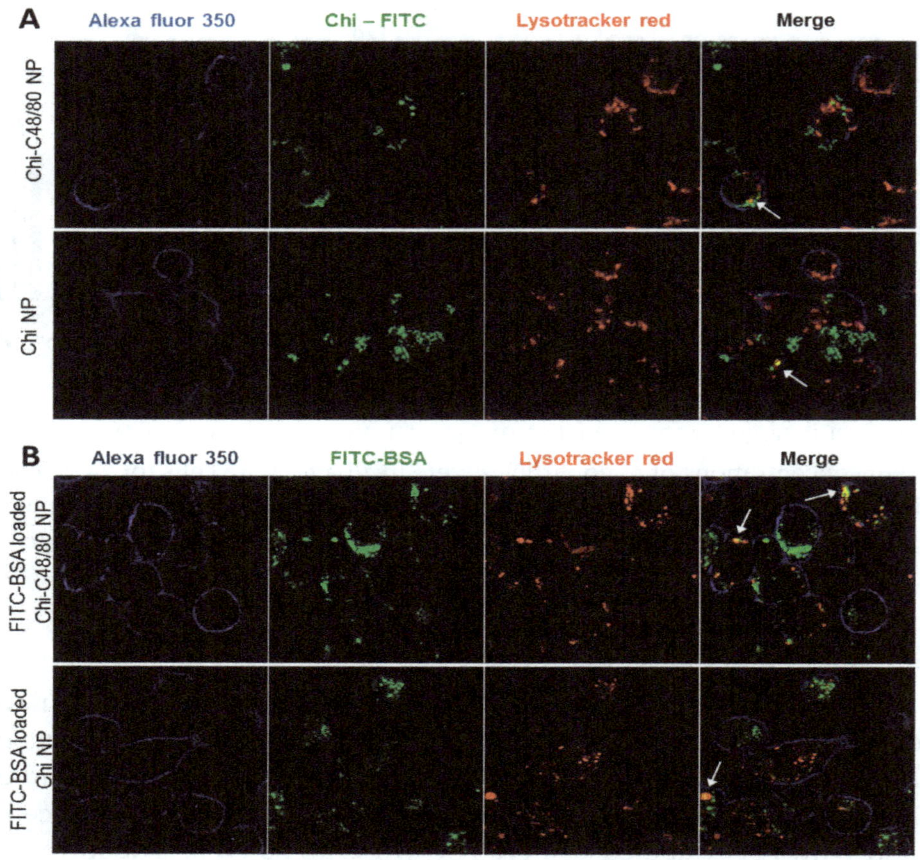

Figure 8. Evaluation of uptake by macrophages. (**A**) Uptake of nanoparticles was assessed by incubating 4 h, 100 μg/mL RAW 264.7 cells with Chi-C48/80 NPs or Chi NPs prepared with fluorescein isothiocyanate (FITC)-labeled chitosan (green). (**B**) Uptake of the antigen loaded on nanoparticles was evaluated by incubating the cells with FITC-BSA loaded Chi-C48/80 NPs or Chi NPs. Cells were labeled with Alexa Fluor© 350 WGA (blue) to identify the membrane, and Lysotracker© Red identifies the acidic endosomes and lysosomes. Arrows in the merge image show co-localization.

3.8. Immunogenicity Study

Chi-C48/80 NPs' ability to act as a nasal vaccine adjuvant for hepatitis B surface antigen was tested and compared with other particulate adjuvants by performing an immunogenicity study using C57BL/6 mice. The immunization schedule comprised a primary nasal immunization followed by two nasal boosts at Days 7 and 21. Therefore, in this study, we included two other established chitosan-based nano-delivery systems developed by our group, Chi-Al NPs [26] and Chi-PCL NPs [27], in order to compare adjuvanticity elicited by the new system.

As depicted in Figure 9A, although all formulations were able to induce detectable IgG titers at Day 21, at Day 42 Chi-C48/80 NPs and Chi-Al NPs induced significantly higher titers than Chi-PCL NPs. All delivery systems tested induced a Th2-type immune response, since the predominant IgG subclass elicited was the IgG1 (Figure 9B). Therefore, Chi-PCL NPs despite being an excellent adjuvant when administered by a subcutaneous route, was shown in this work to have a lower value when used in the intranasal route.

The main reason to develop new and effective mucosal vaccine delivery systems, besides its ease of access and administration, is the possibility to induce mucosal antibodies at the site of entry of pathogens, actively preventing the infection. Our results showed that Chi-C48/80 NPs were able to induce mucosal anti-HBsAg IgA in the vaccinated mice (Figure 9C). Indeed, the nasal washes revealed mucosal IgA titers in 80% of the Chi-C48/80 NP-vaccinated mice, similar to Chi-Al NPs, but vaginal washes revealed 60% of responder mice in comparison to the 40% of Chi-Al NPs. All nanoparticles used in this experiment presented a positive zeta potential, characteristic of a chitosan presence (Figure 9D). Nevertheless, sizes presented a higher variation between formulations, with a Chi-C48/80 NP size about two times larger than the other nanoparticles.

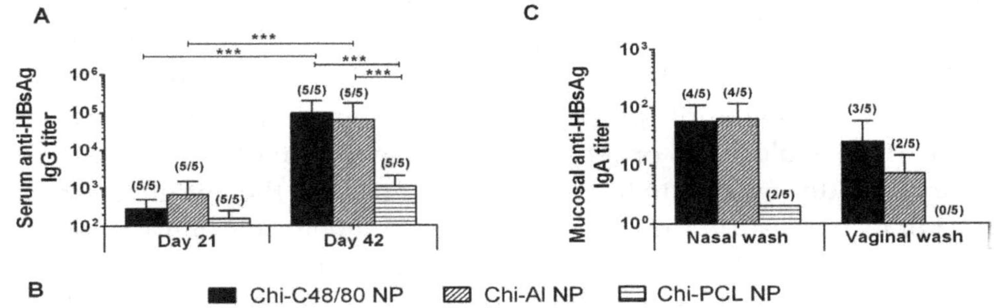

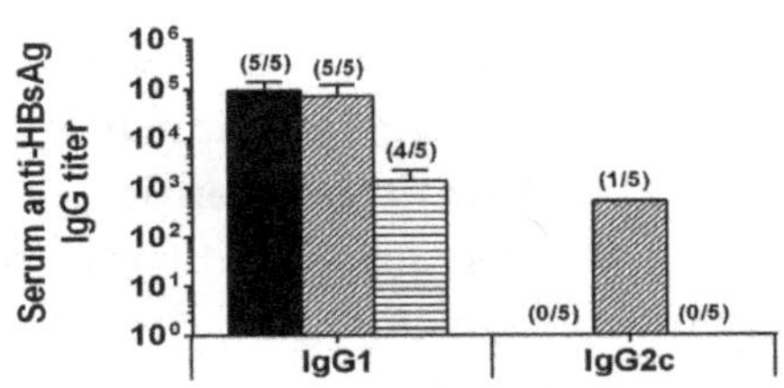

D

Formulation	Size (nm)	PI[a]	ZP (mV)
Chi-C48/80 NP	500.9 ± 65.15	0.161 ± 0.051	+ 23.83 ± 3.76
Chi-Al NP	280.9 ± 32.70	0.255 ± 0.012	+ 30.10 ± 1.90
Chi-PCL NP	208.1 ± 28.70	0.180 ± 0.060	+ 25.70 ± 2.90

Figure 9. Immune profile of C57BL/6 mice after intranasal immunization. Serum anti-HBsAg IgG (**A**), IgG1 and IgG2c (**B**) and mucosal IgA (**C**) titers obtained with 10 μg HBsAg loaded into Chi-C48/80 NPs, Chi-Al NPs, or Chi-PCL NPs. Blood was collected by submandibular lancet method on Days 21 and 42, and nasal and vaginal washes were collected on Day 42. Numbers above bars represent the number of mice in which antibody levels were detected. Data (mean ± SD) correspond to responder mice of each group. Table with summary of nanoparticle size, polydispersity index, and zeta potential of the formulations used during the immunization studies (**D**).

These results suggest that the adjuvant Chi-C48/80 NPs is a valuable strategy to improve the efficacy of nasal recombinant vaccines. Immunoglobulin results were slightly higher than the ones obtained with Chi-Al NPs, which adjuvanticity was already established by our group [26,30,47] and particularly for the nasal route. In fact, Lebre et al. [30] observed Chi-Al NPs complexed with pDNA from HBsAg, were able to induce humoral and mucosal antibodies against HBV. Moreover, in opposition to free HBsAg, Lebre et al. [47] also reported that HBsAg loaded Chi-Al NPs elicited HBsAg-specific IgG in nasal and vaginal washes when the vaccine was subcutaneously administered. On the other hand, when compared to Chi-PCL NPs, Chi-C48/80 NPs demonstrated a superior adjuvant activity. Chi-PCL NP adjuvanticity through subcutaneous and nasal routes was also validated by our group in a direct comparison with free HBsAg [27,48,49]. In detail, through the nasal route, free HBsAg did not induce specific IgG titers, while Chi-PLC NPs elicited a detectable immune response with an HBsAg dose 10 times lower than the control [27]. Moreover, the conclusion that Chi-C48/80 NPs are able to increase the immune response to HBsAg is reinforced when the results are compared to Chi-Al NPs and Chi-PCL NPs, since those delivery systems were already compared in vaccination studies with the commercially available HBV vaccine (Engerix®) [47,49]. In those studies, both delivery systems were able to induce better IgG titers than Engerix® at same dose.

Interestingly, a recent article, published by Schubert et al. [50] observed that the adjuvant activity of C48/80 for the specific immune response against ovalbumin upon intranasal immunization is independent of the MC presence. Therefore, further work aimed to elucidate the mechanistic of action of Chi-C48/80 NPs as a mucosal vaccine adjuvant would be insightful to clarify if its adjuvant activity is related with a C48/80 ability to activate MC, or if it is a mechanism similar to chitosan, that largely stems from the fact that it is a cationic polymer. In fact, chitosan nanoparticles alone are able to activate mast cells, a finding recently made by our group [51].

Overall, the association of C48/80 with chitosan NPs was found to produce a good adjuvant and thus to be a suitable approach to improving the activity of the HBsAg, through mucosal routes of administration.

4. Conclusions

Chitosan is a biomaterial with appealing properties for vaccine delivery. Considering this, we designed and developed a new chitosan-based vaccine delivery system by efficiently incorporating the mast cell activator C48/80 into chitosan nanoparticles. Overall, the data obtained showed that the versatility of chitosan was associated with additional adjuvants without significantly affecting the physicochemical and biocompatible properties of the polymer. This is a characteristic of chitosan that deserves to be further explored in order to support the design of improved delivery systems or immunopotentiators to better modulate the immune response of the antigens. The delivery system was shown to have interesting features for vaccine delivery, namely, the ability to adsorb high amounts of antigen, internalization by antigen-presenting cells, and stability after lyophilization, which can be a useful future development of a cold chain-free vaccine formulation. Chi-C48/80 NPs also demonstrated adjuvant activity for the hepatitis B antigen similar to Chi-Al NPs and superior to Chi-PCL NPs, confirming its feasibility as a vaccine adjuvant through demanding but promising routes, such as the nasal route. To better design nanoparticulate immunopotentiators, it is desirable that the mechanism of the adjuvants be better studied, with the certainty that for each adjuvant we are not talking about a single mechanism, but most likely more than one that, the other way, may be competitive. This knowledge is absolutely essential, so that in the near future it will be possible to design adjuvants with more predictable immunomodulatory action.

Author Contributions: Conceptualization, D.B. and O.B.; investigation, D.B., S.J., and F.L.; writing—original draft preparation, D.B.; writing—review and editing, D.B., T.G., and O.B.; funding acquisition, O.B.

Acknowledgments: We thank Luisa Cortes for expert technical assistance with confocal microscopy.

References

1. Smith, D.M.; Simon, J.K.; Baker, J.R., Jr. Applications of nanotechnology for immunology. *Nat. Rev. Immunol.* **2013**, *13*, 592–605. [CrossRef] [PubMed]
2. De Temmerman, M.L.; Rejman, J.; Demeester, J.; Irvine, D.J.; Gander, B.; De Smedt, S.C. Particulate vaccines: on the quest for optimal delivery and immune response. *Drug Discov. Today* **2011**, *16*, 569–582. [CrossRef] [PubMed]
3. Akagi, T.; Shima, F.; Akashi, M. Intracellular degradation and distribution of protein-encapsulated amphiphilic poly(amino acid) nanoparticles. *Biomaterials* **2011**, *32*, 4959–4967. [CrossRef] [PubMed]
4. Oyewumi, M.O.; Kumar, A.; Cui, Z. Nano-microparticles as immune adjuvants: correlating particle sizes and the resultant immune responses. *Expert Rev. Vaccines* **2010**, *9*, 1095–1107. [CrossRef] [PubMed]
5. Shen, H.; Ackerman, A.L.; Cody, V.; Giodini, A.; Hinson, E.R.; Cresswell, P.; Edelson, R.L.; Saltzman, W.M.; Hanlon, D.J. Enhanced and prolonged cross-presentation following endosomal escape of exogenous antigens encapsulated in biodegradable nanoparticles. *Immunology* **2006**, *117*, 78–88. [CrossRef] [PubMed]
6. Thomann-Harwood, L.J.; Kaeuper, P.; Rossi, N.; Milona, P.; Herrmann, B.; McCullough, K.C. Nanogel vaccines targeting dendritic cells: contributions of the surface decoration and vaccine cargo on cell targeting and activation. *J. Control. Release* **2013**, *166*, 95–105. [CrossRef] [PubMed]
7. Koppolu, B.; Zaharoff, D.A. The effect of antigen encapsulation in chitosan particles on uptake, activation and presentation by antigen presenting cells. *Biomaterials* **2013**, *34*, 2359–2369. [CrossRef]
8. Gao, Y.; Wijewardhana, C.; Mann, J.F.S. Virus-Like Particle, Liposome, and Polymeric Particle-Based Vaccines against HIV-1. *Front. Immunol.* **2018**, *9*. [CrossRef]
9. Barclay, T.; Petrovsky, N. Vaccine Adjuvant Nanotechnologies. In *Micro and Nanotechnology in Vaccine Development*; Elsevier Science: Oxford, UK, 2017; pp. 127–147. [CrossRef]
10. Arca, H.C.; Gunbeyaz, M.; Senel, S. Chitosan-based systems for the delivery of vaccine antigens. *Expert Rev. Vaccines* **2009**, *8*, 937–953. [CrossRef]
11. Amidi, M.; Mastrobattista, E.; Jiskoot, W.; Hennink, W.E. Chitosan-based delivery systems for protein therapeutics and antigens. *Adv. Drug Deliv. Rev.* **2010**, *62*, 59–82. [CrossRef]

12. Baldrick, P. The safety of chitosan as a pharmaceutical excipient. *Regul. Toxicol. Pharmacol. RTP* **2010**, *56*, 290–299. [CrossRef] [PubMed]
13. Mutwiri, G.; Gerdts, V.; van Drunen Littel-van den Hurk, S.; Auray, G.; Eng, N.; Garlapati, S.; Babiuk, L.A.; Potter, A. Combination adjuvants: the next generation of adjuvants? *Expert Rev. Vaccines* **2011**, *10*, 95–107. [CrossRef] [PubMed]
14. Schijns, V.E.; Lavelle, E.C. Trends in vaccine adjuvants. *Expert Rev. Vaccines* **2011**, *10*, 539–550. [CrossRef] [PubMed]
15. Abraham, S.N.; St John, A.L. Mast cell-orchestrated immunity to pathogens. *Nat. Rev. Immunol.* **2010**, *10*, 440–452. [CrossRef] [PubMed]
16. Metz, M.; Maurer, M. Mast cells–key effector cells in immune responses. *Trends Immunol.* **2007**, *28*, 234–241. [CrossRef] [PubMed]
17. Marshall, J.S. Mast-cell responses to pathogens. *Nat. Rev. Immunol.* **2004**, *4*, 787–799. [CrossRef] [PubMed]
18. McLachlan, J.B.; Shelburne, C.P.; Hart, J.P.; Pizzo, S.V.; Goyal, R.; Brooking-Dixon, R.; Staats, H.F.; Abraham, S.N. Mast cell activators: A new class of highly effective vaccine adjuvants. *Nat. Med.* **2008**, *14*, 536–541. [CrossRef] [PubMed]
19. Staats, H.F.; Fielhauer, J.R.; Thompson, A.L.; Tripp, A.A.; Sobel, A.E.; Maddaloni, M.; Abraham, S.N.; Pascual, D.W. Mucosal targeting of a BoNT/A subunit vaccine adjuvanted with a mast cell activator enhances induction of BoNT/A neutralizing antibodies in rabbits. *PLoS ONE* **2011**, *6*, e16532. [CrossRef]
20. McGowen, A.L.; Hale, L.P.; Shelburne, C.P.; Abraham, S.N.; Staats, H.F. The mast cell activator compound 48/80 is safe and effective when used as an adjuvant for intradermal immunization with Bacillus anthracis protective antigen. *Vaccine* **2009**, *27*, 3544–3552. [CrossRef]
21. Wang, S.H.; Kirwan, S.M.; Abraham, S.N.; Staats, H.F.; Hickey, A.J. Stable dry powder formulation for nasal delivery of anthrax vaccine. *J. Pharm. Sci.* **2012**, *101*, 31–47. [CrossRef]
22. Kiyono, H.; Fukuyama, S. NALT- versus Peyer's-patch-mediated mucosal immunity. *Nat. Rev. Immunol.* **2004**, *4*, 699–710. [CrossRef] [PubMed]
23. Neutra, M.R.; Kozlowski, P.A. Mucosal vaccines: The promise and the challenge. *Nat. Rev. Immunol.* **2006**, *6*, 148–158. [CrossRef]
24. Reed, S.G.; Bertholet, S.; Coler, R.N.; Friede, M. New horizons in adjuvants for vaccine development. *Trends Immunol.* **2009**, *30*, 23–32. [CrossRef] [PubMed]
25. Gan, Q.; Wang, T. Chitosan nanoparticle as protein delivery carrier—Systematic examination of fabrication conditions for efficient loading and release. *Colloids Surf. B Biointerface* **2007**, *59*, 24–34. [CrossRef]
26. Lebre, F.; Bento, D.; Ribeiro, J.; Colaco, M.; Borchard, G.; de Lima, M.C.P.; Borges, O. Association of chitosan and aluminium as a new adjuvant strategy for improved vaccination. *Int. J. Pharm.* **2017**, *527*, 103–114. [CrossRef]
27. Jesus, S.; Soares, E.; Costa, J.; Borchard, G.; Borges, O. Immune response elicited by an intranasally delivered HBsAg low-dose adsorbed to poly-epsilon-caprolactone based nanoparticles. *Int. J. Pharm.* **2016**, *504*, 59–69. [CrossRef]
28. Bento, D.; Borchard, G.; Goncalves, T.; Borges, O. Validation of a new 96-well plate spectrophotometric method for the quantification of compound 48/80 associated with particles. *AAPS PharmSciTech* **2013**, *14*, 649–655. [CrossRef] [PubMed]
29. Borges, O.; Cordeiro-da-Silva, A.; Romeijn, S.G.; Amidi, M.; de Sousa, A.; Borchard, G.; Junginger, H.E. Uptake studies in rat Peyer's patches, cytotoxicity and release studies of alginate coated chitosan nanoparticles for mucosal vaccination. *J. Control. Release* **2006**, *114*, 348–358. [CrossRef]
30. Lebre, F.; Borchard, G.; Faneca, H.; Pedroso de Lima, M.C.; Borges, O. Intranasal Administration of Novel Chitosan Nanoparticle/DNA Complexes Induces Antibody Response to Hepatitis B Surface Antigen in Mice. *Mol. Pharm.* **2016**, *13*, 472–482. [CrossRef]
31. Jesus, S.; Soares, E.; Borges, O. Poly-epsilon-caprolactone/Chitosan and Chitosan Particles: Two Recombinant Antigen Delivery Systems for Intranasal Vaccination. *Method Mol. Biol.* **2016**, *1404*, 697–713. [CrossRef]
32. Dudhani, A.R.; Kosaraju, S.L. Bioadhesive chitosan nanoparticles: Preparation and characterization. *Carbohydr. Polym.* **2010**, *81*, 243–251. [CrossRef]
33. Borges, O.; Borchard, G.; Verhoef, J.C.; de Sousa, A.; Junginger, H.E. Preparation of coated nanoparticles for a new mucosal vaccine delivery system. *Int. J. Pharm.* **2005**, *299*, 155–166. [CrossRef]

34. Lim, S.T.; Martin, G.P.; Berry, D.J.; Brown, M.B. Preparation and evaluation of the in vitro drug release properties and mucoadhesion of novel microspheres of hyaluronic acid and chitosan. *J. Control. Release* **2000**, *66*, 281–292. [CrossRef]
35. Zhao, L.; Seth, A.; Wibowo, N.; Zhao, C.X.; Mitter, N.; Yu, C.; Middelberg, A.P. Nanoparticle vaccines. *Vaccine* **2014**, *32*, 327–337. [CrossRef]
36. Foged, C.; Brodin, B.; Frokjaer, S.; Sundblad, A. Particle size and surface charge affect particle uptake by human dendritic cells in an in vitro model. *Int. J. Pharm.* **2005**, *298*, 315–322. [CrossRef]
37. Mudunkotuwa, I.A.; Minshid, A.A.; Grassian, V.H. ATR-FTIR spectroscopy as a tool to probe surface adsorption on nanoparticles at the liquid-solid interface in environmentally and biologically relevant media. *Analyst* **2014**, *139*, 870–881. [CrossRef]
38. Rampino, A.; Borgogna, M.; Blasi, P.; Bellich, B.; Cesaro, A. Chitosan nanoparticles: preparation, size evolution and stability. *Int. J. Pharm.* **2013**, *455*, 219–228. [CrossRef]
39. Sloat, B.R.; Sandoval, M.A.; Cui, Z. Towards preserving the immunogenicity of protein antigens carried by nanoparticles while avoiding the cold chain. *Int. J. Pharm.* **2010**, *393*, 197–202. [CrossRef]
40. Abdelwahed, W.; Degobert, G.; Stainmesse, S.; Fessi, H. Freeze-drying of nanoparticles: formulation, process and storage considerations. *Adv. Drug Deliv. Rev.* **2006**, *58*, 1688–1713. [CrossRef]
41. Dee, K.C.; Puleo, D.A.; Bizios, R. Protein-Surface Interactions. In *An Introduction To Tissue-Biomaterial Interactions*; John Wiley & Sons, Inc.: Hoboken, NJ, USA, 2003; pp. 37–52. [CrossRef]
42. Eyles, J.E.; Bramwell, V.W.; Singh, J.; Williamson, E.D.; Alpar, H.O. Stimulation of spleen cells in vitro by nanospheric particles containing antigen. *J. Control. Release* **2003**, *86*, 25–32. [CrossRef]
43. Grenha, A.; Grainger, C.I.; Dailey, L.A.; Seijo, B.; Martin, G.P.; Remunan-Lopez, C.; Forbes, B. Chitosan nanoparticles are compatible with respiratory epithelial cells in vitro. *Eur. J. Pharm. Sci.* **2007**, *31*, 73–84. [CrossRef]
44. Kean, T.; Thanou, M. Biodegradation, biodistribution and toxicity of chitosan. *Adv. Drug Deliv. Rev.* **2010**, *62*, 3–11. [CrossRef]
45. O'Hagan, D.T.; Valiante, N.M. Recent advances in the discovery and delivery of vaccine adjuvants. *Nat. Rev. Drug Discov.* **2003**, *2*, 727–735. [CrossRef]
46. Yue, Z.G.; Wei, W.; Lv, P.P.; Yue, H.; Wang, L.Y.; Su, Z.G.; Ma, G.H. Surface charge affects cellular uptake and intracellular trafficking of chitosan-based nanoparticles. *Biomacromolecules* **2011**, *12*, 2440–2446. [CrossRef]
47. Lebre, F.; Pedroso de Lima, M.C.; Lavelle, E.C.; Borges, O. Mechanistic study of the adjuvant effect of chitosan-aluminum nanoparticles. *Int. J. Pharm.* **2018**, *552*, 7–15. [CrossRef]
48. Jesus, S.; Soares, E.; Borchard, G.; Borges, O. Poly–caprolactone/chitosan nanoparticles provide strong adjuvant effect for hepatitis B antigen. *Nanomedicine* **2017**, *12*, 2335–2348. [CrossRef]
49. Jesus, S.; Soares, E.; Borchard, G.; Borges, O. Adjuvant Activity of Poly-epsilon-caprolactone/Chitosan Nanoparticles Characterized by Mast Cell Activation and IFN-gamma and IL-17 Production. *Mol. Pharm.* **2018**, *15*, 72–82. [CrossRef]
50. Schubert, N.; Lisenko, K.; Auerbach, C.; Weitzmann, A.; Ghouse, S.M.; Muhandes, L.; Haase, C.; Häring, T.; Schulze, L.; Voehringer, D.; et al. Unimpaired Responses to Vaccination With Protein Antigen Plus Adjuvant in Mice With Kit-Independent Mast Cell Deficiency. *Front. Immunol.* **2018**, *9*. [CrossRef]
51. Bento, D.; Staats, H.F.; Gonçalves, T.; Borges, O. Development of a novel adjuvanted nasal vaccine: C48/80 associated with chitosan nanoparticles as a path to enhance mucosal immunity. *Eur. J. Pharm. Biopharm.* **2015**, *93*, 149–164. [CrossRef]

Permissions

All chapters in this book were first published by MDPI; hereby published with permission under the Creative Commons Attribution License or equivalent. Every chapter published in this book has been scrutinized by our experts. Their significance has been extensively debated. The topics covered herein carry significant findings which will fuel the growth of the discipline. They may even be implemented as practical applications or may be referred to as a beginning point for another development.

The contributors of this book come from diverse backgrounds, making this book a truly international effort. This book will bring forth new frontiers with its revolutionizing research information and detailed analysis of the nascent developments around the world.

We would like to thank all the contributing authors for lending their expertise to make the book truly unique. They have played a crucial role in the development of this book. Without their invaluable contributions this book wouldn't have been possible. They have made vital efforts to compile up to date information on the varied aspects of this subject to make this book a valuable addition to the collection of many professionals and students.

This book was conceptualized with the vision of imparting up-to-date information and advanced data in this field. To ensure the same, a matchless editorial board was set up. Every individual on the board went through rigorous rounds of assessment to prove their worth. After which they invested a large part of their time researching and compiling the most relevant data for our readers.

The editorial board has been involved in producing this book since its inception. They have spent rigorous hours researching and exploring the diverse topics which have resulted in the successful publishing of this book. They have passed on their knowledge of decades through this book. To expedite this challenging task, the publisher supported the team at every step. A small team of assistant editors was also appointed to further simplify the editing procedure and attain best results for the readers.

Apart from the editorial board, the designing team has also invested a significant amount of their time in understanding the subject and creating the most relevant covers. They scrutinized every image to scout for the most suitable representation of the subject and create an appropriate cover for the book.

The publishing team has been an ardent support to the editorial, designing and production team. Their endless efforts to recruit the best for this project, has resulted in the accomplishment of this book. They are a veteran in the field of academics and their pool of knowledge is as vast as their experience in printing. Their expertise and guidance has proved useful at every step. Their uncompromising quality standards have made this book an exceptional effort. Their encouragement from time to time has been an inspiration for everyone.

The publisher and the editorial board hope that this book will prove to be a valuable piece of knowledge for researchers, students, practitioners and scholars across the globe.

List of Contributors

Kieran Burgess, Heyu Li, Yasmin Abo-zeid, Fatimah and Gareth R. Williams
UCL School of Pharmacy, University College London, 29-39 Brunswick Square, London WC1N 1AX, UK

Zhi-gang Huang, Yu Liu, Gang Wei and Wei-yue Lu
Department of Pharmaceutics, School of Pharmacy, Fudan University & Key Laboratory of Smart Drug Delivery (Fudan University), Ministry of Education, Shanghai 201203, China

Feng-mei Lv, Jun Wang and Zhe-peng Liu
School of Medical Instrument and Food Engineering, University of Shanghai for Science and Technology, Shanghai 200093, China

Li-qian Ci
Department of Pharmaceutics, School of Pharmacy, Fudan University & Key Laboratory of Smart Drug Delivery (Fudan University), Ministry of Education, Shanghai 201203, China
School of Medical Instrument and Food Engineering, University of Shanghai for Science and Technology, Shanghai 200093, China

Ling-lin Feng
NHC Key Laboratory of Reproduction Regulation (Shanghai Institute of Planned Parenthood Research), Fudan University, Room 904, No 1 Research Building, 2140 Xietu Road, Shanghai 200032, China

Feng Sun
Chinese Academy of Sciences Shanghai Institute of Materia Medica, Shanghai 201203, China

Shui-juan Cao
Experimental Teaching Center, School of Pharmacy, Fudan University, Shanghai 201203, China

Hazrina AB. Hadi
Department of Pharmaceutical Technology, Kulliyyah of Pharmacy, International Islamic University Malaysia, Kuantan 25200, Malaysia

Saeid Mezail Mawazi
Department of Pharmaceutical Technology, Kulliyyah of Pharmacy, International Islamic University Malaysia, Kuantan 25200, Malaysia
School of Pharmacy, PICOMS International University College, Batu Muda, Batu caves, Kuala Lumpur 68100, Malaysia

Sinan Mohammed Abdullah Al-Mahmood
Pharmacy College, Al-Kitab University, Kirkuk 36010, Iraq

Bappaditya Chatterjee
Department of Pharmaceutical Technology, Kulliyyah of Pharmacy, International Islamic University Malaysia, Kuantan 25200, Malaysia
Department of Pharmaceutics, SPPSPTM, SVKM's NMIMS (Deemed to be University), Mumbai 400056, India

Abd Almonem Doolaanea
Department of Pharmaceutical Technology, Kulliyyah of Pharmacy, International Islamic University Malaysia, Kuantan 25200, Malaysia
IKOP Sdn Bhd, Kulliyyah of Pharmacy, International Islamic University Malaysia, Kuantan 25200, Malaysia

Leticia Martínez-Ortega, Amalia Mira, Asia Fernandez-Carvajal, C. Reyes Mateo, Ricardo Mallavia and Alberto Falco
Institute of Research, Development and Innovation in Biotechnology of Elche (IDiBE) and Molecular and Cellular Biology Institute (IBMC), Miguel Hernández University (UMH), 03202 Elche, Spain

Bianca Peterson, Morné Weyers, Jan H. Steenekamp, Johan D. Steyn, Chrisna Gouws and Josias H. Hamman
Centre of Excellence for Pharmaceutical Sciences (Pharmacen™), North-West University, Potchefstroom 2520, South Africa

Angela Fabiano, Anna Maria Piras, Lorenzo Guazzelli and Ylenia Zambito
Department of Pharmacy, University of Pisa Via Bonanno, 33, 56126 Pisa, Italy

Barbara Storti
NEST, Scuola Normale Superiore and Istituto Nanoscienze-CNR, Piazza San Silvestro 12, 56127 Pisa, Italy

Ranieri Bizzarri
NEST, Scuola Normale Superiore and Istituto Nanoscienze-CNR, Piazza San Silvestro 12, 56127 Pisa, Italy
Department of Surgical, Medical and Molecular Pathology, and Critical Care Medicine, University of Pisa, Via Roma 67, 56126 Pisa, Italy

Kaiqiang Ye, Haizhu Kuang and Xiumei Mo
State Key Laboratory for Modification of Chemical Fibers and Polymer Materials, College of Chemistry, Chemical Engineering and Biotechnology, Donghua University, Shanghai 201620, China

Zhengwei You
State Key Laboratory for Modification of Chemical Fibers and Polymer Materials, College of Materials Science and Engineering, Donghua University, Shanghai 201620, China

Yosry Morsi
Faculty of Engineering and Industrial Sciences, Swinburne University of Technology, Boroondara, VIC 3122, Australia

Roman V. Moiseev, Peter W. J. Morrison and Vitaliy V. Khutoryanskiy
Reading School of Pharmacy, University of Reading, Whiteknights, P.O. Box 224, Reading RG66AD, UK

Fraser Steele
MC2 Therapeutics, James House, Emlyn Lane, Leatherhead KT22 7EP, UK

Rajan Sharma Bhattarai and Rinda Devi Bachu
College of Pharmacy and Pharmaceutical Sciences, The University of Toledo Health Science Campus, Toledo, OH 43614, USA

Sai H. S. Boddu
Department of Pharmaceutical Sciences, College of Pharmacy and Health Sciences, Ajman University, Ajman 2758, UAE

Sarit Bhaduri
Department of Mechanical, Industrial and Manufacturing Engineering, University of Toledo, Toledo, OH 43614, USA
Department of Surgery (Dentistry), University of Toledo, Toledo, OH 43614, USA

Noriyasu Kamei, Hideyuki Tamiwa, Mari Miyata, Yuta Haruna, Koyo Matsumura, Hideyuki Ogino, Serena Hirano, Kazuhiro Higashiyama and Mariko Takeda-Morishita
Laboratory of Drug Delivery Systems, Faculty of Pharmaceutical Sciences, Kobe Gakuin University, 1-1-3 Minatojima, Chuo-ku, Kobe, Hyogo 650-8586, Japan

Dulce Bento, Sandra Jesus, Filipa Lebre and Olga Borges
CNC-Center for Neuroscience and Cell Biology, University of Coimbra, 3004-0504 Coimbra, Portugal
Faculty of Pharmacy, University of Coimbra, Pólo das Ciências da Saúde, Azinhaga de Santa Comba, 3000-548 Coimbra, Portugal

Teresa Gonçalves
CNC-Center for Neuroscience and Cell Biology, University of Coimbra, 3004-0504 Coimbra, Portugal
Faculty of Medicine, University of Coimbra, 3004-504 Coimbra, Portugal

Index

www.ingramcontent.com/pod-product-compliance
Lightning Source LLC
LaVergne TN
LVHW082150200926
848484LV00008B/2133